Validating Automated Manufacturing and Laboratory Applications

Putting Principles into Practice

Guy Wingate

Interpharm Press, Inc.
Buffalo Grove, Illinois

Invitation to Authors

Interpharm Press publishes books focused upon applied technology and regulatory affairs impacting Healthcare Manufacturers worldwide. If you are considering writing or contributing to a book applicable to the pharmaceutical, biotechnology, medical device, diagnostic, cosmetic, or veterinary medicine manufacturing industries, please contact our Director of Publications.

Social Responsibility Programs

Reforestation

Interpharm Press is concerned about the impact of the worldwide loss of trees upon both the environment and the availability of new drug sources. Therefore, Interpharm supports global reforestation and commits to replant trees sufficient to replace those used to meet the paper needs to print its books.

Pharmakos-2000

Through its Pharmakos-2000 program, Interpharm Press fosters the teaching of pharmaceutical technology. Under this program, complimentary copies of selected Interpharm titles are regularly sent to every College and School of Pharmacy worldwide. It is hoped that these books will be useful references to faculty and students in advancing the practice of pharmaceutical technology.

Library of Congress Cataloging-in-Publication Data

Wingate, Guy.

Validating automated manufacturing and laboratory applications : putting principles into practice / Guy Wingate.

p. cm.

Includes bibliographical references and index.

ISBN 1-57491-031-X

1. Pharmaceutical industry—Automation—Quality control. 2. Pharmaceutical technology—Automation—Quality control.

[DNLM: 1. Drug Industry—standards. 2. Drug Industry—instrumentation. 3. Laboratories—standards. 4. Computers. 5. Automation—standards. QV 736 W769v 1997]

RS122.2.W56 1997

6159.19—dc21

DNLM/DLC

for Library of Congress 97-13236

CIP

Commissioned in the UK by Sue Horwood of Medi-Tech. Publications Limited, Storrington, West Sussex, on behalf of Interpharm Press, Inc., USA. General Scientific Advisor: Robin N. Stephens, Manager of International Regulatory Affairs and Clinical Research, AVE Inc., UK

10 9 8 7 6 5 4 3 2 1

ISBN: 1-57491-037-X

Interpharm Press, Inc.
1358 Busch Parkway
Buffalo Grove, IL 60089, USA
Phone: + 1 + 847 + 459-8480
Fax: + 1 + 847 + 459-6644

Author and Editor

Guy Wingate Eutech Engineering Solutions, England

Case Study Contributors

Rob Almond	Glaxo Wellcome, England
John Bianculli	Beckman Instruments, U.S.A.
Peter Bosshard	Hoffmann-La Roche, Switzerland
Peter Coady	P.J. Coady & Associates, England
Tony de Claire	SmithKline Beecham, England
Chris Evans	Eutech Engineering Solutions, England
John Gough	Pfizer, England
Peter Gough	Eli Lilly, England
Thomas Hefti	Hoffmann-La Roche, Switzerland
Ludwig Huber	Hewlett-Packard, Germany
Terry R. Lucy	Glaxo Wellcome, England
Richard Mitchell	Pfizer, England
Peter Owen	Eli Lilly, England
Bob Paige	Eutech Engineering Solutions, England
Chris Reid	Imperial Chemical Industries, England
Owen Salvage	Eutech Engineering Solutions, England
Kate Samways	Rhône-Poulenc Rorer, England
Martin Smith	Zeneca Pharma, France
Hans O. Sucker	Hoffmann-La Roche, Switzerland
Nick Townsend	Beckman Instruments, England
Mark Whitehouse	Yokogawa, England
Guy Wingate	Eutech Engineering Solutions, England
Sion Wyn	Activa Systems, Wales

Foreword By

Anthony J. Trill Medicines Control Agency, England

For Sarah and Katherine

Contents

APPENDICES

PART 2: CASE STUDIES

I. THE VENDOR'S ROLE IN THE VALIDATION OF ELECTRONIC DOCUMENT MANAGEMENT SYSTEMS 423

Sion Wyn

J. VALIDATING ENGINEERING MANAGEMENT SYSTEMS 433

Peter Owen and Peter Gough

Foreword

Tony Trill
Specialist Principal Investigator
UK Medicines Control Agency

As I noted in 1993: "There is extensive literature dealing with theories and concepts, but there is very little published on case histories, possibly due to commercial sensitivity" [1]. Nearly four years on and the paucity of case studies has been addressed. The publication of this book, which records numerous personal experiences and practical issues relating to specific validation projects with automated systems, is a milestone. Compiled by an experienced multi-disciplinary team of practitioners from various pharmaceutical industry sectors, it will provide welcome relief and lessons for developers, suppliers, integrators, purchasers, and regulators alike.

Computer technology is all pervasive. It hides behind the smallest button on domestic appliances, is in smart cards and security devices, mobile phones, cash dispensers, PCs, integrated networks, process plant, automobiles, "jumbo jets", and power plants. Automation is everywhere and is gathering complexity, innovation, and momentum, and we have to rely on it more and more in our everyday lives. The inexorable rise of automation is also seen in the corporate strategies of pharmaceutical manufacturers, calling for investment in new technology to improve business efficiency and competitive edge. When such technology is associated with high risk public safety projects or the production and control of life-saving medicines or devices, we (businesses and regulators) need to know that it is reliable, quality assured, and validated. Easy to say; but the technology (and the terminology) is difficult to understand, let alone prove and qualify, if you are not an electronic systems engineer or a latent Einstein.

Pharmaceutical companies have historically engineered their businesses to be profitable whilst ensuring that quality is built into their medicinal products, or devices, through the observance of GXPs, marketing regulations, and good project management. The GXPs (viz: GCPs, GLPs, GMPs, etc.) essentially require computerised systems in the pharmaceutical sector to be fully documented, defined as to functionality, quality assured, and validated. This book considers the requirements of the various international regulations, guides, and codes in historical perspective and leads the reader into business and project life-cycle issues and activities. This book is invaluable in bridging the gap between theory and practice and is supported by case studies from experienced professional practitioners and engineers who have had to face up to the challenges of proving the quality, structural integrity, and validation of different systems in the "real world" (process control, utility management, to networked control, information and high level business IT and integrated real time applications, etc.). The case studies are organised hierarchically from low level instruments and PLCs through integration to higher level proprietary electronic document and information management systems and beyond.

Pharmaceutical companies, and indeed any profit-conscious businesses investing in automated systems, want quality-assured, robust, reliable computerized systems, delivered on time, within budget, meeting functional, business performance, and cost-related targets. Computer software and systems suppliers, however, in their rush to place new products and versions on the market, have rarely delivered error-free products. In fact, some two thirds of life-cycle costs can be incurred after delivery of the software and system to the users. Pharmaceutical companies do not want lots of downtime, disruption, and escalating costs once a system has been delivered and implemented [3,4]. And, of course, in GXP applications, any deficiencies will be of particular interest during regulatory inspections.

Inspectors and investigators working for the different national regulatory bodies have to apply their national GXPs and regulations when assessing these systems. Whilst these are published, they are not necessarily up to date and, as we all would acknowledge, they are often open to interpretation not only by different inspectors, depending on their background and training, but also depending on the particular computerised system and application. Regulators need to be satisfied that computerised systems installed in pharmaceutical companies are fit for their intended purposes by considering the nature of the application, specifications, quality assurance of the development life-cycle activities, qualification, performance validation, in-use controls, accuracy, and reliability in the context of relevant GXPs. The increasing complexity of (integrated) proprietary computer systems, critical applications, project validation issues, and inspection findings have been considered before, together with the challenge for all parties (as ever) to apply sensible regulations and cost-effective good computer validation practices [2,3,4].

The pharmaceutical industry, suppliers, and developers have also reportedly had some difficulty in ensuring that these projects actually deliver the proposed business benefits and that the systems as built actually meet the specifications, are reliable and validated, quite apart from determining just how much and what type of validation evidence is required to satisfy the different regulatory bodies, and particularly the FDA. Whilst the GAMP Guide [6] and, to some extent, the PDA 18 Report [7] provide the latest interpretation of acceptable development and project guidance in this field (to ensure compliance with the needs of the principle regulatory bodies around the world), and TickIT provides a guide to software quality system construction and certification (using ISO 9001:1994) [8], there has been a lack of papers on practical experiences from pharmaceutical sector project teams seeking to implement new technology.

I believe this book will be welcomed by novices and experts, suppliers, developers, purchasers, and regulators alike, in providing insight into the practical aspects of these complex automation, life-cycle–related projects. Many staff assigned to validation projects could also benefit from sharing the experience of other practitioners. Whether you are looking for the missing piece of the jigsaw for your project or guidance on how to meet the regulations in a practical sense, then this information resource (which puts principles into practice) is a good place to start!

REFERENCES

1. Trill, A.J. (1993), Computerized Systems and GMP—A UK Perspective: Part II, "Inspection Findings", *Pharmaceutical Technology International,* 5 (3), March.

2. Trill, A.J. (1995), EU GMP Requirements and the Good Automated Manufacturing Practice (GAMP) Supplier Guide for the Validation of Automated Systems for Pharmaceutical Manufacturing, *Pharmaceutical Engineering,* May/June, pp. 56–62.

3. Stokes, T., Branning, R.C., Chapman, K.G., Hambloch, H.J., and Trill, A.J. (1994), *Good Computer Validation Practices: Common Sense Implementation.* Buffalo Grove, IL: Interpharm Press, Inc.

4. Wingate, G.A.S. (1995), Computer Systems Validation: A Historical Perspective, *Pharmaceutical Engineering,* July/August, pp. 8–12.

5. Trill, A.J. (1996), An EU/MCA View of Recent Industry Guides to Computer Validation, Including GAMP 1996, PDA Technical Report 18 and the Validation

Toolkit, in proceedings of *PIC/S Seminar,* "Inspection of Computer Systems", Sydney, Australia, September.

6. *Good Automated Manufacturing Practice (GAMP 1996) Supplier Guide for the Validation of Automated Systems in Pharmaceutical Manufacture,* Produced by the GAMP Forum and distributed by ISPE, European Branch Office, Nieuwe Uitleg 21, NL_2514 BR, The Hague, The Netherlands.

7. PDA (1995), The Validation of Computer Related Systems, Technical Report No. 18, *Journal of Pharmaceutical Science and Technolgy*, 49 (1).

8. *TickIT Guide*—A Guide to Software Quality Management System Construction and Certification using ISO 9001, Issue 3.0 (October 1995), London: DISC/BSI TickIT Office, London.

Preface

AIMS, CONTENT, AND AUDIENCE

As a practitioner of pharmaceutical validation, I have often wished for an easy-to-use, comprehensive, practical validation handbook that I could consult for the answer to a question on a point of detail or, perhaps, for an overview of a validation approach appropriate to a particular validation project. Why reinvent the wheel when others have probably already validated similar automation systems? Until now this body of practical experience has been accessible only through personal contacts. This book, I hope, begins to address this need for a validation handbook with case studies. I believe it will prove invaluable to those new to validation, and provide a useful reference text to those wanting to refine their validation skills. Validation is not an exact science, the regulations are interpretive, and there is always scope to improve our understanding of them and how best they can be implemented.

Since 1994, a number of pharmaceutical industry initiatives have supplemented the regulations governing the validation of automated systems with high-level guidelines. The initiatives have been led by the following:

- The joint German Society for Measurement and Automatic Control and Standardisation Association for Measurement and Control in Process Industries (GMA-NAMUR)
- The German Association for Pharmaceutical Process Engineering (APV)
- The International Society of Pharmaceutical Engineering (ISPE)
- The Organisation for Economic Co-operation and Development (OECD)

- The UK GAMP Forum
- The UK Institute for Quality Assurance's Pharmaceutical Quality Group (IQA-PQG)
- The U.S. Environmental Protection Agency (EPA)
- The U.S. Parenteral Drug Association (PDA)

The result has been a broadly accepted industry framework for validating automation systems. This framework encompasses Good Automated Manufacturing Practice (GAMP), Good Automated Laboratory Practice (GALP), and Good Information Technology Practice (GITP). There is a need, however, to bridge the gap between this framework and its practical application. How much validation is excessive, insufficient, or enough for various applications of different automation systems? Recent presentations by representatives of GMP regulatory authorities, pharmaceutical manufacturers, and suppliers at conferences and symposia have called for more case studies. Indeed, Tony Trill, a Principal Investigator with the UK's Medicines Control Agency (MCA) has reiterated this plea in the foreword to this book.

This book deals directly with project problems and their resolution based on the extensive experience of established industry practitioners. It has two parts. I have written the first part of the book to introduce the principles of good practice and why validation is needed. It cites examples (both North American and European) of costs and benefits with profile accounts of non-compliance within the pharmaceutical industry, and it draws lessons from a database of over 350 projects. The various regulatory authorities around the world, including the Australian Therapeutic Goods Administration (TGA), the Japanese Ministry of Health and Welfare, the UK Medicines Control Agency (MCA), and the U.S. Food and Drug Administration (FDA), and their requirements also are introduced. This part goes on to cover organisation, life-cycle approaches, validation requirements of different systems, support programmes, working relationships, validation capabilities, and topical issues.

The second part of the book presents a comprehensive selection of case studies, forming a substantial portion of the book. It is the work of various industry experts, representing both pharmaceutical manufacturers and their suppliers. The aim is to put into practice the principles set out in the first part of the book. The case studies cover the following:

- Instrumentation
- Programmable Logic Controllers (PLCs)
- Industrial Personal Computers (IPCs)
- Supervisory Control and Data Aquisition (SCADA) systems
- Manufacturing Execution Systems (MES)

- Distributed Control Systems (DCS)
- Electronic Batch Record Systems (EBRS)
- Electronic Document Management Systems (EDMS)
- Building Management Systems (BMS)
- Engineering Management Systems (EMS)
- Manufacturing Resource Planning (MRP II) systems
- Laboratory Information Management Systems (LIMS)
- Medical Devices

Emphasis is placed on the practical issues encountered during projects and their cost-effective resolutions.

In addition to the pharmaceutical industry, this book should be of interest to manufacturers of food, biotechnology and cosmetic products, medical devices, diagnostic systems, fine chemicals, bulk pharmaceutical chemicals, and veterinary products. There is no comparable book on the market.

ACKNOWLEDGMENTS

This book was prompted by Sue Horwood of Medi-Tech. Publications (Europe) who thought, and I agreed, that there was a need in the pharmaceutical industry for a book offering practical advice on validating automation systems. Having published numerous validation papers, I had toyed with the idea of writing a book, but it wasn't until Sue approached me that I actually did anything about it. I would like to thank Sue for her enthusiasm and encouragement throughout the project and to thank Amy Davis of Interpharm for offering to publish the book and collating valuable review comments on early manuscripts.

My original concept for a practical book, however, would not have been complete without the provision of case study material. I am indebted to my contributors for their enthusiastic participation and openness in sharing their personal validation experiences with different types of automation systems. I am sure the collection of case studies will prove an invaluable source of advice to other practitioners.

- Rob Almond, Glaxo Wellcome, England
- John Bianculli, Beckman Instruments, U.S.A.
- Peter Bosshard, Hoffmann-La Roche, Switzerland
- Peter Coady, P.J. Coady & Associates, England

- Tony de Claire, SmithKline Beecham, England
- Chris Evans, Eutech Engineering Solutions, England
- John Gough, Pfizer, England
- Peter Gough, Eli Lilly, England
- Thomas Hefti, Hoffmann-La Roche, Switzerland
- Ludwig Huber, Hewlett-Packard, Germany
- Terry R. Lucy, Glaxo Wellcome, England
- Richard Mitchell, Pfizer, England
- Peter Owen, Eli Lilly, England
- Bob Paige, Eutech Engineering Solutions, England
- Chris Reid, Imperial Chemical Industries, England
- Owen Salvage, Eutech Engineering Solutions, England
- Kate Samways, Rhône-Poulenc Rorer, England
- Martin Smith, Zeneca Pharma, France
- Hans O. Sucker, Hoffmann-La Roche, Switzerland
- Nick Townsend, Beckman Instruments, England
- Tony Trill, Medicines Control Agency, England
- Mark Whitehouse, Yokogawa, England
- Guy Wingate, Eutech Engineering Solutions, England
- Sion Wyn, Activa Systems, Wales

Biographies and contact addresses of the contributors are given in Appendix 4 to this book.

Finally, but by no means least, I am indebted to my wife Sarah for her patience, love, and support during the many evenings and weekends I spent preparing this book, especially in the months leading up to and after the birth of our daughter Katherine last summer.

Dr. Guy Wingate
Validation Manager
Eutech Engineering
June 1997

Part 1

Good Practice

CHAPTER 1

Introduction

Over the past 20 years, the pharmaceutical industry has increasingly used automation to support the manufacturing of healthcare products. Within research environments, automation systems are used to speed up product development, reducing the time between the registration of a patent and product approval and, hence, optimising the time available to manufacture product under a patent. Automation systems are also used within the production environment to improve manufacturing performance, reducing production costs, and improving the product quality. Cost and quality are important factors in today's competitive marketplace, especially since national health authorities in North America and Europe are exerting increasing pressure on pharmaceutical manufacturers to reduce the prices of patent drugs. Health authorities who deem patent drug prices to be too high are encouraging their doctors to prescribe cheaper suitable alternative generic drug products. The pharmaceutical industry's investment in automation systems will not be successful, however, unless they satisfy regulatory Good Manufacturing Practice (GMP) requirements.

GOOD MANUFACTURING PRACTICE

Good Manufacturing Practice (GMP) is probably most readily associated with the manufacture of drug products. It is, however, also applicable to the manufacture of food, biotechnology, and cosmetic products; medical devices; diagnostic systems; fine chemicals; bulk pharmaceutical chemicals (BPCs); and veterinary products. The philosophy behind GMP is to ensure that manufactured products

> *are consistently produced and controlled to the quality standards [safety, quality, and efficacy] appropriate to their use* [1].

Aligned with GMP are Good Clinical Practice (GCP) and Good Laboratory Practice (GLP), both of which share the same philosophy.

It is vital that drug products are manufactured to their approved and predetermined specifications because substandard products can be detrimental to health care and, at an extreme, can cause death. Users of drug products include our friends, family, and indeed ourselves. Poor ingredients, incorrect concentrations or quantities, contamination, mislabelling, and inappropriate storage and handling can all cause product deficiencies. The pharmaceutical industry has a "duty of care" to prevent disasters. Corollary headlines, such as "Top-Selling Drug May Have Killed Hundreds" resulting from instances of GMP noncompliance, will destroy the public's trust in the industry.

GMP is based on the premise of Quality Assurance (building in inherent confidence) rather than relying on Quality Control (testing for confidence) and covers both production and distribution. Quality Control should confirm confidence rather than determine confidence. Comprehensive Quality Control, which involves testing all manufactured products, to guarantee standards is prohibitively expensive.

An "onion" diagram is presented in Figure 1.1, showing the layers of Quality Assurance protecting the standard of a manufactured product. This diagram is best explained by an example, such as tablet manufacturing. An incorrect dosage for a tablet may occur during production due to a partially blocked intake of active ingredient into the tablet mix. The manufacturing process will continue to operate if the automation system has not been designed to detect this situation. Independent checks on the usage of active ingredient may only identify the problem after several batches have been produced. The operator will not detect anything unusual if the tablet appearance has not been affected. Quality Control should finally detect the product deficiency by sampling production batches, but only if the sample includes deficient tablets.

Records of the supply chain must also be made and maintained to enable a complete history of a product batch to be traced and, if necessary, substandard product recalled. Such records will include the receipt of raw materials; the manufacture of BPC intermediates and finished products; and the distribution of finished products to hospitals, pharmacies, and wholesalers. An overview of the pharmaceutical supply chain is shown in Figure 1.2. Any deficiencies in the manufacturing process or defects in manufactured products distributed must be investigated and appropriate measures taken to prevent their reoccurrence. Equally, any modifications to the manufacturing process must also be evaluated to determine whether the standard of manufactured product is affected.

The pharmaceutical industry is governed by GMP regulations, such as the World Health Organisation's (WHO) resolution WHA 22.50; the

Figure 1.1. Product Assurance Layers

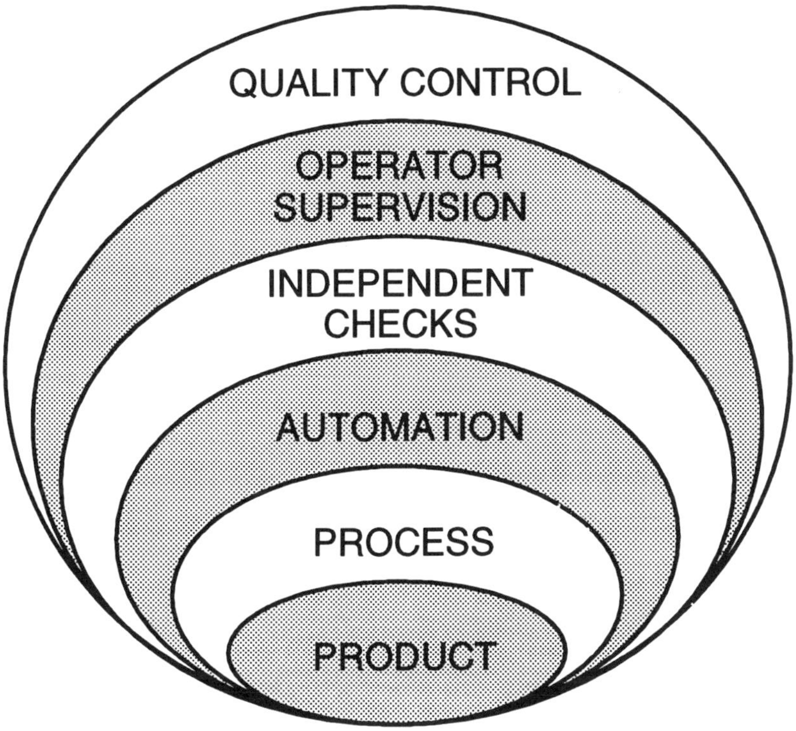

European Union's (EU) Directive 91/356/EEC; the Japanese Manual on Computer Systems in Drug Manufacturing; the U.S. Code of Federal Regulations Title 21, Parts 210 and 211; and Medicinal Products—Part 1 of the Australian Code of Good Manufacturing for Therapeutic Goods. GMP is enforced by national regulatory authorities. Well-known GMP regulatory authorities in the pharmaceutical industry include the FDA (U.S. Food and Drug Administration), the MCA (UK Medicines Control Agency), and the TGA (Australian Therapeutic Goods Administration). The regulatory authorities can prevent the sale of a product in their respective country if they consider its manufacture not to be GMP compliant. To pharmaceutical manufacturers, GMP is a licence-to-operate issue.

The achievement of GMP is the responsibility of senior management in pharmaceutical manufacturing companies. It requires the full participation of staff in many different departments (e.g., research, engineering, production, quality, warehouse) and at all levels within the pharmaceutical company in partnership with the company's suppliers.

Figure 1.2. Supply Chain for Pharmaceutical Products

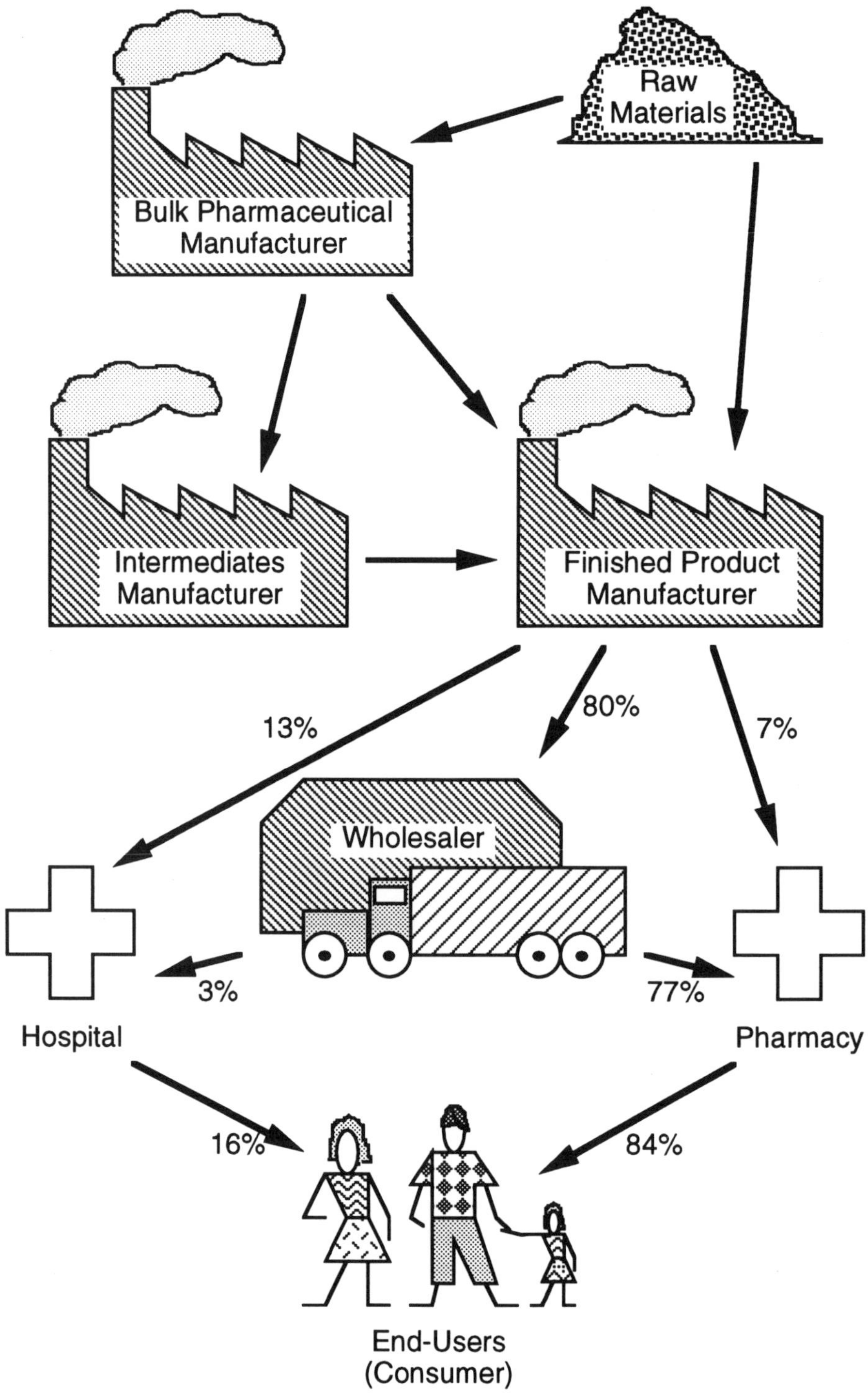

VALIDATION FOR GMP

Demonstrating GMP has become known as *validation* and necessitates

> *establishing documented evidence which provides a high degree of assurance that a specific process will consistently produce a product meeting its pre-determined specifications and quality attributes* [2].

This definition has been widely embraced, with minor modifications, by the various GMP regulatory authorities around the world and encompasses the use of automation systems. Automation systems are sometimes known as computerised systems. Pharmaceutical manufacturers must validate all automation systems used to monitor and/or control drug production whose malfunction could possibly affect the safety, quality, and efficacy (during manufacture) or batch tracking (during distribution) of drug products. Software and hardware must comply with GMP requirements for manufacturing records and equipment respectively [6].

Examples of automation systems include intelligent instrumentation, process computer systems, production support systems, and laboratory systems. Automation systems are based on programmable electronic devices connected to actuators and sensors (and possibly other automation systems) via communication links. A schematic of an automation system is shown in Figure 1.3 and is based on U.S. Pharmaceutical Manufacturers Association's (PMA) schematic for computerised systems [7].

The pharmaceutical industry's duty of care includes the use of automation systems because of their potential impact on the quality of manufactured drug product. Failure in this duty of care implies, at best, negligence or incompetence; at worst, fraud, and may be subject to legal prosecution and liability. Responsible parties may jointly or individually include equipment hardware suppliers, software suppliers, system integrators, and system users. GMP regulators, however, hold the pharmaceutical manufacturing organisation ultimately accountable for GMP compliance. Examples of accountability include deficient design, deficient construction, deficient inspection, deficient user instructions provided by supplier, software installed on an inappropriate hardware platform, system inappropriately used, or operational instructions not followed.

Technological advances that every two years have typically been doubling the complexity of automation systems for the same price, or halving their cost for the same complexity, have made the use of automation systems readily justifiable investments. The complexity of automation systems, however, means that they are susceptible to deficiencies in development and operation (e.g., poor specification capture, design errors, and poor maintenance practice). As the use of automation systems increases, so do the potential problems for pharmaceutical products and public health and safety. It is not surprising, therefore, that regulatory authorities require validation (evidence

Figure 1.3. Schematic Illustrating the Use of an Automation System

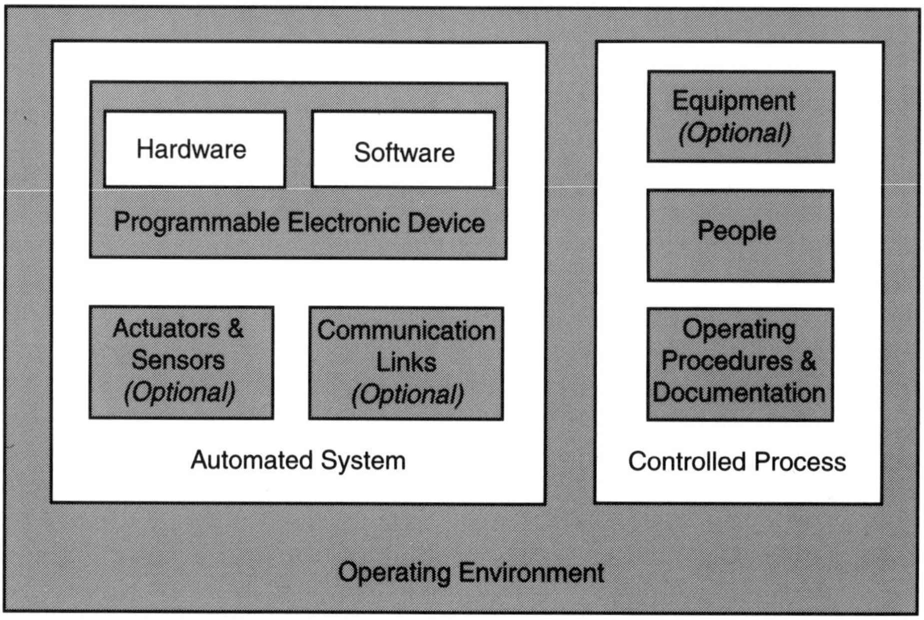

of professionalism concerning the development and operation) of automation systems [1,3]. Even without the requirements for validation, control systems are extremely difficult to implement right the first time. All of this must be achieved without delaying the commissioning and operation of automation systems in what are often fast-track projects with stringent budgets.

A BRIEF HISTORY OF VALIDATION

The concept of validation was developed in 1978 and is widely credited to Ted Byers, who was then Associate Director of Compliance at the FDA. The need to validate automated systems formally began in 1979 when the United States introduced GMP regulatory legislation that specifically referred to automation equipment [3].

The first widely publicised FDA citation for computer validation noncompliance occurred in 1985; however, as early as 1982, the FDA was publicly stating that it was "nervous" if computer systems were unvalidated [4]. In 1983, the FDA issued what became known as the "Blue Book" (because of the colour of its cover) [5]. This publication gave guidance to inspectors on what to accept as validation evidence for computer systems. The Blue Book formally introduced the anticipation of a life-cycle approach to validation. The aim was to build in quality (Quality Assurance) rather than rely on testing-in quality (Quality Control).

Responding to the FDA's proactive position on computer systems validation, the PMA formed a Computer Systems Validation Committee to represent and coordinate the industry's viewpoint. The results were a joint FDA/PMA conference in 1984 discussing computer systems validation and, in the following year, the publication of an industry perspective. The publication presented an alternative life cycle that included an approach for validating both new and existing computer systems [7]. GMP legislation is unusual in that it is equally applied to new production facilities and to production facilities built entirely or partially before the legislation was invoked.

Throughout the 1980s, computer systems validation was debated, primarily in the United States. Ken Chapman has published a paper [8] covering this period, during which the FDA gave advice on the following GMP issues:

- Input/output checking [9]
- Batch records [10]
- Applying GMP to hardware and software [9]
- Supplier responsibility [9]
- Application-specific software inspection [9]
- FDA investigation of computer systems [10]
- Software development activities [11]

In addition, since the end of the 1980s, the FDA and the pharmaceutical industry have debated the GMP requirements and the practicalities of electronic signatures. This has now been resolved by the issue of a new regulation [12].

Complementing the U.S. GMP guidance, the European Commission and Australia both issued GMP codes of practice in 1989 and 1990 [13], respectively. The European code was later issued in 1991 as a directive superseding member state GMP legislation [14].

In most countries, GMP requirements are open to a degree of interpretation. For a court to prosecute a pharmaceutical manufacturer, it must be convinced that the charges reflect the intent to flout governing legislation. In the United States, however, a court's declared judgement determined supplementary GMP information to be substantive. The effect was that the FDA's advisory opinions became binding on the FDA. In August 1990, the FDA announced that it no longer considered advisory opinions binding, on the grounds that such restrictions were unconstitutional. Hence, FDA interpretations of the regulations in Compliance Policy Guides, Guides to Investigators, and other publications by FDA authors are now for guidance only.

Computer systems validation became a high-profile industry issue in Europe in 1990 when two European manufacturers had products temporarily banned from the United States for computer systems noncompliance. The position of the FDA was clear: the manufacturers had failed to satisfy their "concerns" that computer systems should [15]

- Perform accurately and reliably
- Be secure from unauthorised or inadvertent changes
- Provide for adequate documentation of the process

The manufacturers thought that their interpretation of GMP fulfilled the requirements of the existing GMP legislation, but they had not satisfied the FDA's interpretation of GMP. Hence, the modern terminology of cGMP (Current Good Manufacturing Practice) has been introduced to signify the latest understanding of the validation practices and standards expected by regulatory authorities.

In 1991, the UK Pharmaceutical Industry Computer Systems Validation Forum (PICSVF—known as the UK Forum) was established to facilitate the exchange of validation knowledge and the development of a standard industry guide for computer systems validation. At this time, suppliers were struggling to understand and implement the various interpretations and requirements of GMP presented by manufacturers. PICSVF's guide is based on a prototype called V-MAN (Validation Management). In 1994, the guide came to fruition and was launched as a first draft within the United Kingdom and has become known as the GAMP guide (Good Automated Manufacturing Practice). A second draft was published for comment by the European pharmaceutical industry in 1995. An electronic issue (version 1.0) and a further revision in both electronic and paper form (version 2.0) was issued through the ISPE in 1996 [16]. The GAMP guide was complemented in 1995 by two other validation guides produced respectively by the U.S. Parenteral Drug Association (PDA) [17] and a joint committee of two German measurement, automation, and control organisations (GMA-NAMUR) [18]. These initiatives should help manufacturers and suppliers meet the challenge to validate effectively and efficiently all computer systems.

Meanwhile, two experienced GMP regulatory inspectors, Ron Tetzlaff and Tony Trill, published papers presenting the FDA's and MCA's, respectively, inspection practice for computer systems [19,20]. These papers presented a comprehensive perspective on the current validation expectations of the GMP regulatory authorities. Topics covered included the following:

- Life-cycle approach
- Quality management
- Procedures
- Training

- Validation protocols
- Qualification evidence
- Change control
- Audit trail
- Ongoing evaluation

Whilst a common methodology for computer systems validation incorporating these topics has become established within the pharmaceutical industry, the regulatory authorities continue to experience "problems":

> *The major problems observed are in the validation of various manufacturing and control operations. We are seeing more problems now with operations run by computers and the validation of these computer programs* [21].

based on

- Incomplete documents
- Insufficient detail in documentation
- Missing documentary evidence

The regulatory authorities appreciate the difficulty in determining what constitutes sufficient validation for different automation systems. In 1995, the FDA revised their GMP Code of Federal Regulations affecting automation systems, to make allowance for the complexity and reliability of the systems [3]. Pharmaceutical manufacturers can now justify a baseline for validation based on the technology risk and the operational track record of the automation system. This development has been widely welcomed by practitioners.

Recent developments in 1996 include a guideline for computer systems validation, written by the German Association for Pharmaceutical Process Engineering (APV), based on clarifying the requirements of Annex 11 of the EU GMP Guideline. The PICSVF have renamed themselves the GAMP Forum (which is certainly easier to pronounce!), and are planning a third edition of their automation validation guide.

HIGH–PROFILE INDUSTRY INCIDENTS: LESSONS AND IMPLICATIONS

The first high-profile, automation, validation noncompliances were publicised in 1985 and occurred in the United States. The incidents involved a laboratory system at Wyeth's nonclinical laboratory [22] and a computerised dispensing system at Boehringer Ingleheim's production facility [23]. The noncompliances concerned

- Inadequate hardware and software validation
- No revalidation after significant hardware and software changes
- Lack of environmental controls
- No backup power supply to prevent uncontrolled system shutdowns
- Unsecured laboratory computer programs and raw data
- Inadequate security procedures for the HVAC computer system

The potentially devastating outcome of GMP noncompliance of computer systems was demonstrated in 1988 when deficient software in a data management system controlling a blood-plasma bank could have led to the issue of HIV- (Human Immunodeficiency Virus) infected blood [8]. Similarly, computer systems can endanger public health by manufacturing and erroneously releasing drug products with deficient quality attributes.

Automation systems used at production sites in Italy and England belonging to ICI Pharmaceuticals, Glaxo, and other pharmaceutical manufacturers were found to be noncompliant during a foreign inspection programme conducted by the FDA's Ron Tetzlaff in 1991. The automation systems in question were sterilisers and laboratory computer systems. They were the first widely publicised automation validation incidents in Europe and the problems identified included the following [19]:

- No formal plans stating the validation requirements for computer systems.
- Specifications were not available to define the intended software operation.
- No qualification protocols defining testing or acceptance criteria.
- Inadequate accuracy checks, input-output checks, and alarm testing.
- Inadequate change and version control of software.
- No final review of the evidence demonstrating validation.

It was not possible to demonstrate that the particular drug products under manufacture were achieving their respective quality, safety, and efficiacy requirements.

More recent, high-profile instances of GMP noncompliances affecting automation systems occurred in 1995 and involved a water purification plant, an integrated materials control and electronic batch record system, and a tabletting control system at Burroughs-Wellcome in the United States and Ciba-Geigy in Switzerland [24]. Problems discovered by the FDA included the following:

- Technical documents lacked formulae and method details.
- Design documents for systems not maintained in line with plant changes.
- Test parameters changed without authorisation.
- Test procedures not up-to-date with specifications.
- Imprecise specification to vendor led to unrobust system design.

The lesson to the pharmaceutical industry is that the problems identified in the high-profile incidents cited earlier continue to occur. Validation should improve this situation.

COSTS AND BENEFITS

The costs and benefits of validating automated systems is a subject of much debate and many misconceptions. Automation systems can account for up to half the cost of validating a production plant. With such a large investment, it is important to demonstrate not only regulatory compliance but also the benefits of improved manufacturing efficiency and product quality.

Misconceptions

- *Validation is a new development.* In fact, the methodology of validation for automated systems was established by IBM in the 1950s but has only recently received prominence as a requirement within the pharmaceutical industry.
- *Validation of pharmaceutical automation systems has been specially developed by the FDA to protect their domestic markets from foreign competition.* Recent international free-trade agreements should prevent such restrictive trade and have the power, if invoked, to take offending countries to binding arbitration.
- *ISO 9000 accreditation for quality management fully satisfies the requirements of validation for GMP.* This is not true, but ISO 9001 (supply of goods or services) and ISO 9000-3 (supply of software) do provide a good basis for validation.
- *Validation is a one-time event that concludes with a "certification" that the system is validated.* This misconception is usually based on the premise that validation is regulated in the same manner as standards and certification by bodies such as the German TÜV (Technischer Überwachungs-Verein). The GMP regulatory authorities do

not certify validation. Validation is an ongoing activity covering development, operation, and maintenance.

- *Validation incurs unnecessary paperwork—GMP being associated with Great Mounds of Paper rather than Getting More Product.* This is only the case if validation has been poorly implemented.

Cost of Failure

The failure to validate to a regulator's satisfaction can have significant financial implications. All of the noncompliance incidents cited led to the withdrawal or delayed issue of a licence to the pharmaceutical manufacturers to distribute their product in the United States. The PMA has estimated that a company will spend between U.S. $50,000 and U.S. $100,000 for every day of delay during the pharmaceutical submission process [25]. This is a small amount compared to the typical investment of U.S. $250,000,000 to bring a new drug to market. The real financial impact of GMP noncompliance, however, is the loss in sales revenue. For top-selling drugs in production, citations for noncompliance by GMP regulatory authorities can cost their manufacturer upwards of U.S. $2,000,000 per day in lost sales revenue. One of the incidents cited above cost the company concerned over U.S. $100,000,000 in lost sales and revalidation. The challenge is to conduct cost-effectively sufficient validation to ensure GMP compliance and, as illustrated in Figure 1.4, there is always debate over how much is sufficient to fulfil the regulator's expectations. Excessive validation may increase confidence in regulatory compliance but it is expensive. Inadequate validation may be cheaper but, in the long term, the cost of regulatory noncompliance could be devastating. This book aims to clarify how much validation is sufficient, to suggest how it can be cost-effectively organised, and to discuss areas of debate.

There are numerous stakeholders with an interest in successful GMP inspection outcome. GMP noncompliances are likely to reduce public confidence in the pharmaceutical industry and the offending manufacturer. Political pressures may result in improvements for industry practice; the inspection methods of regulatory authorities and the acceptability of validation standards and guides may be reviewed. The standing of regulatory authorities may be affected. There may also be legal liability issues for the regulator and offending manufacturer. The manufacturer's corporate reputation may take years to recover. Drug sales are likely to drop as end users of the products become uneasy about the consistency of supply. Market confidence in the offending manufacturer will be reduced and the brand value affected. The reputation of suppliers may also suffer from association with the offending manufacturer. Insurance premiums for the manufacturer are likely to increase. As an overall consequence, the jobs of all those working for the manufacturer and associated suppliers will be less secure.

Figure 1.4. Good Practice for Validation

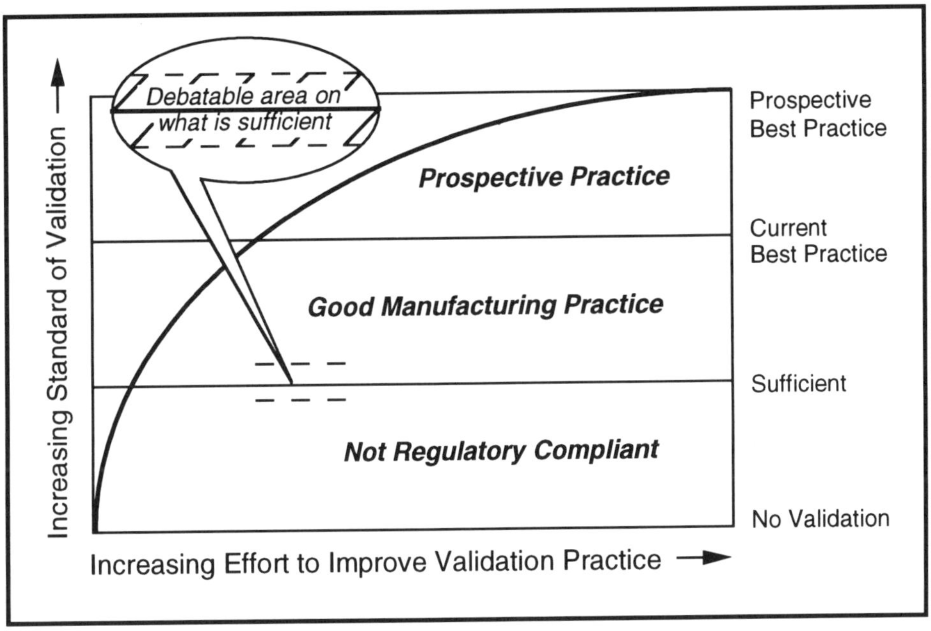

Benefits of Success

Few metrics have been collected to demonstrate the benefits of validation. At a fundamental level, however, the good practices invoked by validation should ensure automation systems are right the first time, every time. Indeed, if the automation system and its plant are already ahead of schedule, it could start production earlier than originally planned and perhaps earn the pharmaceutical manufacturer U.S. $2,000,000 per day in additional sales for a top-selling drug.

Anecdotal evidence of validation benefits includes the case of two tablet manufacturing and filling lines, each controlled by identical automation systems installed by a major pharmaceutical manufacturer [26,27]. The lines were installed on different occasions, one line having been validated from conception to handover, the other line being unvalidated. Figure 1.5 illustrates the benefits of validation in this instance that were wide ranging and included the following:

- Improved productivity
- Waste reduction
- Reduced manpower

Figure 1.5. Anecdotal Validation Benefits

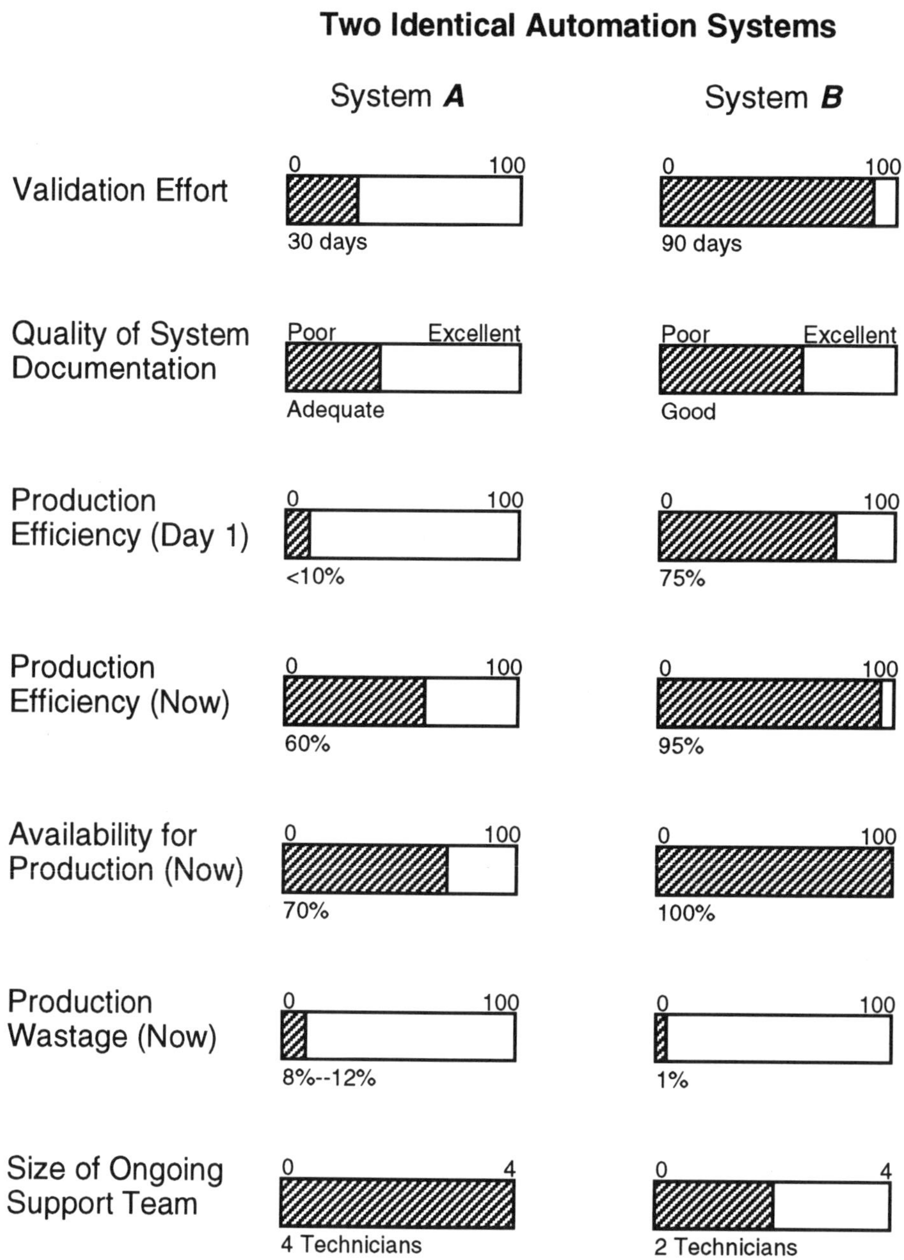

The bottom line to the company was that the investment in validation had a payback of four weeks compared to the unvalidated line! Validation facilitated a change from stock management to just-in-time (JIT) supply to orders. The payback of validation may not be as quick for other projects, but the point is that validation should more than pay for itself in the long term through improved operational efficiencies.

Other anecdotal evidence exists for a *maintenance dividend.* A survey of over 300 applications by Weinberg Associates suggests that the investment in validation is generally offset by maintenance savings within 4 years [28]. An example of the maintenance dividend can be illustrated with a production planning system at ICI which adopted the principles of validation for about half of its 800 computer programs. The quality approach was abandoned by management halfway through the project because there was no perceived project benefit. The total operational life of the system was later examined and maintenance costs for the software adopting the principles of validation was about 90 percent less that the costs for the remainder of the software [29]. Similar examples exist for MRP II systems. With nonquality software typically accounting for 50–60 percent of maintenance costs, validation makes good business sense [30].

Validation also yields intangible benefits. *Production staff* work within a quality environment where fewer unplanned activities reduce stress. Human error is consequently reduced and productivity improved. It would appear that a significant proportion of production problems can be attributed to human error [31]. *Users of drug products* can rely on a regular supply of consistently high quality. A brand loyalty can result. *Regulators* will develop a confidence in the assurance of product standards by a pharmaceutical manufacturer. During GMP inspections regulators will have a positive expectation for compliance rather than an anticipation of noncompliance. *A pharmaceutical manufacturer's* track record of GMP compliance will further enhance the corporate reputation and develop a general industry confidence in the company. *Suppliers* who successfully support GMP within such pharmaceutical companies will also enhance their reputation.

Ultimately, GMP compliance protects public health. The scope of this protection exercise has been indicated by Brian Hartley of the MCA who cited that, on average in 1995, Europeans and North Americans received an average of 10 prescription items and purchased 6 over-the-counter (OTC) medicines [32]. The pharmaceutical industry is by far the most positively viewed of all industries in the chemicals sector, with only 10 percent of the public expressing an unfavourable opinion [33]. This is an impressive figure that has been improving annually by 1 or 2 percent since GMP came to prominence just under 2 decades ago. Validation for GMP would seem to be vindicated.

REFERENCES

1. European Union (1989), *EC Guide to Good Manufacturing Practice for Medicinal Products.*
2. FDA (1987), *General Principles of Process Validation,* Rockville, MD: Food and Drug Administration, Center for Drug Evaluation and Research.

3. U.S. Code of Federal Regulations Title 21: Part 211 (first issued 1979, last amended 1995), *Current Good Manufacturing Practice for Finished Pharmaceuticals.*

4. Fry, C.B. (1982), What We See That Makes Us Nervous, Guest Editorial, *Pharmaceutical Engineering* (May): 10–11.

5. FDA (1983), *Guide to Inspection of Computerized Systems in Drug Processing,* Technical Report, Reference Materials and Training Aids for Investigators, Rockville, MD: Food and Drug Administration.

6. Motise, P. (1996), *Inspection of Computerized Manufacturing Systems,* ISPE European Computer Systems Validation Conference, 24–25 September, Zurich, Switzerland.

7. PMA (1986), Validation Concepts for Computer Systems Used in the Manufacture of Drug Products, In *PMA Proceedings: Concepts and Principles for the Validation of Computer Systems Used in the Manufacture and Control of Drug Products,* Pharmaceutical Manufacturers Association.

8. Chapman, K. (1991), A History of Validation in the United States: Parts 1 and 2—Validation of Computer-Related Systems, *Pharmaceutical Technology.*

9. Compliance Policy Guides, Computerized Drug Processing, 7132a: Input/Output Checking (Guide 07, 1982); *Identification of "Persons" on Batch Production and Control Records* (Guide 08, 1982); *CGMP Applicability to Hardware and Software* (Guide 11, 1984); *Vendor Responsibility* (Guide 12, 1985); *Source Code for Process Control Application Programs* (Guide 15, 1987); Rockville, MD: Food and Drug Administration.

10. Clark, A.S. (1988), Computer Systems Validation: An Investigator's View, *Pharmaceutical Technology,* 12 (1): 60–66.

11. FDA (1987), *Software Development Activities,* Technical Report, Reference Materials and Training Aids for Investigators, Rockville, MD: Food and Drug Administration.

12. Final Rule for 21 CFR Part 11 (1997), Electronic Signatures and Electronic Records, *Federal Register,* 62 (54).

13. TGA (1990), *Australian Code of Good Manufacturing for Therapeutic Goods,* Medicinal Products—Part 1, Woden, Australia: Therapeutic Goods Administration.

14. European Union Guide to Directive 91/356/EEC (1991), *European Commission Directive Laying Down the Principles of Good Manufacturing Practice for Medicinal Products for Human Use.*

15. Masters, G. and Figorole, P. (1988), Validation Principles for Computer Systems-FDA's Perspective, *Pharmaceutical Technology,* 10 (11): 44–46.

16. UK GAMP Forum (1996), *Supplier Guide for Validation of Automation Systems in Pharmaceutical Manufacture,* Second Version, The Hague: International Society for Pharmaceutical Engineers.

17. PDA (1995), Validation of Computer Related Systems, *PDA Journal of Pharmaceutical Science and Technology,* Technical Report No. 18.

18. NE 58: Abwicklung von qualifizierungspflichtigen PLT-Projekten (version 04.06.96); [including . . .] Dannapel, B., Hensel, H., Mockel, B., Muhlenkamp, J., Muller-Heinzerling, T., Otto, A., and Teuchert, V. (1995), Qualifizierung von Leitsystemen: Ein Gemeinschaftsprojekt von GMA und NAMUR zur Validierung, *ATP—Automatisierungstechnische Praxis,* 37 (10): 64–76.

19. Tetzlaff, R.F. (1992), GMP Documentation Requirements for Automated Systems: Parts 1, 2, and 3, *Pharmaceutical Technology,* 16 (3): 112–124, 16 (4): 60–72, 16 (5): 70–82.

20. Trill, A.J. (1993), Computerized Systems and GMP—A UK Perspective: Part 1: Background, Standards and Methods; Part 2: Inspection Findings; Part 3: Best Practices and Topical Issues, *Pharmaceutical Technology International,* 5 (2): 12–26, 5 (3): 49–63, 5 (5): 17–30.

21. International Society for Pharmaceutical Engineering (1994), An Interview with Richard Klug, *Pharmaceutical Engineering,* 14 (3): 26–31.

22. *The Gold Sheet* (1995), January, Boulder, CO: GMP Trends.

23. Branning, R.C. (1986), Experience in an FDA Inspection, In *PMA Proceedings: Concepts and Principles for the Validation of Computer Systems Used in the Manufacture and Control of Drug Products,* Pharmaceutical Manufacturers Association.

24. Trill, A.J. (1996), *The Regulations,* Computer Systems Validation: A Practical Approach, Management Forum Seminar, 26–27 March, London.

25. Weinberg, S., Romoff, R.M., and Stein, G. (1993), *Handbook of System Validation,* Philadelphia, Weinberg, Spelton & Sax Inc.

26. Swift, T. (1996), *Validation—Justifying the Investment to Meet the Business Need,* Process and Computer Validation '96, Spring Innovations, 22–23 April, UMIST Conference Centre, Manchester, England.

27. Selby, D. (1996), *Validation—Value for Money?,* Process and Computer Validation '96, Spring Innovations, 22–23 April, UMIST Conference Centre, Manchester, England.

28. Weinberg, A. (1992), *Case Studies in System Validation: Sixteen Theses,* Philadelphia: Weinberg Associates, Inc.

29. Gilb, T., and Graham, D. (1993), *Software Inspection,* Reading, MA: Addison-Wesley.

30. UK National Computing Centre (1989), *IT-STARTS Developers Guide.*

31. Reason, J. (1990), *Human Error,* Cambridge University Press.

32. Hartley, B. (1996), *International Moves Towards Harmonisation,* Joint PDA/ISPE Conference on Computer-Related System Validation, 2–3 May, Basel, Switzerland.

33. ABPI (1995), *Industry Review 1994,* Association of the British Pharmaceutical Industry.

Chapter 2

Organisation

Legitimate concerns have been raised by pharmaceutical manufacturers concerning the most appropriate way to address the management responsibilities and organisation of validation. This chapter presents a typical approach that satisfies the manufacturer's accountabilities. There is no intent, however, to present this approach as the only acceptable organisation. The needs of the pharmaceutical manufacturer will vary depending on many different factors, including the scope of the validation requirement, the availability of suitably skilled corporate and contract staff, and cost.

ORGANISATIONAL RESPONSIBILITIES

Pharmaceutical manufacturers should appoint a senior management representative with specific responsibility for ensuring that the requirements of GMP are implemented and maintained. This individual must champion the cause of GMP and often takes the job title of validation manager or validation coordinator. The senior manager's authority and responsibility should be clearly defined and recorded.

It is very important that the senior manager has the authority to prevent the release of drug product on the grounds that noncompliant validation can compromise the quality of manufactured drug products. Without this level of authority, the senior manager will have to rely on persuading others who may be under production or sales pressures to authorise the release of drug product. It is taken for granted that quality managers have the authority to withhold drug products when they are deemed to be substandard. The same empowerment should be given to the senior manager responsible for GMP; many companies facilitate this by placing their GMP personnel within their Quality Control/Assurance management hierarchy.

The senior manager is expected to secure adequate numbers of appropriately qualified and experienced staff to conduct validation and ensure they are effectively organised [1]. Specific responsibility for validating automation should be assigned to a manager who is suitably qualified with relevant computer systems experience and appropriate training.

In many organisations, the senior manager responsible for GMP may also have other duties. It must be understood that these other duties do not excuse or relieve the senior manager's responsibility to the GMP regulatory authorities for validation. In the phrase forever associated with John Edgar Hoover, "the buck stops here!"

The expected role of senior managers is indicated by the ISO 9001 standard, which states that management shall

> *define and document [the company's] policy and objectives for, and commitment to, quality and ensure that this policy is understood, implemented and maintained at all levels in the organisation* [2].

Whilst this is useful, more practical guidance is available. Teri Stokes has translated the ISO requirements into five key tasks [3]:

1. Establish a working group to define company policy and objectives for validation.
2. Write a document that states the validation policy, including a statement of commitment to such policies and objectives.
3. Develop an awareness/education programme for delivering this document to all senior managers and to their employees.
4. Prioritise, review, and resource validation projects with funding and work time to implement the policy in an orderly way consistent with its statement of objectives.
5. Establish a validation committee to monitor and support ongoing validation efforts to meet stated objectives within policy guidelines, including procedures.

The working group and validation committee should both be multidisciplinary teams representing research, production, engineering, quality control/assurance, and business support. Members should be sent to internal or external courses so that they understand the basic principles of validation. Alternatively, members can attend a validation conference where they can also meet validation practitioners from other companies. Major conferences are regularly organised by Management Forum, Spring Innovations, and the International Society of Pharmaceutical Engineering (ISPE) throughout Europe and the United States. External consultants with specialist validation knowledge and experience may also be used to support the working group and validation committee, perhaps assisting with internal training courses.

VALIDATION STRATEGY

The aim from the outset must be to make validation as cost-effective as practicable. Several pharmaceutical manufacturers who rushed into the validation of automation systems in the late 1980s and early 1990s have very costly validation programmes that are inefficient and involve more work than necessary.

Members of the working group establishing a validation strategy must appreciate the implications of their policy on working practices. The validation approach to be adopted will be influenced by regulatory GMP legislation and industry guidelines. Wherever possible, the validation approach should also align itself with existing company practices and other regulations governing issues such as operator safety and environmental protection. Particular validation approaches may lend themselves to supporting methods and tools, some of which, such as document control, may be automated. Care must be taken to ensure supporting methods and tools are capable of fulfilling the company's validation requirements. Finally, the form and content of validation evidence to be documented and how it might be handled may also influence the validation approach. A diagram illustrating the interrelationships of these dependencies is shown in Figure 2.1.

VALIDATION POLICY

Validation Policies vary greatly between different companies. There are no set rules governing their content or structure. A Validation Policy should define the corporate intent toward GMP, and may reference a specific policy for validating automation systems. It is suggested that the policy cover the following:

- A definition of the overall principle of validation
- The scope of its application
- A definition of who is responsible
- An outline of how validation will be achieved and maintained
- A statement of commitment
- A glossary defining terminology

Experience has shown that a clear, concise validation policy can be written within a 5- to 20-page document and take 20 days' effort to draft and agree. Typically, most of the effort is spent in consultative meetings in agreeing to

Figure 2.1. Validation Dependencies

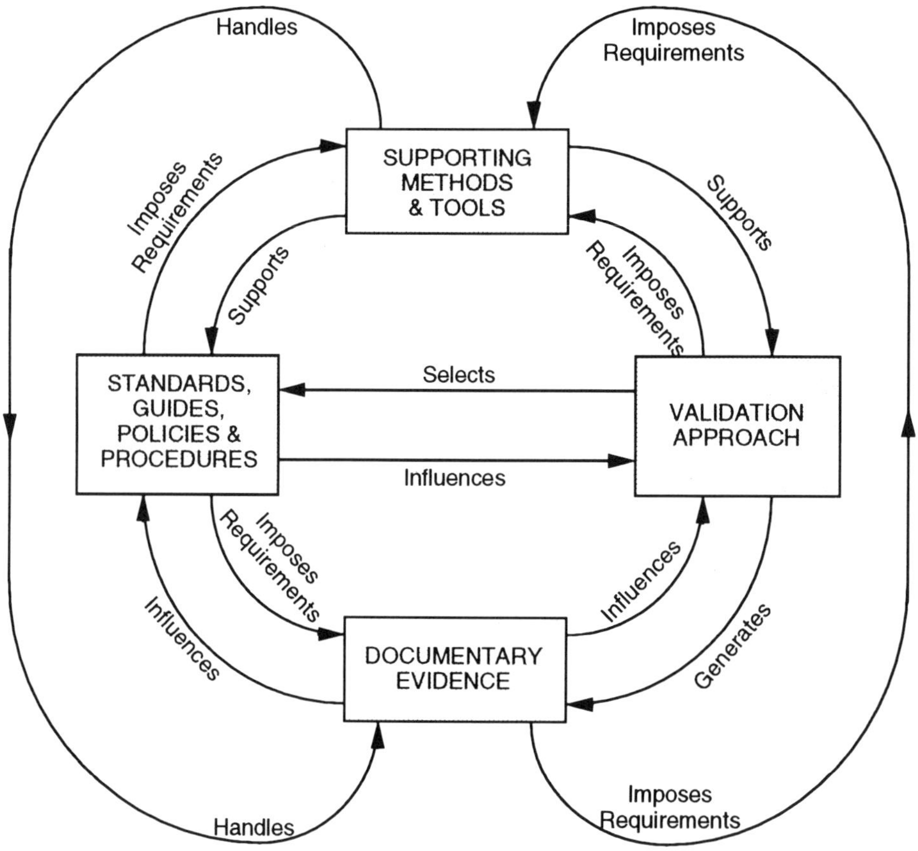

the policy. There is usually one major review of the policy before it is sufficiently refined for release. The policy must be kept up-to-date.

Within any given firm there may be multiple sites, each having different validation requirements and, perhaps, different validation practices. While conforming to overall corporate policies, site policies generally provide more detail on the requirements of a specific site. Policies are intended to establish responsibilities and expectations. Policies do not normally define specific testing requirements.

VALIDATION MANAGEMENT

After a Validation Policy has been formulated, the management of validation can be considered as a cyclical process, as shown in Figure 2.2. The management cycle begins with the development of a Validation Master Plan and its

Figure 2.2. Validation Management Cycle

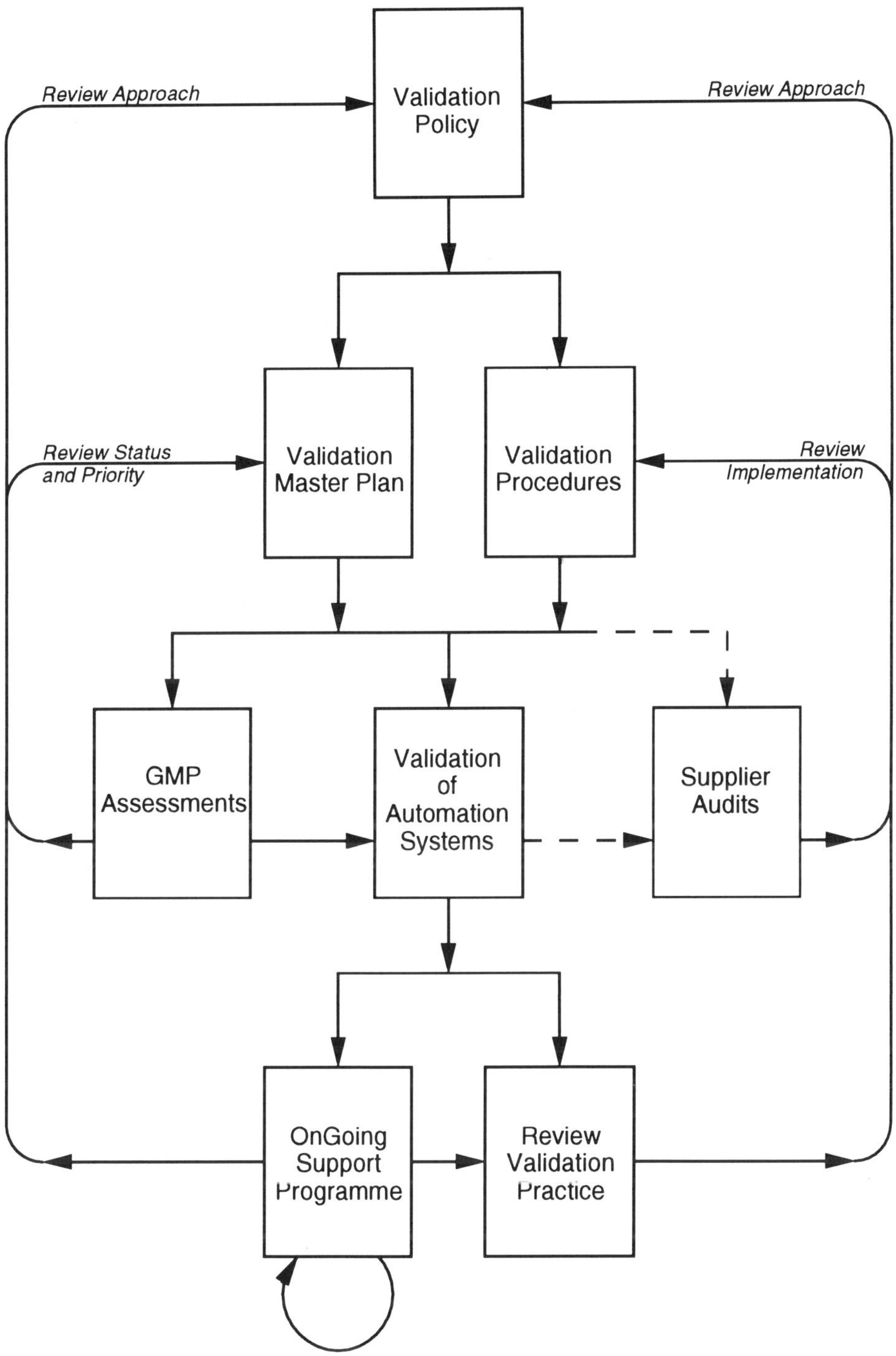

associated inventory of work. This is accompanied by the development of procedures for conducting validation. The validation of individual automation systems then begins and includes preliminary GMP Assessments and Supplier Audits. GMP Assessments survey the validation requirements of automation systems in readiness for preparing Validation Master Plans for each particular system. Supplier Audits assess the capabilities of suppliers in providing automation systems and associated services. Once validation is completed for individual automation systems, the validated status must be maintained by an ongoing support programme. At the end of each project validating an automation system, and throughout the management process, there should be formal opportunities to review validation practices. The status of validation work is likely to change: some existing systems may be decommissioned, new systems may be planned, and the priorities on the current inventory work may vary due to changing company needs. Validation Policy and Validation Procedures may also change as a result of new regulatory requirements or feedback from project experience.

VALIDATION MASTER PLAN

A site usually has a number of Validation Master Plans: an overall site plan complemented by a number of subordinate plans covering individual manufacturing facilities, laboratories, site services/utilities, and so on [4]. Validation Master Plans typically have three main sections. The first section defines the physical buildings and equipment covered by the plan and states how regulatory GMP requirements will be addressed by the pharmaceutical manufacturer's own validation philosophy and policy. The second section justifies which automation systems require validation. All automation systems whose malfunction could possibly affect the safety, quality, and efficacy (during manufacture) or batch tracking (during distribution) of drug products should be validated. A register or inventory of automation systems to be validated is often created. The register is usually attached to the Validation Master Plan as an appendix. Finally, the third section commits the pharmaceutical manufacturer to some basic milestones. These milestones are usually associated with the launch of a new drug product, but may also be timetabled to satisfy anticipated inspections by GMP regulatory authorities. The milestones demonstrate the pharmaceutical manufacturer's intent and may be revised during the course of a validation programme to reflect changing conditions. Senior managers should not be unduly worried about delays so long as the pharmaceutical manufacturer can demonstrate progress to the regulatory authorities and continued commitment to a revised timetable.

Automation systems need only be validated when they are either in direct physical contact with the drug substance or used to measure, monitor, control, or record those critical processing parameters that characterise substandard product (based on [5]). When determining whether or not an automation system should be validated, it is useful to reflect on the advice given by Sam Clark, a former FDA investigator: "If it looks like a duck, flies like a duck, and sounds like a duck, then it's probably a duck". A commonsense approach should prevail. A high-level decision tree for determining a validation requirement is shown in Figure 2.3. It is worth remembering that it is just as important to be able to provide evidence to GMP regulators justifying why certain automation systems cannot affect drug quality as

Figure 2.3. Determining a Validation Requirement

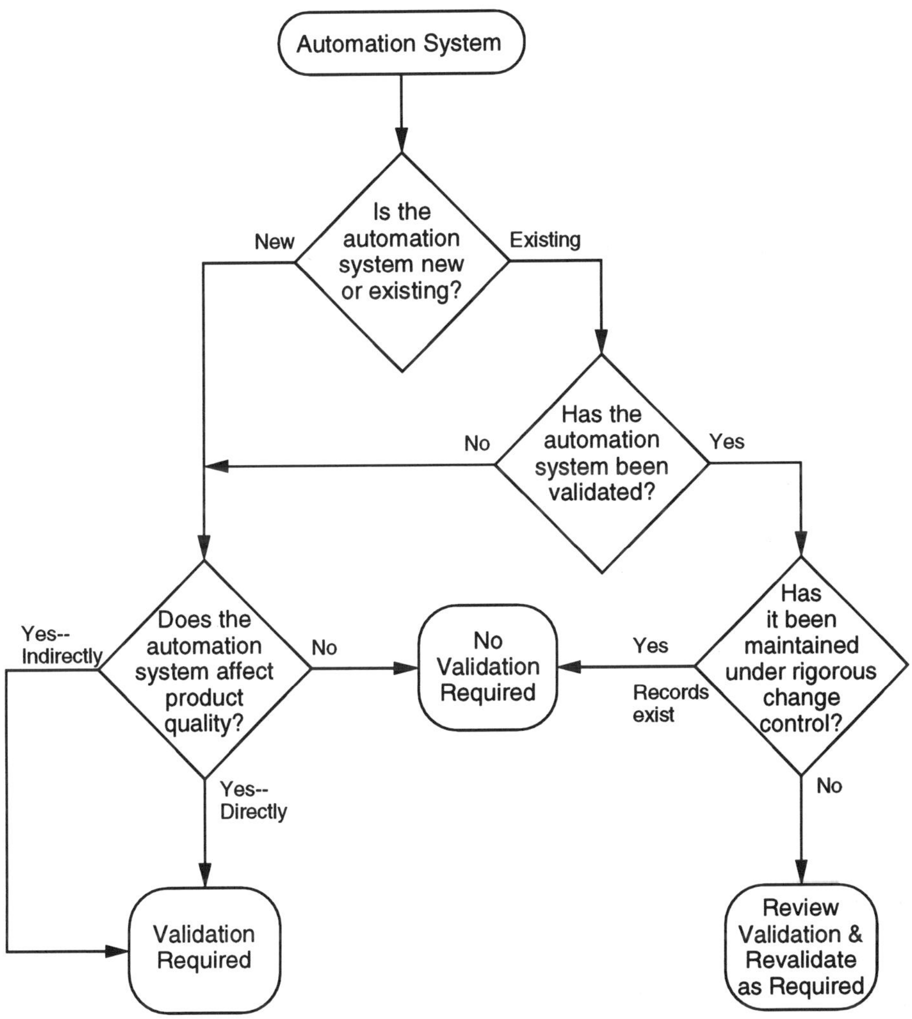

justifying the level and priority of validation needed for automation systems that can affect product quality.

It is often necessary to prioritise validation projects, especially when validating the backlog of existing systems. A register of automation systems will typically assign a priority to each system requiring validation and trace the progress of its validation. Priorities should be set according to a defined strategy. A suitable scheme might assign higher priorities to automation systems associated with shorter management reaction times to deal with situations that could potentially endanger life. The potential impact on an operator, for instance, can be immediate. Substandard BPCs, intermediates, and finished drug products will only impact the end user of a drug product if they are incorrectly authorised as fit for their intended purpose and distributed for use. A pharmaceutical manufacturer can continue to make substandard product, but if there is no alternative use for the product, then there is little sense in continuing production. Finally, current environmental protection is based on containment. Whilst acceptable reaction times to such incidents will vary, they will generally be longer than those associated with the manufacture of substandard drug products.

- Priority 1: Operator safety
- Priority 2: Finished human drug products
- Priority 3: Finished animal drug products
- Priority 4: Intermediates
- Priority 5: BPCs
- Priority 6: Environmental protection

Automation systems should usually be validated with the same priority as the manufacturing processes they support. This includes laboratory systems, utility service automation systems, and business support systems. This scheme will not be appropriate, however, where production sites are biased toward a particular mode of manufacturing: for example, human or animal finished drug products, intermediates, or bulks. In these situations, priorities will normally be set within the context of the relative importance of validation to materials handling, process control (e.g., sterilisation, blending, tabletting), packaging (including labelling), and distribution.

These suggested priorities for validating automation systems may change for particular projects. Some projects may be given a higher priority because a regulatory inspection that is likely to include the system is imminent, or there are outstanding noncompliances from a previous regulatory inspection. Equally, a lower priority may be given to automation systems that are soon to be replaced. Eli Lilly, for instance, when prioritising the validation of their existing automation systems decided not to validate those systems due for replacement within a year [6]. If such a stance is taken, however, it is important that the system is replaced within the stated time frame. It is all too easy to delay the replacement of a system so that it is permanently to be replaced within the year—such situations are not acceptable to the GMP regulatory authorities.

The time to prepare a Validation Master Plan depends on the number, type, and use of automation systems. For a facility with 30 automation systems, a Validation Master Plan with an inventory will normally take about 5 days to write. The length of the document is likely to be between 5–15 pages, depending on its detail. When writing a Validation Master Plan, it is important to minimise the duplication of information with other documents. Sufficient information, however, must be provided so that managers not directly involved in the planning can understand the validation approach in overview. Understandability is important because the Validation Master Plans will be examined by GMP regulators. Guidance on the content of associated validation documents is given in the rest of this book.

GMP ASSESSMENTS

Senior managers may wish to consider using GMP Assessments (also known as Criticality Analyses) to support the planning of individual validation projects for both existing and new automation systems. The aim of a GMP Assessment is to identify the system's overall validation requirements, confirm those aspects of the system which are already GMP compliant, recommend how any necessary validation might be achieved, and outline the necessary resources and engineering skills to conduct that validation. This information can then be used when coordinating the allocation of staff between various validation projects.

GMP Assessments are usually conducted by multidisciplined review committees with expert knowledge of regulatory requirements, the manufacturing process, and the automation system. Assessments appraise and report on the available information (opinion and documentation) pertaining to the validation requirements of an automation system under scrutiny. Information may be excessive, incomplete, inconsistent, or missing. Emphasis should be placed on identifying critical parameters affecting the standard of manufactured drug products and ensuring that aspects of automation systems dealing with these critical parameters receive detailed attention during validation. Figure 2.4 presents a decision tree which should help determine was is and what is not a GMP critical function or components. General validation is still necessary, however, to assure the overall integrity and operability of the automation system.

The outcome of the GMP Assessment is either a report or meeting minutes. Justifications for whether or not functions and components are GMP

Figure 2.4. Identifying GMP Critical Functions and Components

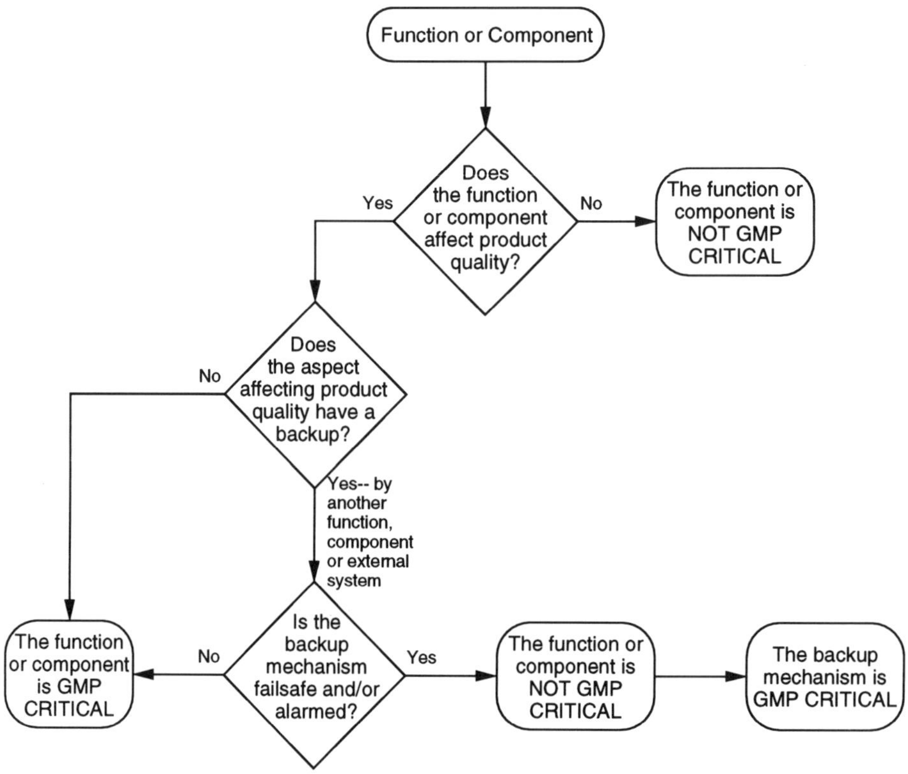

critical must be recorded. GMP Assessments are complemented by project Hazard Studies which identify that the automation system's design has controlled these critical aspects.

Options for assuring GMP that may be applied individually or collectively to an automation system include the following:

- Make an inherent design modification
- Use or amend Standard Operating Procedures (SOPs)
- Use or amend warning messages
- Add an independent protective system
- Use an alternative automation system
- Use an alternative manual system

AUTOMATION SYSTEM VALIDATION

The Information Technology (IT) industry has extensively used life-cycle models to manage the development and operation of computer systems. Initially, these models were developed for cost prediction and cost control, and reflected the observed lifetime development and operation process. More recently, life-cycle models have been used to discipline the validation of automation systems.

A validation life cycle for an automation system is shown in Figure 2.5 and described in chapter 3. It consists of the following phases:

- Validation planning
- System specification
- Supplier Project and Quality Plans
- Design and development

Figure 2.5. Validation Life Cycle

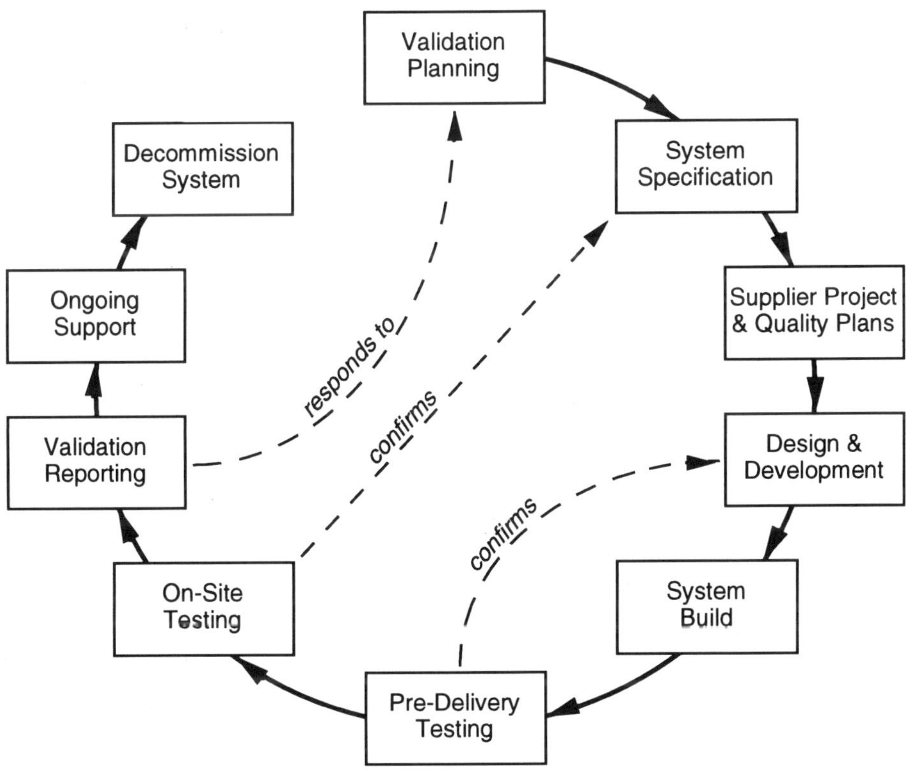

- System build
- Predelivery testing
- On-site testing
- Validation reporting
- Ongoing support
- System decommissioning

The validation life cycle is primarily for new automation systems. The principles, nevertheless, also apply to existing automation systems. This life-cycle framework is consistent with guidance provided by the Australian [7], European [8], Japanese [9], and U.S. [10] GMP regulatory authorities. It is also consistent with guidance provided by the German GMA-NAMUR [11], the U.S. PDA [12], and the UK GAMP Forum [13] industry initiatives.

The steps in the validation life cycle are not necessarily executed in the order indicated. Rather, the steps are usually executed as an iterative process, where various steps may be carried out concurrently; if necessary, steps may also be added. For instance, the Validation Master Plan may be developed after or concurrently with the User Requirements Specification (URS) rather than before as indicated. Equally, a Supplier Audit often involves a series of steps that may not be complete until well into the validation project.

Some of the steps in the validation life cycle will not be needed in some validation projects. For instance, the use of preferred suppliers for software and hardware products or services removes the need for repeated supplier appraisal and selection. Life-cycle steps, however, cannot be removed for equipment with embedded automation systems purchased from or subcontracted to a vendor. The degree of redundancy in the life-cycle model used for validating existing automation systems will be specified in the Validation Master Plan and is discussed further in Chapter 4.

For systems that have been in use for some time, a compilation and review of documentation, and a review of historical data supplemented by a series of functional tests, may be adequate to demonstrate that the system consistently and reliably performs its intended function. Evidence that the software is structurally sound may be provided by a formal evaluation of the supplier's software development and testing procedures and by an analysis of historical, system-related data. Where historical, system-related data is not available, for whatever reason, additional functional testing is required.

During any project, it should be expected that changes and modifications will be made based on progressive project experience. The validation life cycle accommodates changes at all steps, but it requires that such changes be made in accordance with written procedures and that they be documented appropriately. It is important to note that rework or additional validation may be necessary where changed steps affect concurrent or previous steps.

PROCEDURES FOR CONDUCTING VALIDATION

About 20–25 procedures cover the validation life cycle, from prioritising validation and GMP Assessments through validation project activities to validation support activities. These procedures should be prepared by experienced validation practitioners who also have experience in developing procedures. It may be necessary to hire an external consultant to fulfil this role. The consultant should join a team of procedure end users as a ghostwriter to develop the validation procedures. The aim is not impose a set of anonymous validation procedures, but rather to tailor the end user's current working practices into compliant validation procedures with a minimum of change. The end user's personal involvement should ensure the procedures are readily used by them without resentment.

- Prepare a Validation Plan
- Prepare a User Requirements Specification (URS)
- Conduct a Supplier Audit
- Prepare a Functional Specification (FS)
- Prepare a Hardware Design
- Prepare a Software Design
- Conduct a Computer Hazard Study
- Conduct a Good Programming Practice
- Conduct a Software Inspection
- Conduct Software Module Integration Testing
- Conduct an Installation Qualification (IQ)
- Conduct an Operational Qualification (OQ)
- Conduct a Performance Qualification (PQ)
- Prepare a Validation Report
- Hardware and Software Change Control
- Document Control

The effort to produce these procedures is probably in the area of 60 days from an experienced consultant. Where existing procedures are being revised for validation compliance, this estimate of effort can be reduced by about 2 days per procedure. As recommended above, this should be supplemented with about 20 days' effort across all the procedures divided between a team of end users. The team of end users should have a core who are involved in all the procedures to ensure consistency. Other end users on the team, however, can join the team for the development of particular procedures where they have a specific interest. For instance, an end user quality representative may wish to be specifically involved with the Supplier Audit procedure.

Management must approve procedures and any subsequent changes. Approval signatures will be required from at least two individuals representing a quality and technical perspective. Management must then ensure that any deviation from these procedures is properly authorised and documented. Deviations will often be associated with corrective actions; these must also be documented and evidence collated demonstrating their resolution.

SUPPLIER AUDITS AND SELECTION

The pharmaceutical manufacturer is obliged to determine the suitability of proposed suppliers providing products and services, particularly those providing software, to be used in the project.

> *The software is a critical component of a computerised system. The user of such software should take all reasonable steps to ensure that it has been produced in accordance with a system of Quality Assurance* [8].

This is usually achieved through an audit conducted by the pharmaceutical manufacturer that examines the quality assurance attributes of both the supplier's general capability and their equipment or service being used on the project. Suppliers may include equipment vendors, service suppliers, or the manufacturer's in-house capability. Regulators hold pharmaceutical manufacturers accountable for the use of suppliers who are not validation compliant [14].

Supplier Audits may be conducted in advance of validating an individual automation system or as part of an overall strategy to select preferred suppliers. Some pharmaceutical manufacturers mark the capability of suppliers within a rating system. Suppliers might be marked with a numbering system or with a combination of keywords such as "excellent", "satisfactory", "non-compliant", and "ISO certified". Bernard Anderson of Glaxo Wellcome suggested the following rankings [15]:

- The supplier can be used for any type of software development work.
- The supplier can be used for specific types of software development work.
- The supplier can be used for specific types of software development work, subject to *minor* corrective actions being performed.
- The supplier can be used for specific types of software development work, subject to *major* corrective actions being performed.

- A documented quality system must be imposed on the supplier in the event a contract is awarded.
- The supplier cannot be used for systems requiring validation.

Whatever system is used, the ratings must be defined so that users and regulators alike have a unambiguous understanding of their meaning. Project teams can use the rating system to select suppliers without unnecessarily duplicating audits. Companies using this approach, however, must carefully consider how long a rating remains valid until another audit is required, because a supplier's capability will change, and not always for the better.

Audits are usually conducted by an audit team and led by an accredited auditor. Accredited auditors have completed a certified training course and have conducted a number of qualifying audits. Pharmaceutical manufacturers who do not have their own accredited auditors can hire an independent auditor. Names and addresses of accredited auditors can be found in national registers of certified auditors. In the United Kingdom, a register is kept by the Institute of Quality Assurance (IQA).

The audit team's size should be kept to a minimum, but should adequately represent the following areas of expertise [16]:

- Auditing practices
- Computer system engineering
- Computer system quality methods
- Regulatory compliance
- Pharmaceutical industry validation practices

Team members should have a preliminary understanding of auditing before they begin an audit. The ISO 10011 auditing standard [17] provides useful material on audit practice, the qualifications of auditors, and the management of audit programmes.

Many suppliers are certified to one of the ISO 9000 quality management standards [18]. These standards consist of the following:

- *ISO 9000-1*: Guidance on selection of ISO 9000 series standards
- *ISO 9000-2*: Guidance on generic application of ISO 9000 series standards
- *ISO 9000-3*: Guidance on applying ISO 9001 to software
- *ISO 9001*: Covers quality practice for product design, development, production (including inspection and testing), installation, and services
- *ISO 9002*: Covers quality practice for production (including inspection and testing), installation, and services
- *ISO 9003*: Covers quality practice for final inspection and testing

The relationship between these standards and the framework of good practice outlined in this book is shown in Table 2.1. Audits are typically based on the ISO 9001 quality criteria. ISO 9000-3 [19], which is not a standard, gives specific guidance on applying ISO 9000 to software. It must be remembered that ISO 9000 certification does not necessarily imply a validation capability. The auditor should carefully read the ISO 9000 certificate for its qualifying statement and validity duration. Often a system supplier is not actually accredited for software production that may be subcontracted. The audit should identify such circumstances and determine whether the supplier has the necessary safeguards to ensure the quality of subcontracted work.

An audit is usually based on a visit to the supplier's premises, although sometimes a postal audit may be used. A mutually convenient time for the audit is agreed on with the supplier, who should be made aware of the audit's subject and content. It is important that requested documentation and personnel are made available for the audit. The audit will take the form of discussions about, and review of, current and past project documentation. The auditor must be satisfied that the supplier is capable of handling the project. An example checklist for audits is included as Appendix 2A at the end of this chapter. An important factor in selecting a supplier is the track record of the supplier, and references are usually sought from the established customers. Postal audits are only sufficient where the system or software under audit has been widely used without customisation in the pharmaceutical industry. The outcome of the audit is a report, a copy of which is usually sent to the supplier with advice on the resolution of any validation deficiencies. The pharmaceutical manufacturer may organise a follow-up audit to check whether correction actions have been taken. The number and frequency of recommended follow-up audits should be recorded in the audit report.

Table 2.1. Validation Life Cycle Coverage by ISO Standards

	ISO Standards				
Validation Life Cycle	**9001**	**9002**	**9003**	**9000-3**	**10011**
Validation Planning	Yes	Yes	Yes	Yes	No
System Specification	Yes	No	No	Yes	No
Supplier Audit and Selection	No	No	No	No	Yes
Design and Development	Yes	No	No	Yes	No
System Build	Yes	Yes	No	Yes	No
Predelivery Testing	Yes	Yes	Yes	Yes	No
On-Site Testing	Yes	Yes	Yes	Yes	No
Validation Report	Yes	Yes	Yes	Yes	No
Ongoing Support	Yes	Yes	No	Yes	No

ONGOING SUPPORT PROGRAMMES

Once automation systems have been validated, pharmaceutical manufacturers must endeavour to maintain their validated status. There should be formal procedures controlling

- Operation and maintenance procedures
- Documentation management
- Change control
- Security practice
- Contingency planning
- Training
- Performance monitoring
- Periodic review and revalidation
- Decommissioning

These procedures and the automation systems must be periodically reviewed, at least annually according to some regulatory authorities, to ensure ongoing compliance. There have been numerous instances of GMP practices being relaxed by operations staff without the knowledge of senior managers [20]. The cost of maintaining a validated status is estimated to be between 4–20 times less expensive than repeating the validation of automation systems to a standard that is acceptable to regulatory authorities.

MANAGEMENT REVIEW

A management review will usually be conducted periodically, with one or more validation reports being used as feedback on the overall validation programme. Although shown as the last phase of management cycle, reviews can and should take place throughout validation. The review endeavours to draw out lessons from the validation conducted to date, consider the impact of any regulation developments, and report any recommendations. The target is continuous improvement of the manufacturer's validation capability.

Projects can provide a central focus for applying and refining policies and procedures. Feedback from practical experience is vital if a cost-effective validation approach is to be established. An external validation consultant can also be used to provide an independent perspective, to comment on current industry practices, and to provide updates on topical regulatory issues. Management must also effectively address any inspection issues raised by GMP regulatory authorities concerning automation systems [21,22,23].

Validation does not have to be unduly expensive if issues are managed in a timely manner.

Management reviews may make changes to the corporate validation strategy, SOPs, and the automation system register (new or decommissioned systems). Validation rework (additional testing) may also be required. All these issues can have an impact on the Validation Master Plan; thus, the management cycle continues.

RESOURCE PLANNING

Pharmaceutical manufacturers should have adequate numbers of competent personnel to implement validation. Individuals should not be overwhelmed by their responsibilities; the principles of validation should not be compromised. GMP regulatory authorities will not accept staff shortages or deficient training as excuses for noncompliant validation.

Senior managers, however, are often asked by their companies to ensure a successful GMP inspection with minimum resources. It is a difficult task and senior managers themselves often need guidance. ISO 9001 gives the following advice:

> *The responsibility, authority, and interrelation of all personnel who manage, perform and verify work affecting quality shall be defined* [2].

The role of senior management is not limited to validation policies and procedures. Senior managers should also sponsor validation projects and ensure the necessary supporting organisation is established. Project roles will normally include the following:

- *System Owner:* The person responsible for ensuring that the corporate Validation Policy is implemented and that the resultant validated status is maintained.
- *Project Manager:* The person responsible for managing individual validation projects.
- *Validation Expert:* The person responsible for supporting projects with specialist validation knowledge.
- *Project Engineers:* The people responsible for implementing validation procedures on validation projects.
- *Quality Representative:* The person responsible for ensuring project work complies with validation policies and procedures.

Whilst a single individual may fulfil more than one role, it is more likely that some roles will be occupied by more than one individual. System owners sometimes delegate implementation of validation to a supplier. Similarly, maintenance of validation may be supported by a system administrator function that may be internal or external to the company.

GMP regulatory authorities expect to see an organisational chart with the specific duties and job descriptions of individuals recorded. Individuals must be given sufficient authority to fulfil their duties. Duties may be delegated to designated deputies of satisfactory competency. There should be no unexplained gaps or overlaps in duties affecting validation. Senior management is responsible for ensuring personnel assigned to validation work are competent to fulfil their role and arranging any supplementary training requirements. It is not acceptable for senior managers to rely on individuals to fulfil their role without management support. The quality representative should be independent of the project to ensure impartiality.

Eutech Engineering has conducted validation work for several international pharmaceutical manufacturers and has developed a staffing life-cycle model [24]. Eutech's experiences suggest that this model fits most corporate automation validation programmes. This can be used to assess the total validation workload. Figure 2.6 shows that the staffing profile consisting of three phases: preparation, implementation, and maintenance.

The preparation phase reflects a period for developing the Validation Master Plan, the automation systems register, and the SOPs, and sanctioning

Figure 2.6. Staffing Life Cycle

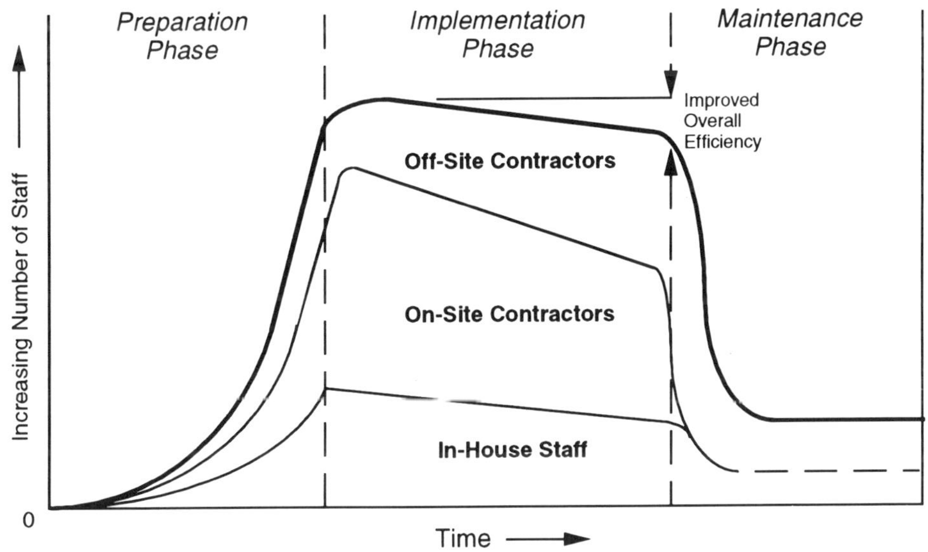

the automation validation programme. This phase will typically involve some external consultancy.

The implementation phase covers the validation of existing automation, which is typically allocated a two- to three-year time frame for completion. The staffing requirements for this phase are usually supplied using a combination of in-house and contractor resources. The in-house staff control the implementation of the validation programme for individual automation systems. Contractors provide an on-site engineering resource for the duration of the validation programme. Contractors can be particularly useful if they are already familiar with automation validation because of their reduced learning curve to understand a new set of validation procedures. Some elements of validation work can be partitioned off into work packages that can be conducted by contractor staff based off-site. It should be the objective of both pharmaceutical manufacturers and suppliers to develop a successful partnership. Contractors are usually used because the extra effort required is temporary, and the pharmaceutical company does not wish to increase its levels of permanent staff.

The final staffing life-cycle phase is entitled "maintenance" and covers the prospective validation of new automation systems and periodic revalidation of existing automation systems. This phase is typically managed in-house, using work packages contracted to suppliers. At this stage, a set of preferred suppliers will have been established who have a successful track record with pharmaceutical manufacturers.

The number of validation staff required will vary depending on site requirements. Some industry metrics presented in Chapter 7 should help practitioners make a preliminary assessment. Staff may be organised into a central group or dispersed between site manufacturing units and departmental functions. Some pharmaceutical manufacturers may even wish to consider outsourcing all of their validation requirements. However staffing is managed, it is vital that sufficient and trained personnel are made available.

REFERENCES

1. OECD (1995), *The Application of the Principles of GLP to Computerised Systems*, No. 10 OECD Series on Principles of Good Laboratory Practice and Compliance Monitoring, GLP Consensus Document, Environmental Monograph No. 116: Paris, Organisation for Economic Co-operation and Development Environmental Directorate.

2. ISO (1994), ISO 9001: *International Standard: Quality Systems—Model for Quality Assurance in Design/Development, Production, Installation and Servicing,* Geneva, International Organisation for Standardisation.

3. Stokes, T. (1994), The Role of Senior Management in Computer Systems Validation, In *Good Computer Validation Practices: Common Sense Implementation* (edited by T. Stokes, R.C. Branning, K.G. Chapman, H. Hambloch, and A.J. Trill), Buffalo Grove, IL: Interpharm Press.

4. PMA (1986), Validation Concepts for Computer Systems Used in the Manufacture of Drug Products, In *PMA Proceedings: Concepts and Principles for the Validation of Computer Systems Used in the Manufacture and Control of Drug Products,* Pharmaceutical Manufacturers Association.

5. ISPE (1996), *Baseline Pharmaceutical Engineering Guide: A Guide for New Facilities,* Volume 1: Bulk Pharmaceutical Chemicals, Developed in Partnership by International Society of Pharmaceutical Engineering and U.S. Food and Drug Administration.

6. Gough, P.H. (1996), *Management of Computer Validation and Culture Change—Experiences at Eli Lilly and Company,* ISPE European Conference on Computer Systems Validation in the Real World, 24–25 September, Zurich.

7. TGA (1990), *Australian Code of Good Manufacturing for Therapeutic Goods,* Medicinal Product—Part 1, Woden: Australia, Therapeutic Goods Administration.

8. European Union Guide to Directive 91/356/EEC (1993), Computerised Systems, Annex 11 of *European Commission Directive Laying Down the Principles of Good Manufacturing Practice for Medicinal Products for Human Use.*

9. Japanese Ministry of Public Welfare (1993), Guideline on Computer Systems in Drug Manufacturing, in *Manual on Computer Systems in Drug Manufacturing.*

10. FDA (1983), *Guide to Inspection of Computerized Systems in Drug Processing,* Technical Report, Reference Materials and Training Aids for Investigators, Rockville, MD: U.S. Food and Drug Administration.

11. NE 58: Abwicklung von qualifizierungspflichtigen PLT-Projekten (version 04.06.96); [including . . .] Dannapel, B., Hensel, H., Mockel, B., Muhlenkamp, J., Muller-Heinzerling, T., Otto, A., and Teuchert, V. (1995), Qualifizierung von Leitsystemen: Ein Gemeinschaftsprojekt von GMA und NAMUR zur Validierung, *ATP—Automatisierungstechnische Praxis,* 37 (10): 64–76.

12. PDA (1995), Validation of Computer Related Systems, *PDA Journal of Pharmaceutical Science and Technology,* Technical Report No. 18.

13. UK GAMP Forum (1996), *Supplier Guide for Validation of Automation Systems in Pharmaceutical Manufacture,* Version 2.0, available from the International Society of Pharmaceutical Engineering.

14. FDA (1985), *Vendor Responsibility,* Compliance Policy Guides, Computerized Drug Processing 7132a, Guide 12, Rockville, MD: U.S. Food and Drug Administration.

15. Anderson, B. (1996), *Vendor Audits,* Computer System Validation: A Practical Approach, Management Forum Seminar, 26–27 March, London.

16. Grigonis, G.J., Jr. and Wyrick, M.L. (1994), *Computer System Validation: Auditing Computer Systems for Quality,* Report on behalf of PhRMA Computer Systems Validation Committee, *Pharmaceutical Technology Europe,* 18 (9): 32–39.

17. ISO (1994), ISO 10011-1 (1990): *Guidelines for Auditing Quality Systems*—Part 1: Auditing, Geneva: International Organisation for Standardisation.

18. ISO (1994), ISO 9000 (1994): *Quality Systems—Model for Assurance in Design, Development, Production, Installation and Servicing,* Geneva: International Organisation for Standardisation.

19. ISO (1994), ISO 9001-3: *Quality Management and Quality Assurance Standards—* Part 3: Guidelines for the Application of ISO 9001 to the Development, Supply and Maintenance of Software, Geneva: International Organisation for Standardisation.

20. Wingate, G.A.S. (1996), Management for Operations' Dependability of Computer-Controlled Chemical Plants, In *Life-Cycle Management for Systems Dependability* (edited by F. Redmil and C. Dale), Springer-Verlag.

21. Trill, A.J. (1993), Computerized Systems and GMP—A UK Perspective: Part 1: Background, Standards and Methods; Part 2: Inspection Findings; Part 3: Best Practices and Topical Issues, *Pharmaceutical Technology International.*

22. Tetzlaff, R.F. (1992), GMP Documentation Requirements for Automated Systems: Parts 1, 2, and 3, *Pharmaceutical Technology.*

23. Clark, A.S. (1988), Computer Systems Validation: An Investigator's View, *Pharmaceutical Technology*, 12 (1): 60–66.

24. Wingate, G.A.S. (1993), *A Life-Cycle Methodology for Computer Systems Validation*, ISPE European Computer Systems Validation Seminar, November, Stuttgart, Germany.

APPENDIX 2A. EXAMPLE SUPPLIER AUDIT CHECKLIST

Audit Details

- ☐ What is the name and address of the firm being audited?
- ☐ Who is the contact at the firm?
- ☐ What are the names and qualifications of the auditors?
- ☐ What is the date of the audit?
- ☐ Is this an initial or follow-up (surveillance) audit?

Business

- ☐ How long has the company existed?
- ☐ How is the company organised?
- ☐ How many pharmaceutical-related customers does the company have?
- ☐ Do they have any customer citations for good work?
- ☐ Is the company's pharmaceutical-related business profitable?
- ☐ What is the long-term pharmaceutical-related business plan?
- ☐ Is the company in any litigation?
- ☐ Does the company hold a recognised quality certification?

Organisation

- ☐ Has a Quality Control System been established? Is it documented?
- ☐ Who is responsible for quality management?
- ☐ Is there a Quality Assurance management structure?
- ☐ Is there a project management structure?
- ☐ Are project work practices documented?
- ☐ How does project work conform to quality standards?
- ☐ Has accreditation/registration been achieved? (ISO 9000, specify other)
- ☐ Is the Quality System audited on a regular basis?

Employees

- ☐ How many permanent, contract, or temporary people does the company employ?
- ☐ How long, on average, do employees stay with the company?
- ☐ What is the company's training policy? Are there any records?

Planning

- ☐ Are project and quality plans produced for projects? Who approves them?
- ☐ Does planning include a contract review?
- ☐ Is there a defined project life cycle? What is it?
- ☐ How are project documents controlled?
- ☐ How is conformance to customer GMP requirements ensured?

System Design and Development

- ☐ Do design considerations cover reliability? Maintainability? and Safety?
- ☐ Do design considerations cover standardisation? Interchangability?
- ☐ Are design reviews carried out? Are they minuted?
- ☐ Are customers invited to attend design review meetings?
- ☐ Are design changes proposed, approved, implemented, and controlled?

System Build

- ☐ Are there guidelines or standards for software programming and hardware assembly?
- ☐ How does the company ensure they conform to current industry requirements?
- ☐ Are there records showing projects conforming to company practices?
- ☐ What third-party hardware or software is used? Are they supplied by reputable firms?

- ☐ How would changes to third-party products affect the customer's end product?

Predelivery Testing

- ☐ Are test specifications produced? Are expected results defined?
- ☐ Who performs the tests? How is testing organised?
- ☐ Are versions of hardware and software inspected?
- ☐ Is software "black-box" (functional) testing conducted?
- ☐ Is software "white-box" (structural) testing conducted?
- ☐ How rigorous is testing? Are abnormal situations tested?
- ☐ How are failed tests documented and corrected?
- ☐ Are test results recorded, signed, and dated? Are these records maintained?
- ☐ Who signs for overall acceptance of testing?

Project Completion

- ☐ What is the mechanism for deciding a project is complete?
- ☐ Is there a certificate of conformity? Is there a warranty?
- ☐ Are project documents handed over to the customer?
- ☐ Are project documents archived?
- ☐ Is there an access agreement for regulatory inspections (e.g., ESCROW)?

Control Procedures and Activities

- ☐ Is there configuration and version control within projects?
- ☐ Does the Quality System provide for the prompt detection of failures?
- ☐ Are all failures analysed? Are correction actions promptly taken?
- ☐ Are regular internal audits carried out? Are auditing procedures documented?
- ☐ Are audits planned? Are corrective actions taken?

- ☐ Are audit records stored and available?
- ☐ Are responsibilities for document review assigned?
- ☐ Are responsibilities for change control assigned?
- ☐ Are obsolete documents withdrawn?
- ☐ Are changes notified to the customer?
- ☐ Are subcontractors audited? How are they managed?
- ☐ Are subcontract documentation standards audited?

General and Housekeeping

- ☐ Are customers solicited for feedback?
- ☐ How are customer responses folded into development plans?
- ☐ Are customers kept informed of development plans?
- ☐ List other customers provided with a similar service/product that is the subject of this audit.
- ☐ Are customers advised of problems found by other users?
- ☐ Who is responsible for ongoing customer support? Is there a support fee?
- ☐ What are the response mechanism and timings for customer problems?

Chapter 3

Validating Automation Systems

The various validation approaches promoted within the pharmaceutical industry by GMP regulators, industry initiatives, and individual pharmaceutical manufacturers all adopt the same basic approach:

- Define what is to be done (plan)
- Define how to do it (procedures and resources)
- Do it, controlling any changes (change control)
- Establish that the end result was what was originally wanted (verification)
- Provide evidence demonstrating the above (audit trail)

This chapter presents the set of life-cycle phases summarising the validation approach typically used within the pharmaceutical industry. Life-cycle phases may be known by alternative names in different organisations. There are no definitive naming conventions or groupings of phases. It is important, however, that all the activities covered by this chapter are included in any alternative scheme.

VALIDATION PROJECT LIFE CYCLE

The life-cycle approach has gained broad acceptance by the pharmaceutical industry and can be refined to meet the needs of particular applications. Different organisations use variants of the life cycle, but the methodology of dividing a life cycle into phases remains the same. For instance, some companies develop the subphases indicated in the phase descriptions above as distinct phases. The specific life-cycle model chosen does not matter. Its constituent phases must, however, be clearly defined in advance, with entry and exit criteria for each phase and appropriate verification procedures to ensure the controlled completion of constituent phases.

The life cycle presented in Figure 3.1 is compliant with the German GMA-NAMUR life cycle [1], the UK GAMP Forum's life cycle [2], and the U.S. PMA's life cycle [3].

An important issue when considering the life cycle is the relative cost of making changes to an automation system as the life cycle progresses. The relative cost of implementing a change is shown in Figure 3.2. Within the system-build phase, the relative cost of implementing a change has been estimated as being up to 3 times as expensive to implement compared to the planning phase, and perhaps higher than 20 times as expensive to implement once the system has completed on-site testing and has been authorised for use. It is very important to clarify incomplete or ambiguous information as soon as reasonably practical, because the longer it is left, the more expensive it will be to correct if a wrong assumption has been made in the interim.

Figure 3.1. Life Cycle V-Model

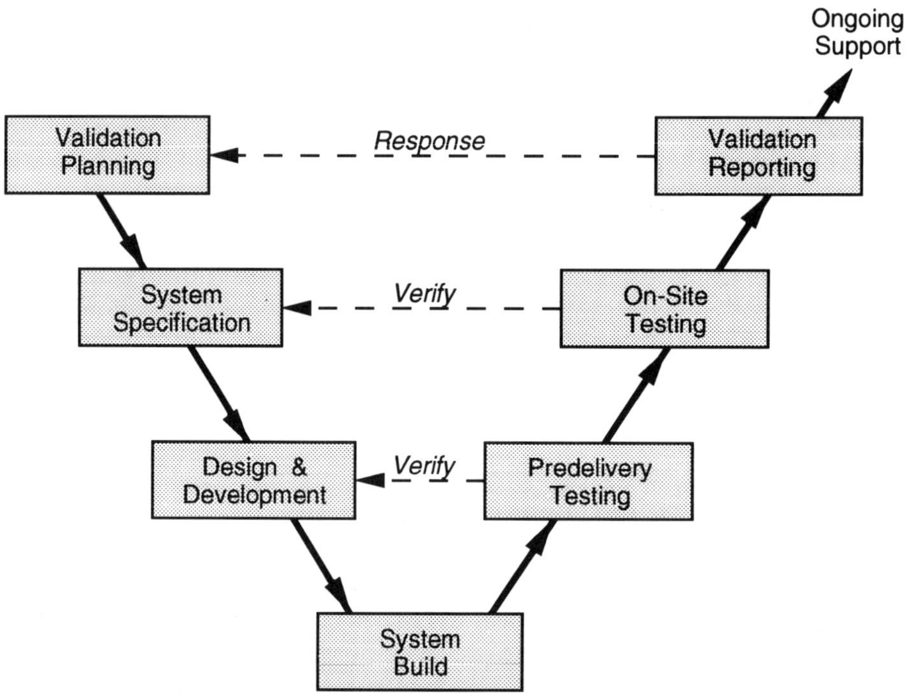

Figure 3.2. Relative Cost of Change

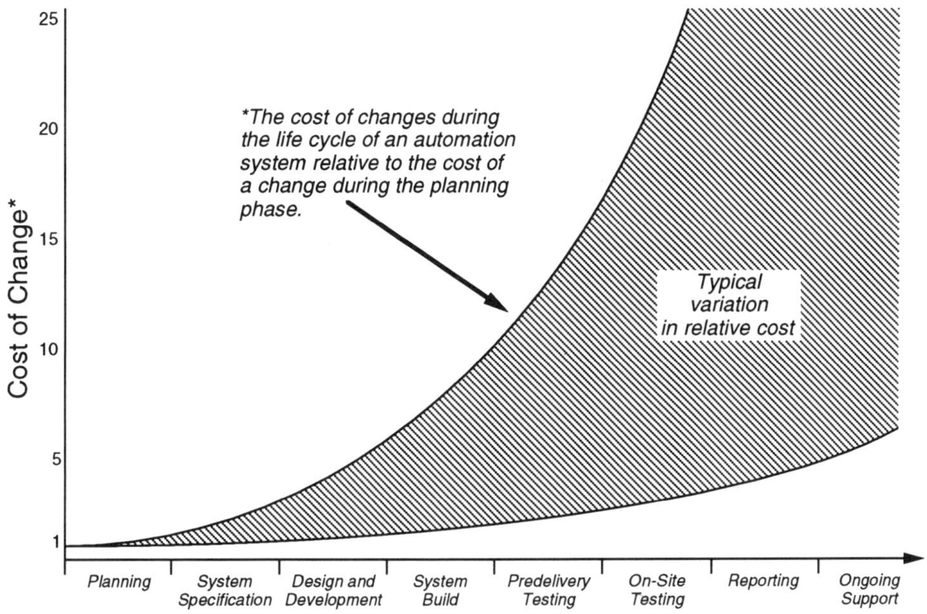

PLANNING

The first life-cycle phase is planning and is the responsibility of the pharmaceutical manufacturer. This phase consists of three main activities that may be conducted sequentially or concurrently: the Validation Plan and User Requirements Specification, which are described below; and the Supplier Audit and Selection, which was described in Chapter 2.

A glossary of terms and acronyms should be collated as an integral part of the planning exercise. There must be a common understanding of terminology used in a project. It is all to easy for individuals to attribute a different meaning to standard terminology without an arbitrating glossary.

Validation Plan

Validation Plans specify how the pharmaceutical manufacturer intends to satisfy the GMP requirements affecting a single automation system or group of automation systems. A Validation Report will be prepared at the end of the project, in response to the Validation Plan, summarising the success or failure of the project, and providing an audit trail for any corrective and outstanding actions. The Validation Plan and Validation Report are often some of the first documents to be examined by GMP regulatory authorities inspecting a manufacturing facility [4]. Without a plan to direct and organise validation activities, missing or substandard validation is likely to go unnoticed. GMP regulatory authorities have frequently found projects where members were incorrectly assuming that each other was providing key validation evidence [5].

Validation Plans often begin by specifying the authority under which they are written (perhaps a Validation Master Plan or on the personal authority of a senior manager) and preview the validation requirements for the project. A brief system description typically follows, covering the system's history (whether it is an entirely new system, a replacement system, or an existing system) and its objective purpose. GMP regulatory authorities expect replacement systems to be as least as reliable as the original manual or automatic system [6]. The aim is to provide a management overview of the project boundaries, defining what is and what is not included within the scope of work.

The roles and responsibilities of both the pharmaceutical manufacturer and any suppliers are then defined and any additional staff training identified. Table 3.1 provides guidance on the assignment of responsibilities. It is important to recognise that the competency of individuals is key to successful validation. A simple organisational chart can prove very useful when describing interrelationships between project staff. Résumés of project staff should be collated and include references to their education and degrees obtained, professional certificates, previous job titles, and responsibilities. Résumés for temporary staff, such as supplier personnel, are often included as an appendix to the Validation Plan. Many pharmaceutical manufacturers, however, prefer to use a central management system to collate the résumés of their own permanent staff.

The validation activities covering System Specification, System Design and Development, System Build, Predelivery Testing, On-Site Testing, and Validation Reporting are then laid out with a description of any issues for specific GMP consideration. The procedures to be adopted and the documentation to be produced must be identified. Planned deviations from validation procedures should be defined in advance within the Validation Plan, to demonstrate management's acceptance and continued control over the project.

Approval signatories for validation documentation should be specified. An individual's job title may not necessarily reflect the reasons and responsibilities implied by a person's signature. On numerous occasions, GMP regulatory authorities have challenged individuals who have signed validation documents and found that the signatories had misunderstood their full responsibilities and performed less thorough reviews than required [5].

Validation procedures and evidence to be provided by suppliers should be distinguished from the pharmaceutical manufacturer's own documentation. The pharmaceutical manufacturer's dependency on suppliers should be

Table 3.1. Assigning Responsibilities

Validation Life Cycle / **Validation Roles**	System Owner	Project Manager	Validation Expert	Project Engineers	Quality Representative	Supplier	Independent Consultants
Validation Planning	A	R	A		A		S
System Specification	R	A	A	S	A	S	S
Supplier Audit and Selection	R	A	A	S	A		S
System Development (including Hazard Study)	 R		S	A S	 A	R S	S S
System Build			S	A		R	S
Predelivery Testing			S	A		R	S
On-Site Testing (inc. Performance Qualification)		A R	A A	S S	A A	R S	S S
Validation Report	A	R	A		A		S
Ongoing Support	R			S	A	S	S
Decommissioning	R			S	A	S	S

Notes: (1) A = Approval; R = Lead Responsibility including Approval; S = Support. (2) Project Engineers will include representatives of the IT and Engineering Departments as necessary. (3) Independent Consultants are not normally employed when the pharmaceutical manufacturer has an available internal Validation Expert.

specified, identifying any necessary Supplier Audits (or reviewing the results of audits already conducted). One important factor to consider is who approves and accepts work as satisfactorily completed. Any requirements for monitoring supplier's work should also be defined.

Finally, a support programme and policy for ongoing evaluation are presented, which will include change control, maintenance and calibration, security practice, contingency planning, operating procedures, training, performance monitoring, and periodic review.

An experienced validation practitioner can produce a Validation Plan for an automation system (usually 10–15 pages long) in about 3 days. The layout of an example Validation Plan is shown in Figure 3.3. Validation Plans may make use of appendices, for instance, project milestones, and résumés of project team members.

Figure 3.3. Example Validation Plan

1. Introduction
2. System Overview
    2.1. Background Information
    2.2 High-Level Functionality
    2.3 Reason for Validating
3. Organisation and Responsibilities
    3.1 Team Structure
    3.2 Training Requirements
4. Validation Approach
    4.1 Scope of Validation
    4.2 Procedures to Be Followed
    4.3 Documentation to Be Produced
5. Supplier Audits
6. Ongoing Evaluation and Control
7. Project Milestones

The Validation Plan must be reviewed and approved before issue. At a minimum, it should be signed and dated by the system owner and quality representative. A Validation Manager may also sign the plan, perhaps as the quality representative if the manager works under the authority of the company's Quality organisation. It is recommended that a senior manager who will ensure that sufficient resources are allocated to the project also signs the Validation Plan to demonstrate the pharmaceutical manufacturer's commitment. The time to review and issue the Validation Plan will vary between different organisations and is primarily dependent on the number of people involved in the review process.

User Requirements Specification

The intent of the automation system is written in a User Requirements Specification (URS) and should provide a firm foundation for the project. If, however, it is not precise, concise, and complete, it may cause major problems later in the project. Project managers should be made aware that whilst inconclusive requirements offer a degree of flexibility to extend the scope of work, they will hinder effective design. An example of a poor requirement was recently cited by Sam Clark, a former FDA investigator:

> *A novice must be able to use the system in a simple manner and a sophisticated user in a sophisticated manner* [7].

Up-front effort should be more than compensated by project pull-through. The cost of modifications and changes later in the life cycle can be 10 or 20 times that of instituting the amendment at this stage. Once the URS has been agreed to, it must be written in a manner that is understandable by both users and the development staff. The manufacturer may request a supplier for assistance in producing this document.

The URS should be written by a multidisciplined team, including production, engineering, and quality assurance staff. End users should be involved as soon as possible and approve the requirements before design and development begins.

URSs can exist as a single document or a number of documents. Information that should be considered is shown in Figure 3.4, which is based on the detailed checklist given in Appendix 3A at the end of this chapter. Diagrams should be used wherever possible to promote greater understanding. Spreadsheets are also useful for defining data and clearly showing missing information.

The level of detail contained in the URS varies depending on its relationship with the Functional Specification (FS). Documents can range between 6 to over 100 pages in length. Shorter URSs are sometimes known as Outline Specifications. Some pharmaceutical manufacturers place few constraints on their suppliers, whilst others may impose particular equipment and design requirements. A close examination of any constraints will usually determine that preferred equipment and design is not critical and this level of detail can be left to the supplier and recorded in the design documentation.

The process control section is typically the largest portion of the URS. This information will be presented in the form of textual descriptions, flowcharts, state transition diagrams, or some similar diagrammatic form; diagrammatic information is often located in appendices. It should include the identification of halt states, error routines, and error recovery. Failure modes should protect both the plant and personnel. Any bespoke software requirements and special calculation requirements should be described. Other important sections in the URS include access security, the human interface, and the process interface. Access security should be considered as a means of reducing the risk of data loss or corruption, inadvertent modification, or unauthorised access. Security may be achieved through the use of passwords, key switches, or other more sophisticated mechanisms, such as biometrics. The human interface should include screen layouts (or prototypes where they have not been finalised) and requirements, such as configuration pages,

Figure 3.4. Specification Topics

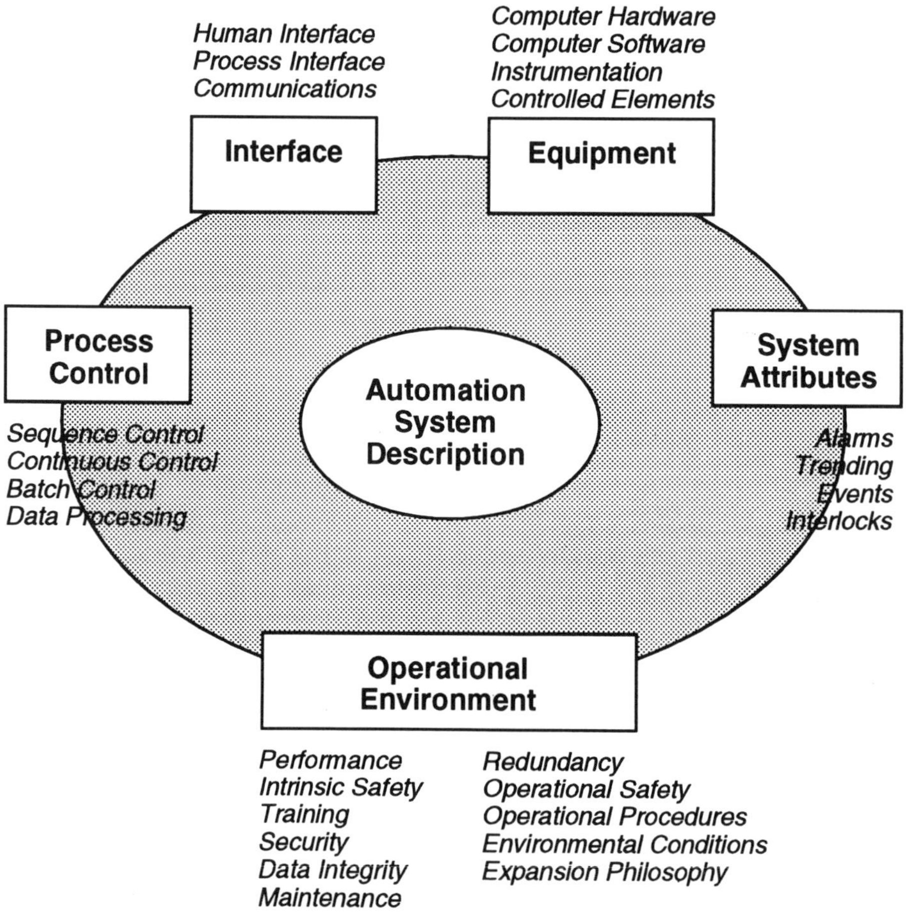

alarm pages, mimics, and system responses to data entry errors. The minimum information for the process interface includes equipment tag numbers, unit references, descriptions, input/output (I/O) types, and any special treatment, such as segregation requirements. Where an automation system replaces an existing system, consideration should be given to the extent of any interface work to commission the new system and identifying any changes in functionality of the system.

Those defining the URS should consider how the requirements can be tested. Alternative phrasing of requirements could considerably clarify Predelivery and On-Site Testing. In response to a poorly written URS, some suppliers have suggested using word searches on "must", "shall", and "will" to determine the minimum set of requirements; vague specifications will lead to vague acceptance criteria! Test protocols and their relationships to the URS, FS, and other development documentation are discussed in more detail later in this chapter.

Within the URS, crucial and desirable requirements should be distinguished. Features that are necessary to validate an automation system should always be considered as crucial requirements. Desired features should be prioritised by their relative importance. The FS should then include a table showing how it complies with the URS. To make this cross-referencing easier to administer, each requirement should be given a unique reference number. A list of known omissions from the current issue of the URS should be highlighted. Any assumptions made by the FS in respect to this missing information should be readily identifiable so that misunderstandings can be clarified before the project progresses too far. Ian Johnson of Glaxo, for instance, recalls an extract fan fitted for operator protection on a powder-filling machine controlled by a Programmable Logic Controller (PLC) that monitored the extract and displayed an alarm to the operator if the extractor failed [8]. The PLC system integrator supplying the application software, however, did not appreciate the potential danger of powder in the operator's working environment and programmed the powder-filling machine to continue working after the alarm was displayed when the extract failed. The URS should have specified the need for an interlock so that if the operator did not notice the alarm, then the powder-filling machine would have stopped.

It is easy to criticise, but much more difficult to write the URS. The first version of the URS is inevitably unstructured, as authors tend to include information as it comes to mind. The generation of a standard format will help, but most authors will still customise the format to their own particular viewpoint. Project managers must accept and plan for restructuring the URS so that a more readable and useful document(s) evolves. Revised issues of the URS, however, must be kept under version control so that project staff are kept informed of information updates.

SYSTEM SPECIFICATION

The second life-cycle phase is system specification and is the responsibility of the supplier. This phase consists of two main activities that are usually conducted sequentially: Supplier Project and Quality Plans, and the Functional Specification.

Supplier Project and Quality Plans

GMP regulatory authorities require work conducted by suppliers for pharmaceutical manufacturers to be formally agreed to in a contract [9] covering:

- GMP requirements
- Responsibilities of parties involved
- Inspections of suppliers
- Customer agreement of subcontractors

The contract usually consists of a supplier's proposal together with a pharmaceutical manufacturer's purchase order. Reference may be made to a URS and other documentation. It is advisable to incorporate or make reference to the Supplier's Project and Quality Plans, which may be separate or combined. These plans share the same purpose as the Validation Plan and define the supplier's approach to their designated validation tasks. Without agreement on validation practices and management, it is unlikely that a project will be completed in full, on time, and within budget. It is not sufficient merely to state that the work must comply with the requirements of various GMP regulatory authorities. Sorting out misunderstandings can be a complex and time-consuming task: "Bad contracts can seriously complicate your life" [10]!

The Supplier's Project and Quality Plans specify project responsibilities, procedures, and deliverable documentation. The supplier's scope of work is frequently centred around System Development, System Build, and Predelivery Testing. The URS and On-Site Testing may also be specified in the plans as requested by a manufacturer. The supplier should be encouraged to include a statement of their capability for the service or equipment they are providing. This statement could be based on a firm's ISO 9000 accreditation. Résumés of key staff should be available to support the capability statement.

Pharmaceutical manufacturers are expected to review the contractual arrangements before beginning a project. The combined information provided in the Supplier Audit and Supplier Project and Quality Plans gives GMP regulatory authorities and pharmaceutical manufacturers alike a good indication of the competency of the supplier and their working relationship with the pharmaceutical manufacturer. A simple checklist might include the following questions [10]:

- Does the customer order reference the final supplier proposal?
- Are the terms and conditions quoted in the customer order or supplier proposal acceptable?
- Are the milestones in the Supplier Project Plan accepted by all parties?
- Is the programme of work in the Supplier Quality Plan accepted by all parties?
- Are the resource requirements available and used on the contract?
- Are you satisfied that the contract can delivered in full, on time, and on budget?

If the answer to any of these questions is "No", then the actions and responsibilities to be taken to resolve the differences should be recorded and verified as complete. The contract should not start until any differences are understood and resolved or accepted. If a checklist is used, then this should be annotated with answers to the questions and signed as complete by the contract reviewer (who may well be the quality manager) and contract manager (who may well be the project manager). In this simple manner, documentary evidence is produced to demonstrate a contract review for a specific project.

Suppliers should also be encouraged to conduct their own contract reviews. They must be satisfied that they can fulfil the contract and that the pharmaceutical manufacturer is aware of and can provide any necessary support.

Contract reviews for automation systems will become increasingly important as manufacturing facilities become more highly automated and dependent on software. Supplier Project and Quality Plans should, therefore, be adopted as a standard working practice for all projects. A combined Project and Quality Plan will normally be 10–15 pages long and follow a standard format similar to that outlined for a Validation Plan in Figure 3.3. An organisation's commitment to Project and Quality Plans is often a good indicator of their commitment to quality management and validation.

Functional Specification

The FS is the supplier's response to the URS, specifying a proposed solution to the URS; therefore, it must be approved by the pharmaceutical manufacturer. In some instances, a URS is not produced; in this case, the FS stands in its own right.

Wherever possible, the FS should follow the same structure of the URS (see Figure 3.4 and the information checklist in Appendix 3A at the end of this chapter) and can make reference to the URS rather than duplicate information. This approach, if adopted for all the documentation, makes it very easy to trace where requirements have been specified and tested (see Figure 3.5). Compliance, omissions, and nonconformances with respect to the URS should all be readily identifiable. Project managers should beware of

Figure 3.5. Audit Trail Through Documentation

User Requirements		Functional Specification		Qualification
1.1 Requirement #1	⟶	1.1 Function #1	⟶	1.1 Test #1
1.2 Requirement #2	⟶	1.2 Function #2	⟶	1.2 Test #2

extensions to the scope of the URS (sometimes referred to as "scope creep") because each modification is likely to lead to a revision on the FS with associated incurred costs and project delays.

The FS should, as far as possible, avoid detailed design and concentrate on defining the operation and user interaction with the automation system. This is generally more difficult than it sounds; in some instances it is not applicable because a URS specifically requests particular equipment or a particular design to be used. Similarly for small projects, it is often more convenient to combine the FS and design documents into what is often referred to as a Functional Design Specification, System Definition, or System Description.

In many circumstances, the supplied system will be based on a standard product and include additional features that are not needed. These features cannot be removed because they are integral to the standard product. The features should be fully defined, noted as unused (and if possible inaccessible), and assurance given that they cannot affect the system's intended operation. Standard documentation available for the standard product can be referenced, if available for inspection by the pharmaceutical manufacturer and GMP regulator, rather than reproduced.

The FS should be written in anticipation of testing. Specifications should be specific, measurable, and achievable, so that testing can clearly demonstrate acceptance. For instance, a sterilising cycle time may be specified to be 90 seconds, when a variation of 5 seconds is quite acceptable. If an acceptable variation of 5 seconds is not recorded, then a test outcome of 89 seconds will fail.

DESIGN AND DEVELOPMENT

The activities associated with this phase vary between projects, but generally follow the established pattern of Software and Hardware Design and Hazard Study. The design is the responsibility of the supplier, whilst Hazard Study is the responsibility of the pharmaceutical manufacturer.

Software and Hardware Design may be split into two activities, as described here, or combined. In either case, the design describes the implementation of the FS in increasing levels of detail until the components of the design (hardware or software) can be mapped directly to a standard product or implemented as bespoke elements of the automation system. The increasing levels of detail may be partitioned into different documents for larger systems. It is important to realise that there will be some feedback of information in the design process as the design is refined. The combined contents of the design documentation should address all the items listed in Appendix 3A at the end of this chapter, and be cross-referenced to the FS to demonstrate how it is being fulfilled. Again, any omissions and assumptions should be unambiguously stated. Once the design is complete, the threats posed by the system and any associated safeguards to the manufacturing process can be assessed as part of a Hazard Study. Hazard Studies are also known within the chemicals and pharmaceutical industries as CHAZOP (Computer Hazard and Operability Study), Vulnerability Analysis, Ts & Cs (Threats and Controls Analysis), or Threats Analysis.

The design must ensure that records generated by automation systems conform to their specified content [15]. Records covering computer inputs, outputs, and data must be accurate [6,15,36]. The automation system should also include built-in checks of the correct entry and processing of data. Manual entry of critical data should have a confirmation check that can be either manual or automatic.

Some organisations conduct a Design Qualification (DQ) as part of the design and development phase. The DQ verifies that all of the URS has been satisfactorily incorporated into the various specification and design documents. In general, a DQ is not necessary for conventional life-cycle projects if the individual review of each document includes a cross-reference check and that there have been no omissions or ambiguities in its relationship to other documents. DQ is appropriate, however, for prototyping projects. With such systems the specification and design documentation rapidly evolve at the end of the design process as an "as-built" description and, therefore, they do not reflect a predefined intent and a design response. The DQ is needed to verify the design suitable for its intended purpose.

Software Design

Automation system software can be split into five categories, as illustrated in Figure 3.6, developed by GMA-NAMUR [1]:

1. *Standard Operating System:* Operating system independent of automation system (e.g., operating system, database)
2. *System Software:* Standard operating software for automation system (e.g., input-output functions, data management software)
3. *Preassembled Software Blocks:* Standard functions (not application-specific) that can be adapted using parameter sets (e.g., standard sequence control, messages, and alarms reporting)
4. *Application-Related Configuration:* Application-specific parameter sets for preassembled software blocks (e.g., sequence control, graphical mimics, trends)
5. *Custom Programming:* Bespoke programming (e.g., special sequence operations, or algorithms)

The Software Design partitions the FS into operational units, referred to as modules. Some modules may be suitable for implementation with standard software packages, in which case the software packages and any

Figure 3.6. Software Architecture

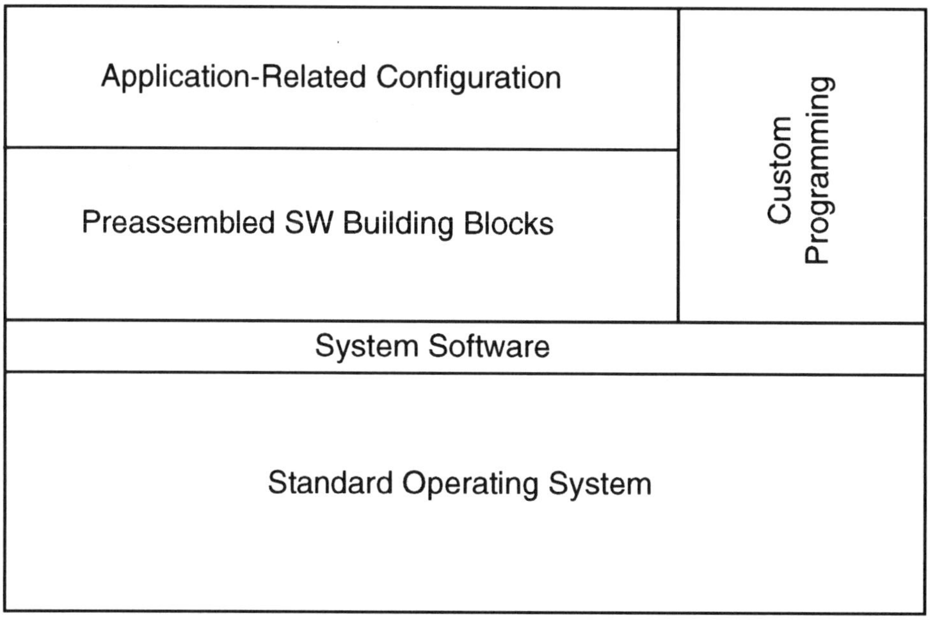

configuration requirements should be defined. Other modules will require bespoke programming. A high-level overview diagram of the software, such as a state transition diagram, is expected by some GMP regulatory authorities [11]. A list of software used should be prepared giving programme names, purpose, version, and language. The list may exist as a document in its own right or as part of another document. For bespoke software, versions may not be known until design and development has been completed, at which point the list of software should be updated.

Care must be taken when developing application software that uses a standard software package. A hospital used a software package to calculate the dosage of a drug based on a patient's height and weight. A student then developed some front-end application software that allowed dispensary staff to calculate dosages based on imperial units rather than the package's metric units. The application software was regularly modified over a number of years, during which there was no change control, no supporting documentation was produced, no comments were embedded in the software code, and no acceptance testing was performed. Only after two years of use was it discovered that the conversion between imperial and metric values was incorrect. It is understandable in such circumstances why suppliers of standard software packages have a limited warranty clause in licence agreements. A typical warranty clause is given below:

> *Although the software producer has tested the software and reviewed its associated documentation, the software producer makes no warranty or representation, either expressly or implied, with respect to the software or documentation, its quality, performance, merchantability, or fitness for a particular purpose. The licensee assumes the entire risk with regard to the use of the software and documentation.*

The design of bespoke modules should start by defining inputs, functionality, and output. Where appropriate, a hierarchy of modules may be described with submodules. Inputs, outputs, and internal module values provide data structures; consideration should be given to the grouping of data items within databases and their access. There may be more than one design document depending on the use of standard software packages and the amount of bespoke programming. Both used and unused aspects of standard software should be defined and include self-test and diagnostic facilities.

In many organisations, the software design process is *ad hoc*. Given the FS, usually written in a natural language, an informal design document is prepared. Coding commences and the design intent is modified as the system is implemented. When the software is complete, the design has usually changed so much that it bares little resemblance to the original software design document. In such circumstances, the design document must be rewritten to fully reflect the final design. The design document must not be too brief. This is often the case when the design evolves through a prototyping exercise. Programmers who develop prototypes are often very reluctant to fully document their resultant designs. Sam Clark, a former FDA investigator, recalled an inspection where the entire design description for one computer program consisted of *"This program modifies standard errors"* [7]. The design description for a category of computer programs in another system was defined as *"Those collating data each time a unit is tested or whatever"*. The project manager must control this tendency in programmers so that a meaningful and complete design is produced.

More methodical design approaches are available from "structured methods" which are sets of notations and guidelines that orchestrate a finished software design before coding begins. Some examples of widely used structured methods include the following:

- Yourdon, Jackson System Development, and MASCOT, which can be used for real-time system development
- Shlaer Mellor Object-Oriented Analysis for batch control

A particular design methodology is not advocated here. When selecting a suitable design methodology, the skills and experience of the project team applying the methodology must be taken into consideration. Further, the availability of Computer-Aided Software Engineering (CASE) tools and Integrated Project Support Environments (IPSEs) supporting the methodology must be considered. It is recommended that development tools, such as CASE and Real-Time System-Analysis System-Design (RTSASD), used to support validation, be examined to establish confidence in their capability [12]. The reasons for selecting a particular design methodology should be clearly documented; perhaps they offer Computer-Aided Design (CAD) with built-in design rules for configuring sequence function charts.

Aspects of Statistical Process Control (SPC) are increasingly used to control production. Key process variables affecting product quality should be identified and acceptable operating limits specified [13]. Parameters affecting yield that cannot affect product quality should be carefully distinguished. Messages recording acceptable production deviations of key process variables should be differentiated from alarms raised by unacceptable situations [14].

Hardware Design

The Hardware Design describes the equipment constituting the automation system and its configuration in readiness for installation and commissioning. A high-level schematic of the system's equipment is expected by some GMP regulatory authorities [11]. The equipment will include instrumentation, computer-related hardware, including communication links, and any interface devices to the manufacturing process, other automation equipment, or operations staff. The Hardware Design is likely to consist of a number of documents and make reference to preassembled information from suppliers providing standard models of equipment.

Instrumentation will include field instruments used in the manufacturing process and other instruments with associated tasks, for instance, of monitoring laboratory or computer room environmental conditions. The accessibility of instruments must allow cleaning and maintenance. Siting is also important and instruments should be installed as close to the point of measurement as possible. The placement of flowmeters in piping deadlegs should be avoided. Careful consideration should also be given to the appropriate position of other instruments, such as thermometers and thermocouples, so that they too can fulfil their measurement and control function [14,15]. Construction materials that contact the pharmaceutical process stream must not contaminate or affect the manufactured product. Instrument lubricants and coolants must not contact in-process product or equipment. The reliability of instruments should also be considered; for instance, a pressure transmitter that uses atmospheric pressure as its reference may suffer poor reliability [16]. A draft calibration schedule may also be prepared.

Computer hardware includes all equipment making up the computer system: processing units, user screens, keyboards, printers, and network interfaces. Some automation systems may have elements of computer hardware distributed at a central site or computer room. User screens and keyboard inputs are often placed at distributed locations to be closer to the operator's place of work. Intrinsically safe user screens and sealed keyboards may be required in some classified areas. Automation systems may need an Uninterruptible Power Supply (UPS), or protection from electrical interference, such as Electro-Magnetic Interference (EMI), Electro-Static Discharge (ESD), and Radio Frequency Interference (RFI). Sometimes, chart recorders will be needed to monitor the temperature and humidity of the installation site. The accumulation of dust is another danger that can lead to the inoperability of equipment. Even fire and flood should be considered. The operational limitations of hardware and other key parameters for individual items of equipment must be specified, along with any calibration or special maintenance requirements. Designated spare and redundant parts should be included in the Hardware Design documentation.

The performance of computer hardware must not constrain the effectiveness of the Software Design. The traffic loading of communication links should not diminish any real-time processing requirements. This will include any Local Area Networks (LANs) and Wide Area Networks (WANs). Databases should not operate at capacity, and access contentions between multiple processes or users should also be examined. Additional memory and memory management software may be needed to improve the operating speed of any computer system.

Hazard Study

System development should include a Hazard Study to identify threats to the process automation system's integrity and operability. The manufacturing process being controlled by the automation system must be brought into a safe condition to protect the quality of the manufactured product [17]. The Hazard Study checks or proposes methods of protection against identified threats. An important factor to consider is the time to resume full integrity and operability or switch to manual operation. Recovery times are very important for delay-sensitive manufacturing processes.

Hazard Studies usually take the form of a team meeting. Team members are selected for their particular knowledge of the manufacturing process, the computer system, and the software program. During the Hazard Study meeting, the team will go through diagrammatic representations of the system by considering all links between different components of the system. Other information may also be used to drive the process, such as sequence charts. The experience of the review leader will guide the review team through the configuration of the automation system, the software control scheme, the effect of GMP-related functions on the process, and the general operability and security of the automation system.

Some example questions for the Hazard Study are given in Appendix 3B at the end of this chapter. Of particular interest to the study is the effect of partial or catastrophic failures, recovery mechanisms (e.g., roll-back and roll-forward), and the general usability of the system (e.g., the need for multiple screens to access data, screen refresh times, meaningful information displays). The list of questions can be expanded with operational and regulatory experience. For instance, Eutech Engineering has collated a database of over 350 operational incidents that it uses to refine its Hazard Study process, as illustrated in Figure 3.7 [18].

Guidewords can be used to expand the Hazard Study questions, but care must be taken to ensure that all review participants understand their precise meaning and whether or not they are suitable in the context they are being used. Some guidewords are given below based on examples already used within the chemical industry [19]:

- on, off, interrupt
- as well as, only, other than, part of
- no, not, wrong
- less, none, more
- reverse, inverse
- more often, less often
- early, late, sooner, later, before, after

The Hazard Study meeting must be minuted, possibly using report forms, and any actions that arise from the review agreed to and owned by a member of the review team. The actions must be described in detail in the meeting

Figure 3.7. Hazard Study Feedback Loop

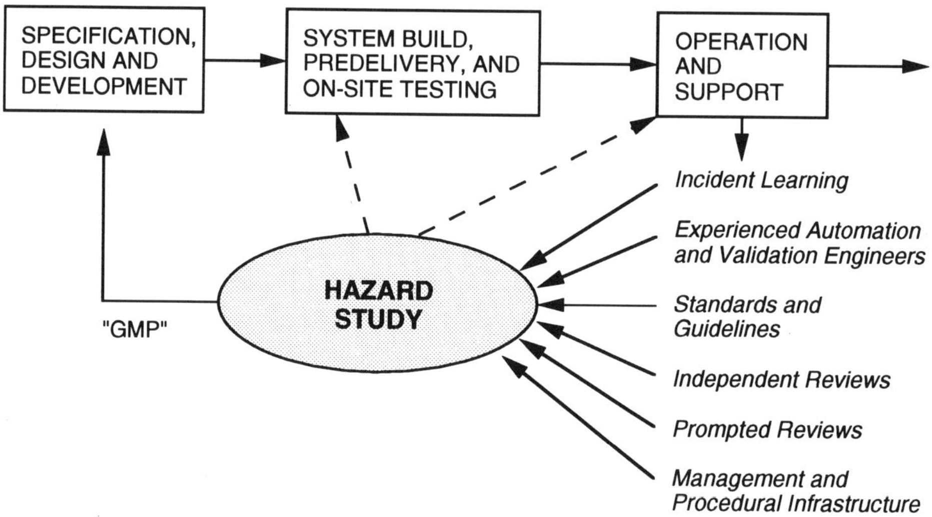

record, with a proposed completion date. The actions must only be signed off and dated as accepted when evidence of their completion is made available. Some actions may require modification in the system design and associated documentation. Other actions may identify specific Predelivery or On-Site Tests for inclusion in the qualification protocols. Alternatively, operating procedures may need to be developed or refined. A final report detailing the personnel involved with the review, the topics considered, and the findings of the review is usually written when all of the review actions are completed. The report should be kept under change control.

Ian Johnson reports several design problems concerning a fluid bed dryer, a tablet press, and a water deioniser system, all of which could have benefited from a Hazard Study [8]. The alarms in the fluid bed dryer were not latched by the embedded PLC. Alarms should have remained until acknowledged by an operator pressing the "alarm reset" button. Four alarm conditions in the same fluid bed dryer did not sound a horn or flash warning lamps because they were wrongly dependent on another status condition being present. The tablet press had a PLC compression force monitoring system with a compressed-air–driven reject mechanism that, when the compressed-air supply failed, no alarm or warning was initiated (flashing lamp, audible horn, or displayed message on an operator terminal). With this particular tablet press, a tablet that should have been but was not rejected went down the accept chute—presenting a direct threat to product quality. The PLC–controlled deioniser did not isolate its water supply if the PLC failed. There were no hard-wired alarms or interlocks to alert operations staff and protect the body of deionised water already in the plant, thereby directly threatening drug product quality. A Hazard Study would have provided early warning of these deficiencies before the automation systems were implemented.

SYSTEM BUILD

Once the automation system has been designed, it can be built. The activities associated with this phase are the responsibility of the supplier and cover Software Programming, Software Inspection, and System Manufacture and Assembly.

Software Programming

GMP regulatory authorities expect software to be programmed and maintained under version and change control [20]. They also encourage the use of good programming practices [12,21]. Such programming practices should be defined and cover the following:

- Software structure (file organisation: including comments, headers, and trailers)

- Naming conventions (including variables and filenames)
- Revision convention (configuration/change control)
- Code format (style including indentation, labels, and white space)
- Controls on the complexity of code (modules should aim to be in the range of 150 to 250 lines long [38])
- Ensuring that there is no redundant code
- Role of compilers (configuration switches and optimisation)

The quality of software programming is directly related to the effort required to maintain it. Convoluted software often signifies a history of change, perhaps involving the integration of bits and pieces of code from other systems. It is hard to understand, not only to the developer, which will often result in poor documentation, but more especially to those maintaining the system. In the short term, it may not appear practical to rewrite such "spaghetti" software, in which case, the supporting documentation should be strengthened with a detailed software inspection. If the software has a longer lifetime, and especially if portions of the code are put into future products, then the maintenance costs will make it cost effective to rewrite the code. This latter scenario is often the case with large business systems, such as MRP II.

The selection of a programming language can also have a significant impact on the effectiveness of a piece of software. Data-driven languages tend to lead to data-oriented solutions whilst formula-driven languages, such as FORTRAN and COBOL, tend to lead to algorithm-oriented solutions. A poor choice of a programming language could well impose an inappropriate solution and consequential deficiencies. It is very important, therefore, that the programming language is selected to complement the software's design.

Programming Approach

The implementation of programming practices should be tailored to the particular characteristics of different programming languages and take into account their known deficiencies. For instance, the main problems associated with conventional ladder logic include the following [22]:

- Poor facilities for structured or hierarchical program decomposition
- Limited facilities for software reuse
- Poor facilities for addressing and manipulating data structures
- Limited facilities for building complex sequences
- Cumbersome facilities for arithmetic operations

Error-prone features within other programming languages, such as BASIC, C++, and RTL/2, include the following [23]:

- GOTO, Assigned GOTO, and GOSUB
- Floating-point numbers
- Pointers
- Parallelism (concurrent processing)
- Recursion
- Interrupts
- Dynamic allocation of memory

It has been suggested in the past that some programming languages are more prone to errors than others, but recent research indicates that errors are more likely to be due to the programmer than the language used [24]. Potential programming problems can, therefore, be circumvented by careful programming. Disciplined programming standards, such as IEC 1131-3 and ISA-S88, and defensive programming techniques can help in this regard.

Redundant Code

It is not uncommon to find up to 20 percent of the code being redundant when code is developed from an earlier version with a slightly different functionality. GMP regulatory authorities have expressed concern that redundant code might be unintentionally accessed during system operation and recommend its removal [25]. Redundant code can include the following:

- Superseded code from earlier software versions
- Residue code from system modifications
- Unused features of standard software packages

Wherever possible, redundant code should be removed and the software recompiled. Care, however, must be taken to ensure that rarely used code is not wrongly classified as redundant, such as

- Apparently unused modules in large configurable systems
- Diagnostic features that are intended to be inactive until needed
- Test programs that are intended to be inactive until needed

There should not be any executable code in unused areas of memory (sometimes referred to as firmware). Inadvertent jumps to these memory locations can result from transient faults induced by EMI, ESD, and RFI. Unused areas of memory should be initialised to contain logic patterns that, if erroneously interpreted as a program instruction, will cause the system to revert to a known and predefined safe state [26]. All overlays of reserved memory should be filled with similar logic patterns. A number of hardware and software system-level techniques including "error-capturing instructions" and "capability checking" are available that are suitable for implementation within a variety of design constraints [27].

Compilers

Many compilers offer configuration options for various compile time and run time checks (e.g., underflow, overflow, array bound checking, range checking). All compiler checks should be activated unless it is not possible to leave them switched on for the final version. Some compiler checks may slow down compilation to an unacceptable degree; this is especially so for very large programs.

It has been suggested that the most error-prone area of compiler operation is code optimisation [23]. This facility manipulates the software's structure in an attempt to improve its overall functional efficiency. Incorrect optimisation could have a devastating effect on the software's desired functionality. Therefore, it is strongly recommended that this compiler option be switched off for GMP critical software.

Software Inspection

The operational dependence of automation systems on software is not disputed, and the importance of professionally developed software is widely appreciated. GMP regulatory authorities hold pharmaceutical manufacturers accountable for the "suitability" of automation systems, including software [28], and expect them to take "all reasonable steps to ensure that it [software] has been produced in accordance with a system of Quality Assurance" [6]. One GMP regulatory authority is quoted as stating that "there is no room in the pharmaceutical industry for magic boxes" [29].

Source Code Reviews have been promoted to assess independently the accuracy and quality of software [30]. Source Code Reviews have four basic objectives:

1. Detect possible coding errors
2. Determine adherence to design specifications, including affirmation of process sequencing, I/O handling, formulae, algorithms, and message and alarm handling
3. Determine adherence to programming practices (e.g., headers, version control, change control)
4. Identify redundant code

The UK GAMP Forum has responded with a review procedure (referred to here as Software Inspection) covering software design, adherence to coding standards, software logic, redundant code, and critical algorithms [2].

The Software Inspection must be recorded and systematically cover all aspects of the software, with particular attention to GMP elements of functionality. If no deficiencies are identified regarding a functional element, then this should be minuted in the review records. A report for the Software Inspection should be prepared, summarising the scope of work that might include more than one program. Specific statements on software structure, programming practice, GMP–related functionality, information transfer with other portions of the system or other systems, error handling, redundant code, version control, and change control should be made before an overall conclusion on the suitability and maintainability of the software is drawn. The Software Inspection is particularly useful when verifying calculations that during the systems operation are being updated too quickly to check. The report may identify some software modifications; in this case, evidence of their completion of intended implementation should be given.

It is generally considered that widely distributed off-the-shelf (OTS) software does not need Software Inspection if it is produced by a reputable developer and it requires no more than an application parameter configuration [31]. In most automation systems, therefore, Software Inspections are limited to bespoke software and configuration within OTS software products. New version releases of OTS software should be reviewed to determine the acceptability of the supplier's software development. Pharmaceutical manufacturers should consider waiting until the software has developed some kind of track record. A typical waiting period might be six months for a widely used piece of software. Where a pharmaceutical manufacturer consciously decides to be an early adopter, then additional Predelivery and On-Site Testing is likely to be required to establish confidence in the software.

Examples of real problems identified in Software Inspections are listed below. Software Inspections will typically require about four days' effort, split between an independent reviewer and the software programmer, for a PLC or configuration of a small Distributed Control System (DCS). The time saved by identifying problems before Predelivery or On-Site Testing is considered by many to more than compensate for the time and effort to conduct a Software Inspection.

- Version and change control not implemented in so called "industry standard" PLC and DCS software.
- Functions and procedures in MRP II software not having a terminating statement so the execution erroneously runs into the next routine.

- Incorrectly implemented calculations: moving averages in Supervisory Control and Data Acquisition (SCADA) systems, material mixing concentrations in DCSs, and shelf-life date calculations in Laboratory Information Management Systems (LIMS).
- Duplicated error messages because cut and paste used without required edit.
- Interlocks and alarm signal inputs used by PLC software labelled as unused on electrical diagrams.

Whilst rarely invoked, some GMP regulations require reasonable regulator access to application-specific software, including any Software Inspection records [30,32]. For the purpose of regulatory GMP inspections, pharmaceutical manufacturers should, therefore, agree on inspection access to application-specific software with its suppliers. A typical agreement might require software to be made available within 24 hours. Some manufacturers have established escrow accounts with suppliers, but this is not mandatory. A lack of cooperation from the software supplier is an acknowledged problem, and in such circumstances, it is recommended that pharmaceutical manufacturers use other suppliers for future projects [5,12].

System Manufacture and Assembly

Many automation systems are assembled at the supplier's premises; any assembly problems are resolved before the system is delivered to the pharmaceutical manufacturer's site. Special equipment may need to be manufactured or constructed and this should be built as specified in the Hardware Design. More complex systems are usually assembled at the pharmaceutical manufacturer's site. In either situation, it is important to assemble and install the automation system in accordance with defined procedures. Any risk posed to the pharmaceutical manufacturing process by poor assembly must be minimised [14]. Assembly practices should, therefore, be governed by a review of industry standards and the original equipment manufacturer's (OEM) recommendations. Automation systems are likely to incorporate equipment from a number of OEMs. Wiring and earthing practices must be safe.

The quality of assembly work should be monitored. Many organisations use visual inspection and diagnostic testing to confirm that the automation system's hardware has been correctly integrated and that its software has been correctly installed. Some companies tag equipment that has passed such a quality check so that it can be easily identified.

PREDELIVERY TESTING

Predelivery Testing is the responsibility of the supplier and includes Modular and Integration Testing and System Prequalification in preparation for

On-Site Testing. Some organisations refer to Predelivery Testing as Factory Acceptance Testing. Predelivery Testing is based on verifying, within the practical constraints of being at the supplier's premises, the automation system's specification and design and development documentation (see Figure 3.8). The pharmaceutical manufacturer will often endeavour to include as many tests as possible in the Predelivery Testing. Evidence of a supplier's testing can reduce the amount of On-Site Testing expected by GMP regulatory authorities. It should also reduce the time needed to commission the automation system on the pharmaceutical manufacturer's site, as qualification can focus on confirming an already established operational capability.

The supplier will normally invite the pharmaceutical manufacturer to observe their testing. This is particularly important if the pharmaceutical manufacturer is reducing On-Site Testing based on the premise of successful Predelivery Testing. Many pharmaceutical manufacturers use Predelivery Testing as an opportunity for informal operator training before the automation system arrives on-site. If specific training is required for On-Site Testing or the on-going operation of the automation system, then formal training is needed and this should be documented in personnel training records.

Modular and Integration Testing

Modular Tests exercise the components and sub-systems of the design in isolation, using known inputs to generate actual outputs that are compared to expected outputs (see Figure 3.9). Modular Testing, also known as unit testing, does not need to be exhaustive; remember, the aim is to develop a high degree of confidence in the key functionality of modules. Modular Tests must

Figure 3.8. Testing Protocols

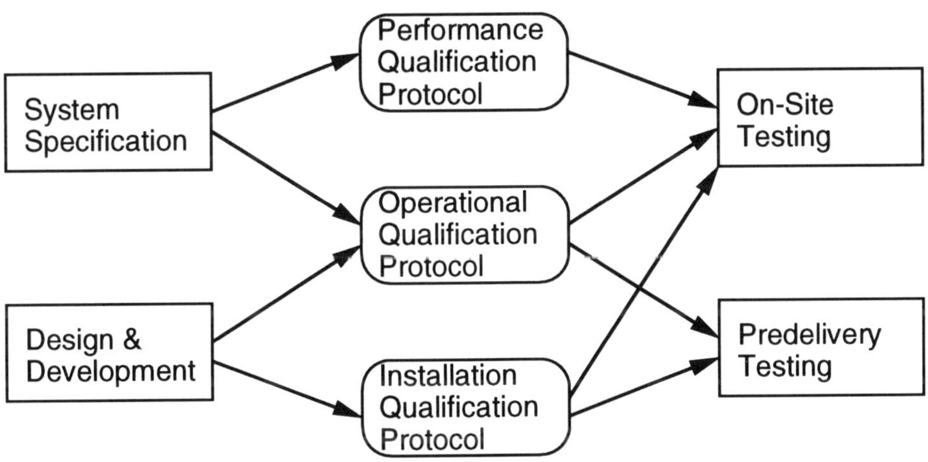

Figure 3.9. Modular Testing

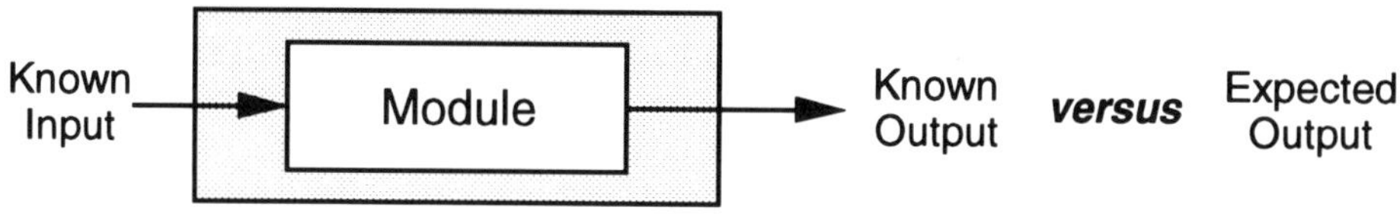

be accompanied by Integration Testing [14]. Together, Modular and Integration Testing are often referred to as structural (or "white box") testing.

Integration Testing exercises the interfaces between components and typically ensures subsystems that have been separately developed work together correctly (see Figure 3.10). Testing should ensure high coverage of internal control flow paths, error handling, and recovery procedures, which are difficult to test in the context of functional (or "black box") testing.

It is important that the pharmaceutical manufacturer has confidence in the structural testing as well as the functional testing of the automation system. Records of Modular and Integration Testing (including test specifications and results) should be kept by the supplier and retained for inspection, if requested, by the pharmaceutical manufacturer. Any test harnesses, emulations, and simulations used during testing must be specified and assurance in their capability demonstrated.

System Prequalification

System Prequalification tests are conducted by the supplier to verify the automation system's specification and design. System Prequalification is sometimes called alpha testing. In particular, it should address the items listed in the example system description given at the end of this chapter (Appendix 3A). Instrumentation to be used on a pharmaceutical manufacturer's site must be calibrated before use, either as a predelivery exercise or after its arrival on-site. Calibration records must be kept [14,15]. Tests not addressed as part of the System Prequalification must be included in the On-Site Testing.

Automated testing tools can be used to great effect during Predelivery Testing and are discussed in more detailed in Chapter 8. The use of any automatic testing tools must be agreed with the pharmaceutical manufacturer and agreed on in the Supplier Project/Quality Plan.

Test specifications should be documented and approved before testing begins. Each test should individually reference the system's requirements that, as recommended earlier, should have been itemised in the specification and design. If the pharmaceutical manufacturer wants to use these tests to justify a reduction in the amount of On-Site Testing, then the manufacturer

Figure 3.10. Integration Testing

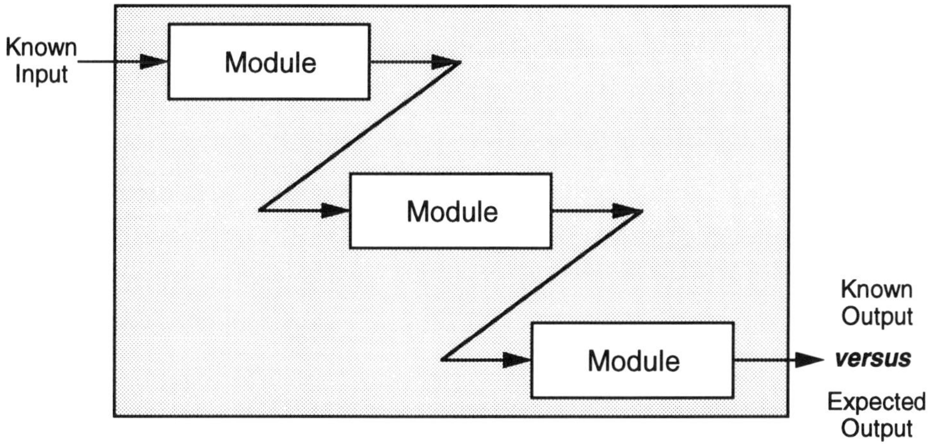

should be invited to review the test specifications. An example test script format is shown below:

- Project title
- Unique test reference and run number
- Reference documentation
- Space for name, date, and signature of the tester and witness
- Objective of the test
- Test procedure
- Acceptance criteria for a successful test outcome
- A section noting "pass", "pass with reservation", or "fail"
- A space for observations to be recorded during testing

Tests should aim to find errors, not prove they do not exist. Testing is not debugging or snagging. It has been suggested that perhaps more than half of the tests conducted on an automation system should challenge its operational capabilities [5,11,12]:

- Boundary Values *(Guidewords: Minimum, Zero, Maximum)*

  Many problems arise when the design fails to take account of processing boundaries, such as data entry, maximum storage requirements, and maximum variables scanned at highest scan frequency.

- Invalid Arguments *(Guidewords: Alphanumeric, Integer, Decimal)*

  Includes operator data entry, acknowledgements, state changes, open circuit instruments, instruments out of range, and instruments off-scan.

- Special Values *(Guidewords: Null-Entry, Function Keys)*

  Includes totally unexpected operator input.

- Calculation Accuracy *(Guidewords: Precision, Exceptions)*

  Includes precision to a number of decimal places, underflow and overflow, division by zero, and other calculation exceptions.

- Performance *(Guidewords: Sequence, Timing, Volume of Data)*

  Includes execution of algorithms, task scheduling, system load, performance of simultaneous operations, data throughput, I/O scanning, and data refresh.

- Security and Access *(Guidewords: User Categories, Passwords)*

  Includes access controls for normal and privileged users, multiuser locking, and other security requirements.

- Error Handling and Recovery *(Guidewords: Messages, Alarms)*

  Includes software, hardware, and communication failure. Logging facilities are also included.

- Call Coverage *(Guidewords: Call Tree, Decision Tree)*

  As a general principle, all calls to routines, functions, and procedures should be exercised at least once during testing. In addition, all decision branches should be exercised at least once during testing.

The test outcomes are documented as a "pass", "pass with reservation", or "fail" test result accompanied by raw data evidence and record content verified by an independent witness. The outcome of each test is compared against acceptance criteria to ascertain whether the result fulfils the criteria without deviation.

- PASS—signifying that the test meets the acceptance criteria as detailed in the test script in full without deviation from the test procedure.

- PASS WITH RESERVATION—signifying that the test does not meet the acceptance criteria, but that the actual result is acceptable to both the tester and the witness. The deviation from the acceptance criteria and the reason for accepting the test outcome must be recorded or referenced in the observations portion of the test script.

- FAIL—signifying that the test does not fulfil the acceptance criteria.

Test records are collectively reviewed and a conclusion is drawn from the overall outcome of testing. Satisfactory testing is signified by approval of the completed work. Unsatisfactory testing may lead to (individually or in combination)

- The abandonment of single or multiple tests
- Corrective actions affecting automation or documentation
- A concession on the acceptability of test outcomes
- Retest of single, several, or all tests

A successful overall testing outcome releases the automation system for delivery to the pharmaceutical manufacturer.

The success of Predelivery Testing should be based on identifying and correcting deficiencies rather than merely looking at the initial pass rate. After all, it is far more important to detect deficiencies now than be misled into thinking the system is fully functional, only to be embarrassed during On-Site Testing or to be noncompliant during live operation. Common testing problems observed by GMP regulatory authorities include the following [7]:

- Poor choice of test cases
- Failure to define intent of tests
- Failure to document test results

Ian Johnson [8] recalls a PLC–controlled granulator that succumbed to the challenge of operators entering inappropriate values for control parameters. Inputting zero for run duration or stopping torque would run the granulator forever. Inputting zero revolutions per minute for motor speed would still enable the motor to run. Unfortunately, no memory was available to implement warning messages, editing, or rejection of "bad" input. As the granulator would not run without the PLC, the whole system was abandoned.

ON–SITE TESTING

On-Site Testing is the responsibility of the pharmaceutical manufacturer, although suppliers often assist. This phase consists of four sequential activities, as illustrated in Figure 3.11: Site Preparation, Installation Qualification (IQ), Operational Qualification (OQ), and Performance Qualification (PQ). Site Preparation ensures that the setup requirements for the automation system are complete; IQ verifies the configuration and calibration of delivered equipment to the Software and Hardware Design; OQ verifies the operational capability to the System Specification; and PQ verifies the intent of the

Figure 3.11. On-Site Testing Timeline

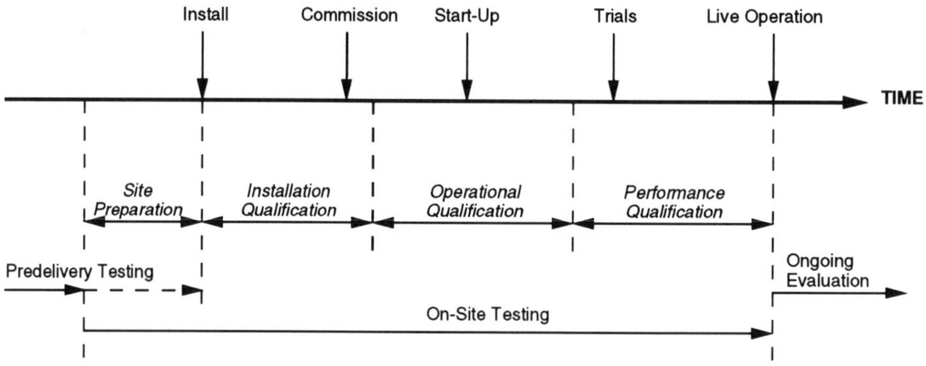

system to the URS. The inclusion or exclusion of tests between these qualification activities is usually based on convenience.

Qualification should follow the same principles outlined for the automation system's prequalification within Predelivery Testing. Test specifications (also known as qualification protocols) must be reviewed and approved before testing begins; it is especially important that the qualification is *S.M.A.R.T.* [33]:

- *Specific:* test objectives address documented requirements.
- *Measurable:* test acceptance criteria are objective, not subjective.
- *Achievable:* test acceptance criteria are realistic.
- *Recorded:* test outcome evidence is signed and, where available, "raw data" are attached.
- *Traceable:* test records, including subsequent actions, form a repeatable audit trail.

Test specifications can, in theory, be written during system development. In practice, however, whilst they may be drafted during development, they often need details confirmed with information that is only available after system development and Predelivery Testing is complete.

A report is prepared for each qualification activity, summarising the outcome of testing. Any failed tests, retests, and concessions to accept tests must be discussed. Not every test need pass without reservation in order to allow the next qualification activity to begin, as long as this situation is justified in the reports and corrective actions to resolve any problems are initiated. Each report will typically conclude with a general statement authorising progression to the next qualification activity.

Some pharmaceutical manufacturers agree to conduct beta testing for suppliers, whereby they take delivery of a system for use in its intended operating environment and report any problems experienced back to the supplier. Beta systems cannot be considered as "standard" or fully tested. More information on standard systems can be found in Chapter 8. Pharmaceutical manufacturers must not use betaware as part of a validated automation system.

Site Preparation

The physical site of the automation system is prepared. The suitability of the site's operating environment for the specified automation system [6] is checked. It should be compliant with any manufacturer's or system integrator's recommendations. The placement of the system, including the building of any special rooms or housing, associated wiring, and power supply voltages, must be confirmed as adequate. Instrumentation must be accessible to facilitate operations and be covered by maintenance and calibration schedules [15]. Environmental requirements outlined in the System Specification and Design, such as temperature, humidity, vibration, dust, EMI, RFI, and ESD, should also be checked in comparison with their acceptable bounds. In-situ testing of the automation system can now begin.

Installation Qualification

The integration of the automation system—hardware, software, and instrumentation—must to be confirmed in readiness for the OQ. Some practitioners have referred to this as testing static attributes of the automation system.

All of the specified components of the system should be present and correct, including printers, and the Visual Display Units (VDUs), including touch screens, keyboards, and computer cards. The correct version of firmware must also be checked and may include a physical inspection of an Electronically Programmable Read Only Memory (EPROM) to verify its label data. As part of this process, the pharmaceutical manufacturer typically repeats the integrated automation system testing conducted prior to delivery [6]. Simulation and emulation support of On-Site Testing should be avoided [34].

The automation system's computer hardware requires its electrical earths and signal earths for intrinsic and nonintrinsic safety to be checked. Any system clocks also require checking. The identifying serial numbers and model numbers of all cards should be checked against the Hardware Design. The automation system's signal routing must be checked. Confirm the identity of I/O signals (both digital and analogue) as presented on the user interface with any database configuration and interface. The interface may be supported by one or more cards. Confirm signal continuity between field terminations and the computer hardware's interface.

The correct versions of software must be installed and appropriate backup copies should exist. The storage medium for the software must be labelled with the software reference name and version. Facilities should exist to store the backup files in a secure place [15]. Any software diagnostic tests will be conducted. Software drivers, such as communication protocols, will also be tested. The configuration of databases, and the content of any library information, should also be checked.

Instrumentation should have its predelivery calibration verified and any remaining calibration set. Calibration should be conducted with at least two known values. Loop checks should be made for the entire system. Inputs and outputs must be checked to provide strong assurance of accuracy [15].

Stage 1: Verify identification of instrumentation. Confirm suitability of any materials of construction in product contact and supplier's recommended operating conditions. Confirm wiring and field cabling of instrumentation from the field to the automation system termination panels (loop checks). Confirm field instrumentation in calibration. Check any signal conditioning. Confirm immunity to electrical interference.

Stage 2: Verify input and output signals from the automation system termination panel to the operator console via any database configuration. Check output actuator signals from automation system and verify output signals driving actuators. Signals can be generated by manipulating the environment around the device (e.g., chiller spray) or by injecting a signal close to the field device (e.g., high value for limit switch). Any corresponding equipment helping to generate artificial signals must be referenced.

Stage 3: A total check of I/O should be made—drive motors, open and close valves, and so on—from the operator interface.

All documentation provided by the supplier should be present. User manuals, as-built drawings, instrument calibration records, and procedures for operation and maintenance (including calibration schedules) of the system should all be checked to verify that they are suitable. Confirm Contingency Plans and any Service Level Agreements (SLA) are in place. Any training requirements necessary before qualification should have been completed.

The importance of completing IQ before commencing OQ is illustrated by a recent incident where a pharmaceutical manufacturer had over 35 percent of the instrumentation for a multiproduct plant but did not have available calibration certificates. There were various reasons for this situation, but none were recorded—some instruments were no longer used, some had extended recalibration periods, some had been undergoing calibration for several weeks. The nett effect was that the automation system under qualification was clearly not in a controlled state suitable for OQ and, as a consequence, it was not ready for manufacturing.

Operational Qualification

After installation, it is necessary to demonstrate that the automation operates in accordance with the FS and Design. Some practitioners have referred to testing dynamic attributes of the automation system. Tests will include the following:

- Confirming the functionality (standard and configured) of application software and software packages
- Checking network integration
- Testing alarm and message handling—all error messages should be checked
- Testing interlocks and trips
- Checking reports and displays
- Verifying GMP operations—all critical decision paths must be checked and challenged
- Checking procedures for start-up and shutdown
- Checking procedures for backup and recovery
- Testing security and access

The robustness of the installed automation system in its operating environment should also be covered by the OQ. Tests must demonstrate that the continuity of correct functionality is not disrupted by acceptable variations in

- Power supply
- Temperature
- Humidity
- Vibration
- Dust
- EMI, RFI, and ESD

This list of operational environment requirements is not exhaustive and may be extended or reduced depending on the defined needs of the system. Electro-Magnetic Interference (EMI) and Radio Frequency Interference (RFI) might be tested with the localised use of mobile phones (walkie-talkies), arc welding equipment, and electronic drills. The aim is to test the automation system in situations that are considered normal working conditions. Options for testing low and high temperature operability include the use of freezing sprays (normally used in microelectronic manufacturing) and hair dryers. Variations in temperature and humidity might also be monitored over a period of time using a portable chart recorder as part of the PQ. Electro-Static Discharge (ESD), vibration, and dust are more difficult to test and it may be possible to only periodically review whether or not they have had an impact during live operation. If this is the case, then it should be clearly stated and followed up as part of the ongoing support programme for maintaining validation described in Chapter 5.

Test specifications can make use of operating procedures, where they have been prepared, to define test methods and, thereby, concurrently confirm system functionality and any associated procedures. Operations personnel must be able to use all operating procedures before the automation system is used for live manufacturing. Any training required to conduct these tests should be verified before testing begins.

Additional tests mandated or recommended by the Supplier Audit, Software Inspection, Hazard Study, and IQ should be included. The testing requirements for different categories of software are outlined in Table 3.2. As recommended earlier in this chapter, the URS, the FS, and the Hardware Design and Software Design documentation should have unique reference numbers for each feature to be tested. Test specifications can cross-reference to these numbers and, thereby, make it easier to identify if any features have not been tested by Predelivery Testing or IQ.

The OQ may be based on a repetition of a chosen sample of Predelivery Tests. As discussed earlier, this is only allowable where extensive testing has

Table 3.2. Categories for Software Qualification

Automation System Software (Supported by Documentation & Supplier Audit	Testing Requirements for Pharmaceutical Manufacturer			
	Record Version	Record Configuration	"Black Box" Acceptance Testing	"White Box" Acceptance Testing
Standard Software	Yes	Not Applicable	Yes Sample only	Not Applicable
Configurable Software	Yes	Yes	Yes	Yes Macros only
Custom-Built Software	Yes	Yes if appropriate	Yes	Yes

Notes: (1) All software, including firmware, should be categorised as either standard, configurable, or custom built. (2) The table assumes that the pharmaceutical manufacturer does not have to supplement OTS software products with "white box" testing because the supplier already has sufficient evidence of such testing.

been successfully conducted and recorded. The test sample must include, but not be limited to, those tests originally conducted as emulations and simulations. If the sample of repeated tests do not fulfil their acceptance criteria, then the cause of failure must be investigated and an extended sample of tests must be repeated once again. The advantage to this approach is that commissioning time on the pharmaceutical manufacturer's site is reduced, and the system can become fully operational sooner. It might be argued that repeating the supplier's Predelivery Testing does not add any value, but practical experience suggests that crucial deficiencies are often discovered in the system's functionality even at this late stage in the life cycle. Here are just a few examples:

- Backup copies of application software for a freeze drier PLC did not work.
- A SCADA system froze when too many concurrent alarms were raised.
- The operator of a control system would never be aware of concurrent alarm messages because the graphic pages had banners that only displayed the last alarm.
- When clamping and unclamping buttons were pressed together in a fluid bed drier, embedded PLC software initiated clamping [8].
- PLC software allowed the drum of a tablet coater to turn, even when side doors were not sealed [8].

Testing can concentrate on critical drug manufacturing parameters or functions, but care must be taken not to select too few parameters or functions. It is unlikely that a manufacturing process is only dependent on one or two key parameters. It should also be recognised that each key parameter may be related to a dozen or more process variables, each of which should be validated. The pharmaceutical manufacturer must be able to provide GMP regulatory authorities with documentary evidence justifying why some parameters are critical and others are not critical. Evidence is usually supplied in the form of minutes from a review meeting (possibly supplementing an earlier GMP Assessment) between engineering, operations, and quality representatives considering the issue.

A testing strategy called thread testing is useful for real-time automation systems [35]. Real-time systems are difficult to test because of the subtle, time-dependent interactions between different functions of the system. Testing consists of tracking the processing of external events as it "threads" its way through the system's functionality, and checking that the threads comply with System Specification and Design. State transition diagrams are often very useful in this respect. Complete thread testing may not be practical because of the large number of I/O combinations. In such cases, the most commonly exercised threads in the automation system should be identified and selected for testing.

Performance Qualification

At this stage, the pharmaceutical manufacturer must demonstrate that the completed site installation ("as-built") of the automation system is operating to the intent of the URS. Verifying whether or not the automation system is fit for its intended purpose necessitates specifying tests related to the manufacture of an individual drug product. In particular, the influence of the automation system on the consistent manufacture of three product batches (five batches for biological applications), batch records, media fill trials, labelling, and cleaning should be investigated. The degree of testing will be influenced by the amount of OQ testing already conducted. Testing may include the following:

- Confirm applicability of operating procedures.
- Check production records against plant logbooks for inconsistencies.
- Monitor GMP critical parameters.
- Monitor alarms and messages.
- Confirm security access procedures.
- Confirm operator interface is fully functional.
- Start-up and close-out batch.
- Confirm collection and check reproduction of batch records.
- Confirm batch records are correct.
- Identify any additional procedures or training requirements.
- Check viability of contingency plan.
- Check backup and restoration procedure.

Automated batch records must provide accurate reproduction of master data [15] and equivalent assurance to a double manual check, noting that manual checks can identify and record unexpected observations [11,15]. Automated systems releasing batches need authorisation for each batch, and the responsible person should be recorded against the batches [6,15,37]. All batch records require quality control inspection and approval prior to release and distribution of the product [15]. The identity of operators entering or confirming data should be recorded. Authority to change data and reasons for change should be recorded in an audit trail.

VALIDATION REPORT

The Validation Report is prepared in response to the Validation Plan to provide a management summary of the success and concessions arising from the validation exercise [5]. The objective of the report is to justify the completion and acceptance of the validation conducted. Recommendations may be made and include a follow-up audit or additional testing. Some organisations refer to the issue of the Validation Report authorising use of the automation system for live manufacturing as certification.

The report should be prepared by the person identified in the Validation Plan, usually the pharmaceutical manufacturer's project manager. Where this is not the case, then the authority under which the report is written should be stated.

The report usually follows the same format as the pharmaceutical manufacturer's Validation Plan, to provide an easy cross-reference for compliance. The report should review the documentation associated with the various phases of the validation project (see Figure 3.12) and preview the ongoing support required to maintain validation of the automated system. The review should, therefore, cover the Supplier Audit, System Specification, System Development and Design, System Build, Software Inspection, Predelivery Testing, and On-Site Testing. Any deviations and interventions to the pharmaceutical manufacturer's Validation Plan or Supplier's Project/Quality Plan must be recorded and their impact on validation investigated. Deviations and interventions may include changes to SOPs during validation, concessions on the acceptability of test results, or modifications to the life-cycle model to make it more appropriate. Corrective actions needed to resolve any outstanding issues must be identified. Test metrics summarising qualification are sometimes included, such as the percentage of successful tests meeting acceptance criteria and the number of modifications required. Suppliers may, similarly, supply a report summarising their validation work, which can also be referenced by the Validation Report.

Where there are a number of similar automation systems, it may be useful to establish a User Group. This group could meet regularly to exchange user experiences, disseminate support information, and organise any collective training. Later, when the systems require replacement, the User Group can develop a migration strategy. The User Group may be limited to a pharmaceutical manufacturer's own organisation, perhaps on the premise of confidentiality, although there are benefits for wider consultation between different companies including suppliers.

The Validation Report authorising use of the automation system should not be issued until all support requirements, including document management, calibration, maintenance, change control, security, and so on have been put in place. It is essential that the validation status of the system is not compromised. Revalidation will be required if validation controls are not being implemented. The costs of revalidation can be in excess of 5 times more expensive than ensuring validation controls are available and used in the first place. Management must ensure that their organisation's investment in validation is not effectively thrown away.

Figure 3.12. Life-Cycle Documentation

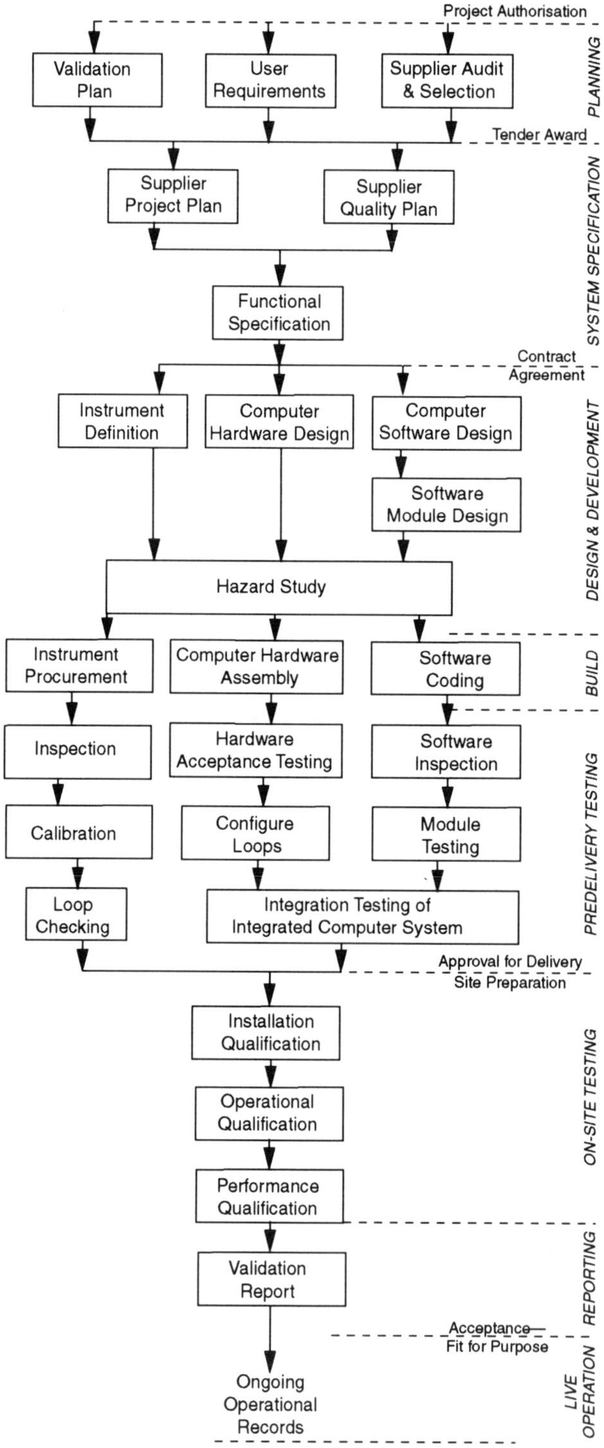

REFERENCES

1. NE 58: Abwicklung von qualifizierungspflichtigen PLT-Projekten (version 04.06.96); [including . . .] Dannapel, B., Hensel, H., Mockel, B., Muhlenkamp, J., Muller-Heinzerling, T., Otto, A., and Teuchert, V. (1995), Qualifizierung von Leitsystemen: Ein Gemeinschaftsprojekt von GMA und NAMUR zur Validierung, *ATP—Automatisierungstechnische Praxis,* 37 (10): 64–76.

2. UK GAMP Forum (1995), *Supplier Guide for Validation of Automation Systems in Pharmaceutical Manufacture,* Second Draft, available for the International Society for Pharmaceutical Engineering, The Hague, Netherlands.

3. PDA (1995), Validation of Computer Related Systems, *PDA Journal of Pharmaceutical Science and Technology,* Technical Report No. 18.

4. Trill, A.J. (1996), Regulatory Requirements for Computer Validation, *Computer Systems Validation: A Practical Approach,* Management Forum Seminar, 26–27 March, London.

5. Tetzlaff, R.F. (1992), GMP Documentation Requirements for Automated Systems: Parts 1, 2 and 3, *Pharmaceutical Technology,* 16 (3): 112–124, 16 (4): 60–72, 6 (5): 70–82.

6. European Union (1993), Annex 11—Computerised Systems, European Union Guide to Directive 91/356/EEC.

7. Clark, A.S. (1995), *Inspection of Software System,* ISPE European Computer System Validation Seminar, 20–21 September, Zurich.

8. Johnson, I. (1995), *Validation of Finished Product Equipment,* ISPE European Computer System Validation Seminar, 20–21 September, Zurich.

9. European Union (1991), *Work Contracted Out,* Article 12 EEC/356/91.

10. Wingate, G.A.S. (1996), Resource Requirements, Costs and Benefits, *Computer Systems Validation: A Practical Approach,* Management Forum Seminar, 26–27 March, London.

11. TGA (1990), *Australian Code of Good Manufacturing for Therapeutic Goods,* Medicinal Products, Part 1, Therapeutic Goods Administration, Woden, Australia.

12. Trill, A.J. (1993), Computerised Systems and GMP—A UK Perspective, Part 1: Background, Standards and Methods; Part 2: Inspection Findings; Part: 3 Best Practices and Topical Issues, *Pharmaceutical Technology International,* 5 (2): 12–26, 5 (3): 49–63, 5 (5): 17–30.

13. FDA (1987), *General Principles of Process Validation,* Rockville, MD: Food and Drug Administration, Center for Drug Evaluation and Research.

14. European Union Guide to Directive 91/356/EEC (1991), *European Commission Directive Laying Down the Principles of Good Manufacturing Practice for Medicinal Products for Human Use.*

15. U.S. Code of Federal Regulations Title 21, Part 211 (last amended 1995), *Current Good Manufacturing Practice for Finished Pharmaceuticals.*

16. ISPE (1995), *Bulk Pharmaceutical Chemicals, Baseline: Pharmaceutical Engineering Guide for New Facilities,* Volume 1 (First Draft), International Society for Pharmaceutical Engineering, Tampa, Florida.

17. FDA (1983), *Guide to Inspection of Computerized Systems in Drug Processing* (Blue Book), Reference Materials and Training Aids for Investigators, Rockville, MD: Food and Drug Administration, Center for Drug Evaluation and Research.

18. Lucas, P.R. and Wingate, G.A.S. (1996), Threats Analysis for Computer Systems, Special Issue on Computer Systems Validation, *Pharmaceutical Engineering,* 16 (3).

19. Chung, P. and Broomfield, E. (1995), Hazard and Operability (HAZOP) Studies Applied to Computer-Controlled Process Plants, in *Computer Control and Human Error* (Edited by T. Kletz), Institute of Chemical Engineers.

20. FDA (1984), *CGMP Applicability to Hardware and Software,* Guide 11, Compliance Policy Guides, Computerized Drug Processing, 7132a, Guide 11, Rockville, MD: Food and Drug Administration, Center for Drug Evaluation and Research.

21. FDA (1987), *Software Development Activities,* Technical Report, Reference Materials and Training Aids for Investigators, Rockville, MD: Food and Drug Administration, Center for Drug Evaluation and Research.

22. Lewis, R.W. (1995), *Programming Industrial Control Systems Using IEC 1131-3,* Control Engineering Series 50, Institution of Electrical Engineers, London.

23. Senior, M. (1996), *Software Programming Guidelines,* Supplier Guide for Validation of Automated Systems in Pharmaceutical Manufacture, Version 2, International Society of Pharmaceutical Engineering.

24. Hatton, L. (1997), Unexpected (and Sometimes Unpleasant) Lessons from Data in Real Software Systems, *Safety and Reliability of Software Based Systems,* Springer-Verlag.

25. Leveson, N. (1995), *Safeware: System Safety and Computers,* Reading, MA: Addison-Wesley.

26. Wingate, G.A.S. and Preece, C. (1993), *Software Implemented Fault Tolerance for Microprocessor Controllers,* IEEE Proceedings of the Reliability and Maintainability Symposium (RAMS '93), Atlanta.

27. Sosnowski, J. (1994), Transient Fault Tolerance in Digital Systems, *IEEE Micro,* (February).

28. FDA (1985), *Vendor Responsibility,* Guide 12, Compliance Policy Guides, Computerized Drug Processing, 7132a, Guide 12, Rockville, MD: Food and Drug Administration, Center for Drug Evaluation and Research.

29. Fry, C.B. (1982), What We See That Makes Us Nervous, Guest Editorial, *Pharmaceutical Technology,* (May–June): 10–11.

30. FDA (1987), *Source Code for Process Control Application Programs,* Compliance Policy Guides, Computerized Drug Processing, 7132a, Guide 15, Rockville, MD: Food and Drug Administration, Center for Drug Evaluation and Research.

31. Chapman, K. (1991), A History of Validation in the United States: Parts 1 and 2 —Validation of Computer-Related Systems, *Pharmaceutical Technology.*

32. U.S. Federal Food, Drug, and Cosmetic Act, Section 704, Factory Inspection.

33. Wingate, G.A.S., Smith, M., and Lucas, P.R. (1995), *Assuring Confidence in Pharmaceutical Software,* Safety and Reliability of Software Based Systems, First Annual European Network of Clubs for Reliability and Safety of Software (ENCRESS) Conference, September, Brugge, Belgium.

34. Clark, A.S. (1988), Computer Systems Validation: An Investigator's View, *Pharmaceutical Technology,* 12 (1): 60–66.

35. Sommerville, I. (1992), *Software Engineering,* Fourth Edition, Reading, MA: Addison-Wesley.

36. FDA (1982), *Input/Output Checking,* Compliance Policy Guides, Computerized Drug Processing, 7132a, Guide 7, Rockville, MD: Food and Drug Administration, Center for Drug Evaluation and Research.

37. FDA (1982), *Identification of "Persons" on Batch Production and Control Records,* Compliance Policy Guides, Computerized Drug Processing, 7132a, Guide 8, Rockville, MD: Food and Drug Administration, Center for Drug Evaluation and Research.

38. Hatton, L. (1997), Software Failures—Follies and Fallacies, *IEE Review,* 43(2): 49–54.

APPENDIX 3A. EXAMPLE CHECKLIST FOR SPECIFICATION AND DESIGN OF AUTOMATION SYSTEM

System Description

- ☐ Overview of the process with which the automation system will interact (e.g., laboratory, manufacturing, packaging, labelling, business)
- ☐ High-level description of the role of the automation system
- ☐ Operational boundaries and interface requirements
- ☐ Development Tools: CASE tools, Computer Aided Design (CAD)
- ☐ List of constraints including working language affecting automation system

Equipment

- ☐ Computer hardware: Central Processing Unit (CPU), Random Access Memory (RAM), memory devices (hard-disk, CD-ROM, and so on), storage devices, communication interfaces to equipment and other automation systems, operator terminals
- ☐ Computer software: operating system, communication drivers, network controllers, system software, configurable programs, application programs, databases
- ☐ Instrumentation: number, type location; model numbers, software versions; tagnumbers, data types, valid range
- ☐ Controlled elements: valves, heaters, motors and motor starters, relays, solenoids, and so on
- ☐ Power requirements with tolerable operating range

Interface

Human Interface

- ☐ Number, size, and location of screens (mimic backgrounds and foregrounds)
- ☐ Input devices (keyboards, mouse, tracker ball, touch screen, and so on)
- ☐ Number, type, and location of printers (alarm, colour, report)

- ☐ Interface features (information pages, visual/audible alarms, mimics/graphics)
- ☐ Security features (levels of access authority, passwords, key switches, biometrics, logging unauthorised access attempts, and so on)

Process I/O Interface

- ☐ Operator intervention
- ☐ I/O specification for different devices
- ☐ Installed spare capacity, including fail-safe redundancy features
- ☐ Future expansion with any implications for reduced performance
- ☐ Plant external I/O signals (type, format, range, accuracy, timing)
- ☐ System-derived inputs (calculated variables: totalisers, analogue-digital converters, interposing relays, frequency, period, validity)

Communications Interface

- ☐ Protocols, buffer, cable specifications, line drivers, termination, loading, traffic density, automatic error correction

Process Control

- ☐ Sequence control: text, flowcharts, and state transition diagrams
- ☐ Continuous control: automatic and control loops, database storage, scan frequencies, complex control schemes (cascade, ratio, predictive)
- ☐ Batch control: batch initiation, process decomposition, continuous monitors, recipe handling (timers, volumes, weights, temperatures, pressures, download, and sequence interaction), logging
- ☐ Data processing: derived values, data conversions, scaling, frequencies, periods, calculations, algorithms, validity checks, error correction

System Attributes

- ☐ Alarms: number and priorities, groups, response times, escalation, annunciation, presentation (including colour and colour changes), conditioning, acknowledgments, viewing, printing and storage capacity, segregation

- ☐ Trending: real-time and historical data, histograms, balance sheets, who can configure and view trends, printing and storage capacity
- ☐ Events: number, categories, notification, viewing, logging, printing and storage capacity
- ☐ Interlocks: hard-wired interlocks, scan rates, suppression, logging, reporting, acknowledgment, automation system handshakes and watchdogs, avoid deadly embrace

Operational Environment

- ☐ Performance: response times (e.g., screen refresh rates, cycle times, and critical control response times), Mean-Time-to-Failure (MTTF), system remedial action, power failure recovery, start-up, shutdown
- ☐ Redundancy: dual operation, segregated I/O on dedicated cards, peripherals, interfaces, internal networks, power supplies, hard discs
- ☐ Intrinsic safety: equipment for zoned areas
- ☐ Operational safety: fail-safe mechanisms, error handling, database integrity, operator timeouts, fault tolerance, watchdogs, contingency plans, internal and legislative safety compliance
- ☐ Operational procedures: operator commands, override control, process monitoring, parameter modification, load scheduling, start-up and shutdown, fault-finding instructions, user manuals, and documentation
- ☐ Training: formal courses, hands-on training, manuals
- ☐ Security: levels, means of access, parameter modification, programme access, data security
- ☐ Data integrity: archiving, buffer storage, device storage, data recovery, backup, restoration
- ☐ Environmental conditions: earthing, filtering, loading, surge protection, temperature, humidity, vibration, electrical interference (ESD, EMI, RFI), fire, flood, hygiene
- ☐ Maintenance: spares, special handling practices and tools, cleaning, media backups and restoration, service contracts, service instructions, calibration schedules
- ☐ Expansion philosophy: tuning variable demand, functional changes, spare capacity, performance, physical size restrictions

APPENDIX 3B. SOME EXAMPLE HAZARD STUDY QUESTIONS

Configuration of Automation System

- ☐ Is the system implemented according to the intent of its specification?
- ☐ Are there sufficient I/O to enable plant/process to be operated as intended?
- ☐ Are all sensors and equipment working correctly as designated?
- ☐ What is automatic? What is manual?
- ☐ Does the design consider expansion requirements?
- ☐ Does the design consider the possibility of performance degradation (e.g., disk full)?
- ☐ What is the integrity of the power supply?
- ☐ Will the system be affected by electrical interference or poor earthing?
- ☐ Will the system be affected by ambient temperature or humidity?
- ☐ Will the system be affected by dust, contamination, or corrosive materials?
- ☐ Have precautions been made for fire, flood, vibration, and shock?
- ☐ Have precautions been made for environmental needs and hygiene standards?
- ☐ Is the system intrinsically safe?
- ☐ To which mode do instruments fail?
- ☐ How does the system know if equipment is faulty (instrument, computer, and manufacturing equipment)?
- ☐ Is there any redundancy built in to cover equipment failures?
- ☐ What is the system response to and recovery from utility failure?
- ☐ How are these facilities controlled?
- ☐ Are there hard-wired trips and interlocks? Challenge them.
- ☐ How are redundant and standby systems tested?
- ☐ Are off-line test or bureau systems used as a source of spares?

☐ How can the validity of these spares be assured?

☐ Do suppliers have necessary spares, and equipment?

☐ Can suppliers back up, re-create present software configuration, and restore it?

☐ Is the equipment still supported by its original manufacturer? Are parts still available?

☐ Are other automation systems connected to this system?

☐ What happens if the connection between systems is lost?

☐ How are these connections controlled?

☐ Are the maximum length of communication lines exceeded?

Software Control Scheme

☐ Has the software been reviewed, is there a backup, and can it be restored after a fault?

☐ Is the software documented, with all documents kept in a safe place?

☐ Will the system recover to a safe state after a power outage?

☐ Examine all sequence charts.

☐ Examine summary software flowcharts.

☐ Examine database structure and content.

☐ Challenge software functionality for incorrect user input, corrupted data, and incorrect decision.

☐ Ask what the consequences will be for erroneous operation.

☐ How are hazardous situations notified to operations staff?

☐ Can software recover automatically, and has this been tested?

GMP–Related Functions

☐ Who is responsible for directing operations?

☐ Does supplied documentation adequately cover abnormal plant/process states?

- ☐ Are there safe states for operation (start-up, shutdown, holds, normal running, emergency shutdown, maintenance)?
- ☐ What happens to the pharmaceutical product in the event of a failure?
- ☐ Can the pharmaceutical product be recovered in the event of a failure?
- ☐ When it is safe to resume operation?
- ☐ Is there an operating procedure to cover recovery after partial failure?
- ☐ Is there an operating procedure to cover recovery after full failure?
- ☐ Is there a contingency plan?
- ☐ Challenge all reasonable planned scenarios.
- ☐ Is the contingency plan periodically reviewed and updated?
- ☐ Has the contingency plan ever been tested?
- ☐ Is there a copy of all system parameters and settings?
- ☐ Can in-process changes to equipment operating parameters be made?
- ☐ How many product rejects are needed to halt equipment operation?
- ☐ Is there product reject verification?
- ☐ How are batch records controlled?
- ☐ Investigate alarms associated with all failure modes. Are they useful?
- ☐ What happens when large numbers of alarms are raised together?
- ☐ Is there a hard copy of valid alarm settings?
- ☐ Can an interlock be left in an incorrect state?
- ☐ Identify and challenge event logging and trending.
- ☐ Are regular (annual?) service reviews conducted?
- ☐ Are trends in equipment performance and failures monitored?

Operation of Automation System

- ☐ Is the plant/process operating philosophy fully defined and understood?
- ☐ Are all plant/process operation phases defined (start-up, shutdown, abort, recovery)?
- ☐ Are there operating procedures in place for the automation system?
- ☐ Are procedures updated and personnel retained after changes to plant/process?
- ☐ Was appropriate training given to all personnel associates with system operation?
- ☐ Are standards and recommended manufacturers' practices followed?
- ☐ How does the operator know what equipment is under automation control at any point in time?
- ☐ Can the operator accidentally change key parameters?
- ☐ Can the automation system tolerate invalid operator input?
- ☐ How does the operator know that a production problem has occurred?
- ☐ How does the operator know what to do (procedures and training)?
- ☐ Has allowance been made for colour-blind operators?
- ☐ Is the accuracy of data displayed consistent with control needs?
- ☐ Are standard names, colours, units, symbols, and abbreviations defined?
- ☐ Are alarms and messages recorded in more than one location in case of printer failure?
- ☐ How do we know if any equipment has failed during operation?
- ☐ Is a fault reporting procedure in place?
- ☐ Are system reliability and failure rates regularly reviewed for trends?
- ☐ How frequently are relief instruments used and tested?

- ☐ Can equipment be operated from more than one location? Could this lead to errors?
- ☐ Is a service agreement in place?
- ☐ Are response times defined?
- ☐ Is equipment maintained and calibrated regularly?
- ☐ Are maintenance and changes controlled by a procedure?
- ☐ How are changes between summer and winter times controlled?

Security

- ☐ Do procedures for physical access exist?
- ☐ Can software be modified without authorisation?
- ☐ What authorisation is needed to modify software?
- ☐ Have access levels been used to define/enable different levels of access?
- ☐ Are passwords/keylocks used to define/enable different levels of access?
- ☐ Are all changes to software automatically recorded?
- ☐ Can alarms be suppressed, and readings taken off-line or out-of-scan?
- ☐ Are there special security arrangements for critical items?

Chapter 4

Validation Strategies

This chapter offers some specific guidance on how to implement the validation life-cycle approach presented in the last chapter for a range of automation systems that can be found supporting pharmaceutical manufacturing. Strategies are outlined for the

- Validation of new automation systems based on the particular characteristics of different automation systems and the critical parameters associated with individual applications.
- Validation of existing automation systems based on the different life-cycle requirements for systems that can and cannot be taken off-line for testing.

Further practical details for validating different automation systems are covered by the collection of case studies presented in Part 2 of this book.

MANUFACTURING SYSTEMS

Automation systems are widely used within manufacturing operations, and there is an increasing drive to link these systems into what is commonly referred to as a Computer Integrated Manufacturing (CIM) environment. Figure 4.1 divides the CIM environment into four levels:

1. Field Management
2. Process Management
3. Production Management
4. Business Management

Figure 4.1. Manufacturing Pyramid

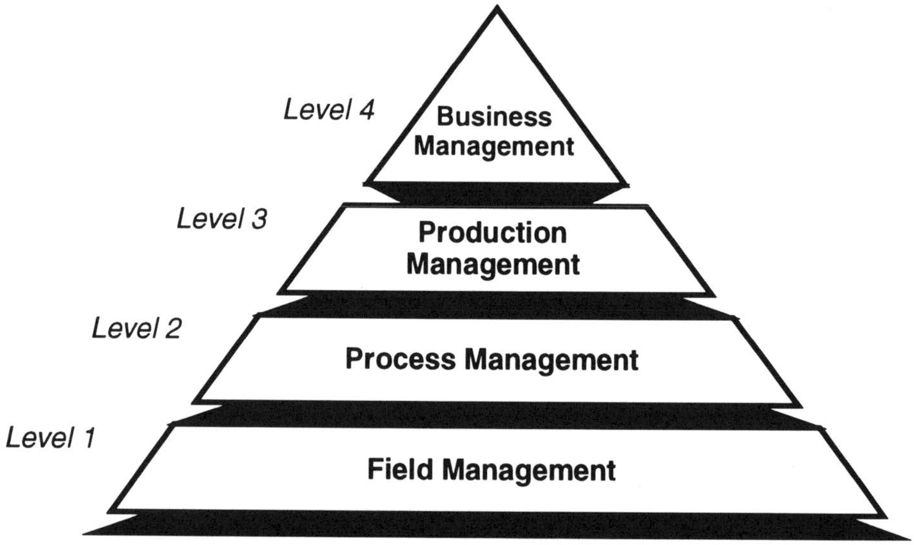

The automation systems used within each of these levels tend to have common characteristics that will influence their validation. For instance, field management systems are generally configurable instruments. Process management systems, meanwhile, are more complex than field management systems, providing real-time operability, and often include bespoke programming. Examples of process management systems include PLCs, SCADA systems, and DCSs. Both field management systems and process management systems are generally dedicated to a manufacturing unit, although that unit may be a multiproduct facility.

Production management systems include Manufacturing Execution Systems (MESs), LIMS, and Engineering Management Systems (EMSs). These systems are not necessarily dedicated to a particular plant or laboratory and may be shared, for instance, between several manufacturing units on a site. Whilst production management systems may have response-time dependencies, these are generally much less stringent than the real-time operations required by process and field management systems. Business management systems include Manufacturing Resource Planning (MRP II) Systems and Electronic Document Management Systems (EDMSs) and are typically based on large IT packages. These packages often claim to be configurable, although such configuration may be extensive and almost akin to bespoke programming. Unlike automation systems in other CIM levels, business management systems are often implemented to coordinate operations across different sites, possibly in different countries. Figure 4.2 shows where different systems fit within the CIM environment.

Figure 4.2. Integrated Manufacturing Systems

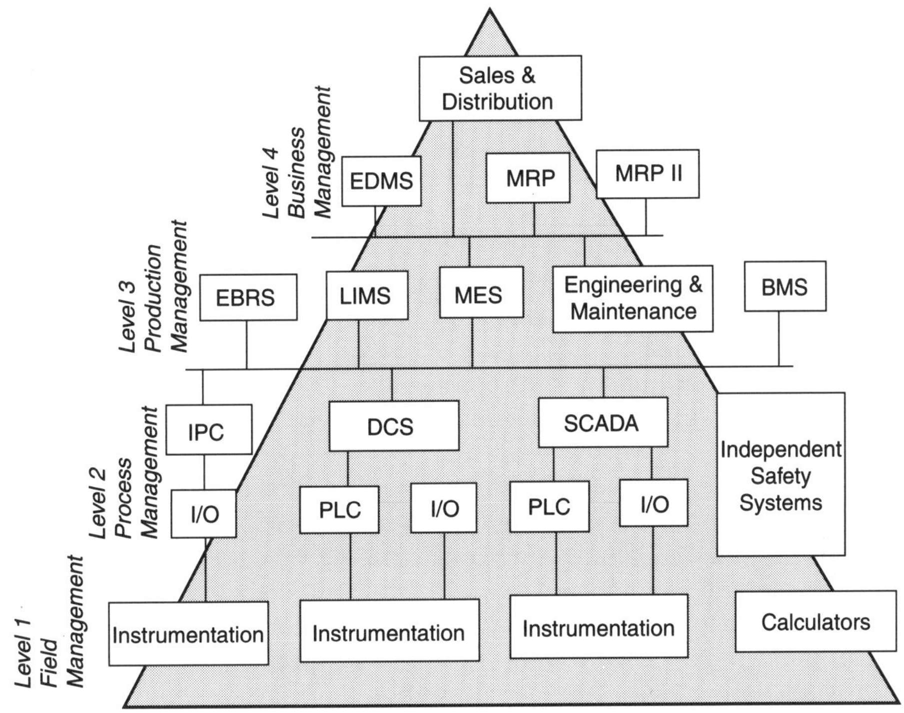

PUTTING EFFORT WHERE IT IS NEEDED

From a technical perspective, with the possible exception of some expert systems, all automation systems can be validated. Validation is about building confidence in the correct operation of a system. The degree of confidence that can be built for different systems may vary, but a case can always be developed. Beware of using the term *unvalidatable*. It is far more likely that cost is prohibiting validation rather than technicalities, and there are usually alternative validation approaches that can assist in making the exercise more cost-effective. Whatever the cost, however, GMP regulatory authorities will not excuse pharmaceutical manufacturers from using automation systems without any needed validation.

So, how much validation is insufficient, enough, or too much? Pharmaceutical manufacturers and suppliers alike must resist rushing into validating their automation systems without carefully considering the implications of consistently implementing their validation practice across all their systems. Too little validation may not necessarily be identified on a first inspection by a GMP regulatory authority. However, the longer it goes unnoticed as deficient, the higher the price to bring it up to standard. Practitioners must avoid being complacent. Meanwhile, too much validation may delight inspectors, but it is costly in unnecessary time and effort. Once identified as excessive, it may also be difficult to justify a lowering of standards to GMP regulatory authorities.

So how much is enough validation? There is no panacea, but a key step is concentrating effort where it is needed. As described in Chapter 2, whilst validation is required for the whole system, tailored to the type of automation system, emphasis should be placed on validating the GMP aspects of the system. There are often just a few critical functions and/or components that affect product quality, supported by a collection of measurements and manual interactions. The nature of any manual interactions will have a significant impact on the amount of validation required. Automation systems that only record the manual control of a process will require less detailed validation than those that directly control a process. The collection of batch data is another important factor in assessing the degree of control taken by an automation system.

Critical process functions and components can be identified as part of a distinct exercise, as discussed in Chapter 2, or as a task integrated within the development of a Validation Plan. Concentrating validation on critical process functions and components can realise a considerable savings compared to a detailed blanket of validation so often implemented as a precaution against noncompliance. Of course, there may be specific business needs that direct validation to err on the side of caution and include too much detail, for instance, the validation of a key drug product. Practitioners should restrain from needless validation; GMP regulatory authorities will discuss issues and options for validating automation systems and practitioners should not be shy or worried about asking their advice. The cost of validation should always be challenged. Other automation systems may be available that are easier to validate, or hard-wired systems or manual systems may be an option. Impartial corporate experts or consultants can be used to help develop the most cost-effective validation strategy.

FIELD MANAGEMENT SYSTEMS

Process Instrumentation

Instrumentation requires validation. This includes instruments based on microprocessor technology and referred to as intelligent or smart instruments, such as bar-code readers and vision systems. Validation necessitates

- Confirming that the instrument is the equipment manufacturer's standard catalogue item, noting any configuration or customisation details. If the instrument is bespoke, then it should be fully defined.

- Checking to a recognised standard that the instrument has adequate immunity to static electricity, electro-magnetic disturbances, and supply voltage or frequency disturbances. It should be tested for this immunity to a recognised standard.
- Examining any diagnostics and watchdogs that cover essential GMP functions. Regularly calibrate the instrument, investigating any operational discrepancies identified.

A Supplier Audit is necessary to confirm a pharmaceutical manufacturer's confidence in an instrument. Bespoke elements of an instrument must have been fully defined and tested before delivery. Critical algorithms and calculations should have been subject to documented Software Inspections. Firmware should be defined in the manufacturer's specification data sheets and validated as outlined in the last chapter. Some modern instruments use Fieldbus™ communication modules, and these too should be defined in specification data sheets.

The IQ must verify the identity and physical location of the instrument as part of an automation system. The instrument must be appropriate for its intended purpose. The OQ must verify that the instrument's tuned and calibrated functionality is compared to its manufacturer's specification. Verify that where necessary for GMP failures there is an output signal to shutdown a system and that this signal is a simple on/off or analogue signal. The instrument itself should fail to a specific safe state. Check that the performance of the power-up and power-down sequence is suitable for the intended application. The PQ must verify continuing correct operation under calibration.

Loop specifications, instrument switch configurations, and any user accessible software configurations must be kept under strict change control. Calibration schedules must also be maintained to ensure ongoing operational GMP compliance.

Analytical Laboratory Equipment

It is a basic requirement of Good Laboratory Practice (GLP) that analytical equipment must be fit for its intended purpose, and appropriately calibrated. The validation approach is broadly the same as for process instrumentation regardless of whether we are dealing with a complex instrument, such as a High Performance Liquid Chromatography (HLPC), or a simple instrument, such a pH meter. Unlike process instrumentation, however, analytical laboratory equipment is usually stand-alone.

A validation life cycle for analytical laboratory equipment, based on a standard OTS product, is shown in Figure 4.3. The supplier's System Specification must be complemented by analytical methods specified for the particular needs of the equipment's application. Critical components of the

Figure 4.3. Schematic Overview of Process Control System

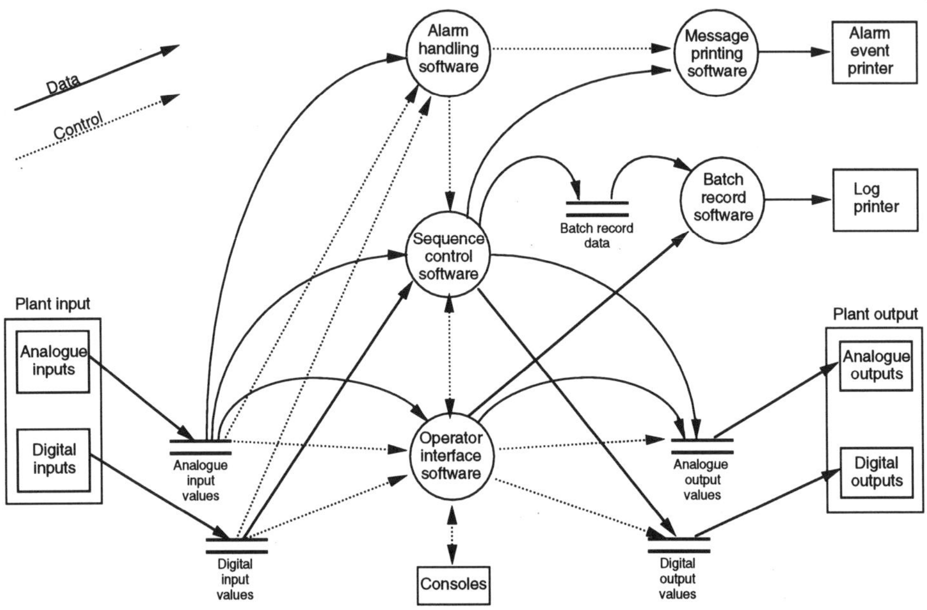

equipment must then be identified (perhaps using a decision tree such as that presented in Chapter 2) so that their procedural calibration requirements can be addressed. Any macros and configuration parameters must be defined. Where the equipment is not a standard OTS product, then a full specification and design must be prepared. IQ and OQ are then conducted, and may be combined into a single activity. Method-specific setup tests particular to the equipment's application, including calibration of the critical components, will form the basis of the PQ. This portion of the PQ is also conducted every time the equipment is used [1] and is sometimes referred to as the Performance Verification (PV) [2]. All critical components in a piece of equipment must be identified and covered by the PV; examples include wavelength accuracy checks, oven temperature tests, bath stirrer speed tests, sipper volume checks, and stray light tests. The remaining content of the PQ compromises those tests which do not focus on analytical methods.

Independent Monitoring Systems

Independent monitoring is usually implemented as a safety feature. Hardwired links, such as those to safety-critical equipment, should be defined and tested separately as part of an integrated system. Independent monitoring, however, is sometimes also used to support an automation system whose validation does not give sufficient confidence that it will operate consistently and reliably. Where independent monitoring systems support a primary automation system, there is an obligation to validate both the primary system and the independent monitoring system. The MCA has indicated that the primary system

> *must be supported with full acceptance testing for functionality, calibration, correct maintenance, and control of the primary computerised device and routine challenge testing* [3].

It is not acceptable to GMP regulatory authorities to abandon or avoid validating the prime automation system because reliance is still being placed in its normal operation; independent monitoring systems usually function as watchdogs for abnormal operation. Validation should aim to establish evidence that the combined system fulfils the need for dependability.

Calculators

Staff using calculators for batch data should not unquestionably accept the calculator's output, since there may have been a human error on data input. The best solution is to purchase calculators with a printer facility and to attach a printout of the calculation to the batch record, ensuring that the printout has been signed and dated. There should also be a record of the calculator's model and manufacturer. Calculators that are used for non–GMP-related activities need not be validated.

PROCESS MANAGEMENT SYSTEMS

Process Control Systems

Process control systems are used for continuous and batch manufacturing. Examples include PLCs, Industrial Personal Computers (IPCs), SCADA systems, and DCSs. IPC–, PLC–, SCADA–, and DCS–based batch control systems perform similar functions, but some of their characteristics, such as capacity, fault-tolerance, and operator interface, vary significantly. IPC solutions are generally least expensive and offer very effective Windows-based operator interfaces but offer little or no fault tolerance. PLCs are well suited to logic control, permissives, and fast interlocking. SCADA and DCS solutions can coordinate a number of IPCs and PLCs as well as connect directly to plant equipment and instrumentation. DCSs are most expensive but can cope with more complex manufacturing operations. Other selection considerations will include the capability of these systems to support change management, access security, historical record keeping, batch audit trails, data acquisition speeds, and Statistical Process Control (SPC).

The strategy for validating these different process computer systems is largely the same. It is important to recognise, however, that the application of this strategy will vary between different systems depending on how they are used and what the GMP Assessment identifies for special attention. Some example manufacturing stages for which process control systems are used include the following:

- *Preparation:* ensuring that the vessels are clean and ready for use, that the ingredients are available, and possibly that the reactor is preheated.
- *Charging:* the introduction of the ingredients to the appropriate vessel(s).
- *Reaction:* the main production stage where the chemistry is controlled to produce the active ingredient.
- *Separation and/or purification:* the product is extracted from its reaction medium and unreacted ingredients. Product may be purified. Waste may be recycled.
- *Transfer:* the finished product leaves the processing plant leaving it free to make another batch.
- *Packaging:* the finished product is packaged and labelled ready for distribution.

A schematic overview of a typical process control system is shown in Figure 4.4. It is important to define and control any system configurable parameters and variable switch settings that can vary process functions, such as "high/low limits", "range", "enable/disable", and "alarms/messages", to avoid invalid control sequences during the drug product's manufacturing process, and the possible adverse quality results or lost batches of product. The data acquisition capability of these systems should be twice as fast as the fastest incoming analogue signal [4]. SPC features must also be addressed, and critical process parameters must be validated and their acceptable ranges justified. Software Inspections, Hazard Studies, and qualifications must cover all these items. Other tests should cover batch data, access security, and trending historical data.

Software standards are available that offer a consistent approach to programming and the promise of significantly better software quality. IEC 1131-3 is primarily for PLCs, although it can be used for other industrial control systems. ISA-S88 provides a standard modular approach for batch control and is often used for DCSs. The benefits claimed by these standards include the following [5]:

- Robust identification and definition of user requirements
- Improved communications between users and suppliers

Figure 4.4. Validation Approach for Analytical Laboratory Equipment

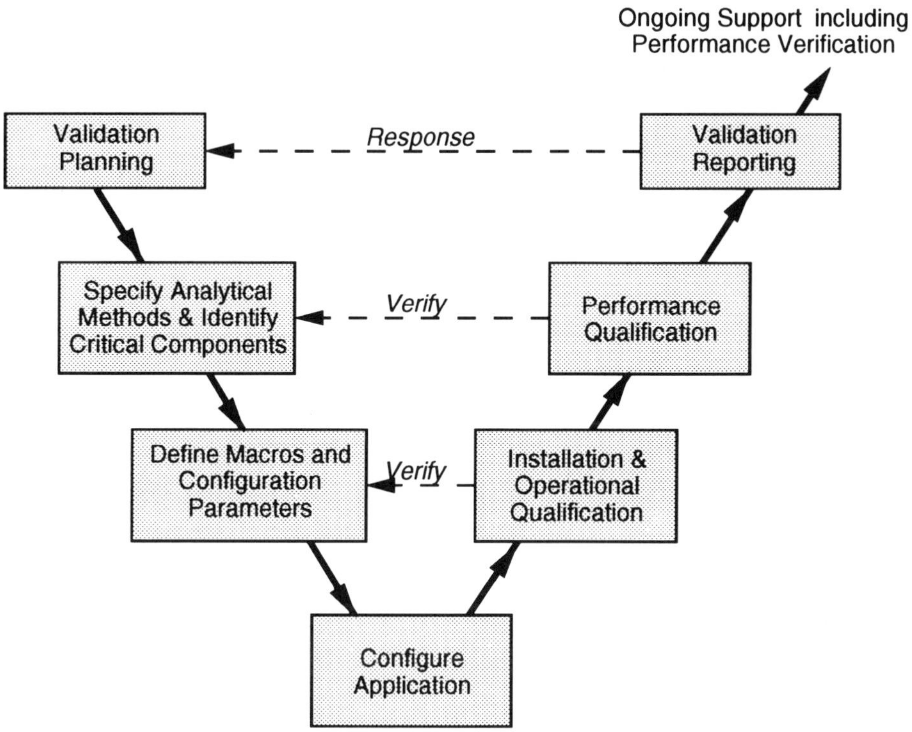

- Simplified recipe development
- Reduced overall design and development costs
- Lower engineering and maintenance costs over life cycle

It should be noted that these benefits may not always be appropriate for specific process control systems. Where standards are used, software designers and programmers may need training.

Process computer systems normally coordinate their PQ activities with the OQ of the manufacturing process. Some organisations incorporate PQ tests for the automation system within the OQ protocol for the manufacturing process. Where this approach is adopted, the aspects of the automation system tested should be clearly identified. Testing involving the manufacturing process should, wherever practically possible, avoid the use of expensive active ingredients. Placebo and water trials will generally provide sufficient confidence in the PQ of the automation system.

Utility Control Systems

Support systems, such as heat transfer systems, electric power, and non-process contact water for cooling, are not critical and need not be validated. The control of critical parameters that these systems affect, however, should be validated. An example based on a heat transfer system is given by ISPE [6]. This system would not be considered critical, but if the temperature parameters on the reactor that it affects are critical, their control would be validated, and they would be monitored continuously.

Automation systems controlling or monitoring utilities that come into contact with pharmaceutical products (e.g., compressed air during packing, Heating, Ventilation, and Air-Conditioning [HVAC] systems for sterile production areas, and pure water supply) require full validation, because failure in their service could adversely affect the quality of manufactured product.

A slightly different situation exists for utilities that purely provide an auxiliary service, such as reactor jacket chillers. The option of validating instrumentation monitoring the supply of a utility at its point of use and not validating the control of the utility should be carefully considered. Where reliance is placed in monitoring instrumentation, then the following points must be addressed:

- Position of instruments fully meets requirement to monitor utility at point of use (justify assumptions and any derived measurements).
- Measurements are taken at an appropriate frequency (chart recorders are generally preferred).
- Instruments in contact with utility do not affect quality of service (similar situation to materials in contact with process materials do not affect the quality of pharmaceutical product).

In many instances, it may be easier and cheaper to validate the utility's controlling automation system than to implement and validate an independent monitoring system.

Some organisations have justified not validating Building Management Systems (BMSs) because they have implemented independent monitoring. This approach is not recommended, because independent monitoring is essentially testing for assurance, and the basis of validation is building in assurance of correct operation. Reliance on BMSs should, therefore, only be acceptable where the automation system has been validated. If the cost of validating these systems is prohibitively high, then the pharmaceutical manufacturer should consider replacing them with independent monitoring.

Embedded Systems

Many process control systems are now supplied embedded within manufacturing equipment. Care must be taken to examine the software, as this is not often developed by the equipment supplier, but rather provided by contract staff or subcontractor organisations.

Supplier Audits should review subcontractor arrangements and provisions should be made for Software Inspection. Software often has a history extending over several previous applications, each with a slightly different functionality. If contract programmers have been used, it is unlikely that the supplier has an overall understanding of the system's functionality and development history. Pharmaceutical manufacturers must understand the capabilities of their system; many use validation to build up their own expertise in the absence of adequate supplier support.

Pharmaceutical manufacturers must beware of unstructured prototype developments with little or no supporting documentation. The danger is that unnecessary code is never removed and the application becomes very complex. There have been numerous accounts of embedded systems incorrectly displaying operator messages from earlier versions, some of which may be in a different language from the current application. Comments embedded in the software may also be in different languages.

PRODUCTION MANAGEMENT SYSTEMS

Manufacturing Execution Systems

There is some confusion between practitioners on what constitutes an MES. For the purpose of discussion, MESs are considered here to provide process control of an entire facility or factory and usually involve the management and control of electronic batch records. They also offer the opportunity to link process management systems and business management systems into a CIM environment.

The validation approach for an MES should combine the approach outlined in this chapter for process management systems and Electronic Batch Record Systems (EBRSs). Careful attention should be placed on identifying critical parameters and conducting a Hazard Study. Validation should endeavour to partition the complexity of an MES into components that are more readily validated. This may mean that a number of validation projects are initiated, each with a Validation Plan and Validation Report, and collated under an overall Validation Master Plan.

Engineering Management Systems

EMSs can provide a variety of functions. Preventive maintenance scheduling (including calibration) and control of work orders, permits to work, and job plans all require validation. It should be possible to trace the authorisation, working procedures for the work, and acceptance of work completed. Some systems may also control spares lists, and these must be checked to determine the suitable control of parts and serial numbers and reference to supporting documentation detailing specifications and any certification. Similarly, control of maintenance, repair, and change control records, and the linking of procedures to work, should be validated. Guidance on document control is given in the section dealing with EDMSs. Financial information does not need validation unless it is used to identify parts or work.

Laboratory Information Management Systems

Automation systems are being increasingly used by laboratories to support regulatory drug submissions and drug manufacturing operations. These systems are being used for data capture, processing, and storage. Examples of laboratory systems include programmable analytical instruments, Personal Computers (PC), and LIMS, so the validation of these systems should specifically address the requirements of Good Laboratory Practice (GLP) and include the following [7]:

- Identification and functional definition of systems (including hardware, system software, application software, programming languages, and databases).
- Control procedures (including qualification, change control, periodic testing, maintenance, contingency plans, and security).
- Evaluation of effectiveness of GLP specific functions (including archive and retrieval of experimental and other data).
- Quality assurance (including compliance monitoring of procedures, performance of staff, and review adequacy of documentation).
- Staff training (including on-the-job training, external training courses, training schedules, and training records)

These requirements concur with the general validation principles outlined in this book. Further details of specific GLP requirements for computerised systems can be found in OECD's draft guide on the topic [8]. In addition, two case studies are presented in Part 2 of this book on validating automated laboratory systems from the perspective of a pharmaceutical company and a supplier.

Performance Qualifications will vary with the type of automation system. For instance, it is normal practice to repeat the PQ for laboratory systems as part of the equipment setup for individual laboratory studies.

Data Processing Systems

Examples of data processing systems include clinical trial databases, statistical analysis packages, and blood bank management systems. These systems should be validated in compliance with GCP, GLP, and GMP regulations as required by their application. For instance, the GCPs for clinical systems mandate [22]

- The system is fit for its intended purpose.
- Documentation is complete and accurate.
- Full audit trail for all data changes.
- Data protection against unauthorised changes.
- Safeguard blinding during data entry and processing.

Care must be taken not to casually exclude data processing systems from validation. If a decision is made not to validate a particular system, then the justification should be clearly documented.

BUSINESS MANAGEMENT SYSTEMS

Business Systems (Including MRP II)

Business systems are used to coordinate the management and planning of resources supporting the manufacture of drug products and, as such, are often business critical—failure to operate as required could close down an operating company faster than any adverse inspection by a GMP regulatory authority. Examples of business systems include Enterprise Resource Planning (ERP), Materials Requirements Planning (MRP), Manufacturing Resource Planning (MRP II), and Sales and Operations Planning (S&OP) systems.

A typical business system consists of a huge core of standard configurable software based on a mainframe or client-server hardware platform servicing potentially a very large number of users, possibly on different sites (even different countries!), connected via terminals on a communications network. The functionality of the systems is often described as consisting of a number of modules. For each module, a validation strategy should be developed listing all processes, transactions, and functions and recording with a justification which will and will not be validated. The following list of elements that often require validation is given for guidance:

- Production planning
- New product development
- Sales (including export)
- Purchasing (approved materials from approved suppliers)
- Receiving inventory (including rework)
- Warehouse movements

- Stock checks (e.g., perpetual inventory)
- Manufacturing (including work order generation)
- Despatch and distribution (including packaging and labelling)
- Quality control (including laboratory reports)
- Security (including access authorities)
- Data hygiene (including master materials, batches, and vendors)
- Personnel (e.g., training records)

This list is not exhaustive and each element should be carefully examined to check the degree (if any) of validation needed. Forecasting, marketing, wages, and finance should not require validation unless they impact on the checklist above. A checklist of GMP–sensitive data items, such as that presented in the MRP II case study in part two of this book, can be used to help identify validation requirements. In practice, about 10 percent of an MRP II system can be described as GMP critical, that is, between 100 and 200 processes, transactions, and functions for a single-site application.

A validation approach for business systems based on the life-cycle model presented in the last chapter is shown in Figure 4.5. The size and complexity of business system applications often necessitates a phased roll-out of the system elements, which will complicate any project approach. A cut over the whole system at once is usually considered too risky. Phases are usually based around firstly financials, then customer services, and finally manufacturing. Each phase will follow a life-cycle validation approach, adding to the evidence supporting validation. During the implementation, practitioners must ensure they do not

- Unwittingly compromise the standard nature of a configurable OTS product by too much customisation.
- Lose control of quality during what are often fast-track projects (there are often large numbers of project staff from a variety of backgrounds, not all of which are necessarily conversant with either IT or validation). The MCA has suggested that MRP II systems have not been validated or well documented in the past [22].
- Unacceptably increase project risk by business process re-engineering instead of limiting the implementation to current established ways of working.
- Ignore known shortcomings with the core supplier product (rememeber to document how they are being tackled).
- Disregard the potential financial and validation impact of upgrading/intregrating their current IT infrastructure (networks, workstations, etc.) to support the business system implementation.

Figure 4.5. Business Systems Validation Approach

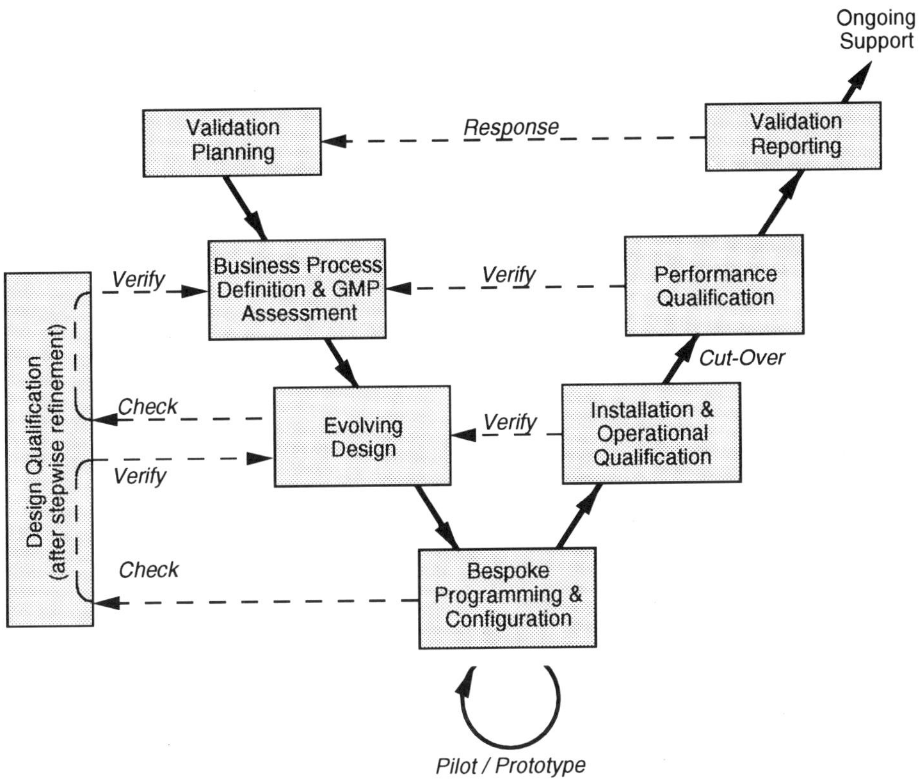

Business systems applications are often based on descriptions of the application (business processes, transactions, and functions) coupled to documentation provided by the supplier of their software products, many of which are standard OTC solutions. The degree to which confidence can be placed in the dependability of a supplier's standard product (yet to be configured or customised) will be determined through a Supplier Audit. Documentation supplied with that standard system, however, is likely to need enhancements if it is to be used to support validation. Supplementary records can be developed by the application integrator supplying the system or the pharmaceutical manufacturer. Business system applications are often designed, developed, and tested on-site using a prototyping (piloting) approach, and this means that the final design will not be frozen until just before cutover. Documentation is, therefore, likely to require updating at the end of the project.

Software Inspections will be needed for bespoke application-specific aspects of the system developed for the pharmaceutical manufacturer (e.g., menus, reports, and forms). The Supplier Audit should confirm that the supplier had relevant code review procedures in place for the development of their standard product and that these were used. It is recommended that the pharmaceutical manufacturer complement their supplier's Software Inspection with their own quality checks on the standard product software (use of headers, comments, and so on), but a detailed Software Inspection is not worth undertaking.

The distinction between Predelivery and On-Site Testing phases, described in Chapter 3, often becomes blurred because both are conducted on the pharmaceutical manufacturer's site. In such situations, testing can be based on the following activities:

- IQ (of delivered system for prototyping and final application)
- Unit Configuration Testing (e.g., business scenarios, module operability)
- Testing Bespoke Aspects (e.g., reports, macros)
- Interface Testing (interconnections with associated systems)
- Incremental Testing (integration testing of combined units)
- OQ (functional testing of combined units)
- Data Migration (from legacy system or test bed to live environment)
- PQ (i.e., user acceptance testing for consistent operation)

The testing activities outlined above up to and including the OQ will normally be conducted off-line in a development or test environment that requires some limited system data population. SOPs are often used to supplement tests in the OQ with final revisions to the procedures being made and approved prior to the OQ.

A prerequisite to the PQ is the data migration of "live" data for on-line operation. Validation requires that the live system with the live data is exactly similar to that used for testing and that the data have integrity. Live data may come from existing systems, perhaps electronically transferred, or from manual input. For either origin, a check on the data's integrity should be conducted and erroneous data corrected. Where a complete check of the data is not practical, a directed sample should be taken to include a 100 percent check of GMP critical data and a sample of other data. Sample sizes for non-GMP data checks often range between 5 percent and 20 percent, but the size needs to be justified. If a sample uncovers unacceptably high levels of erroneous data, then the sample should be extended to establish overall confidence in the data. It is extremely important that data have high integrity, otherwise the system will suffer from GIGO (Garbage In, Garbage Out).

The PQ will monitor system operation (e.g., data errors, system availability, and user enquiries—see Figure 4.6) and often is only possible after

Figure 4.6. Example PQ Criteria for Business System Validation

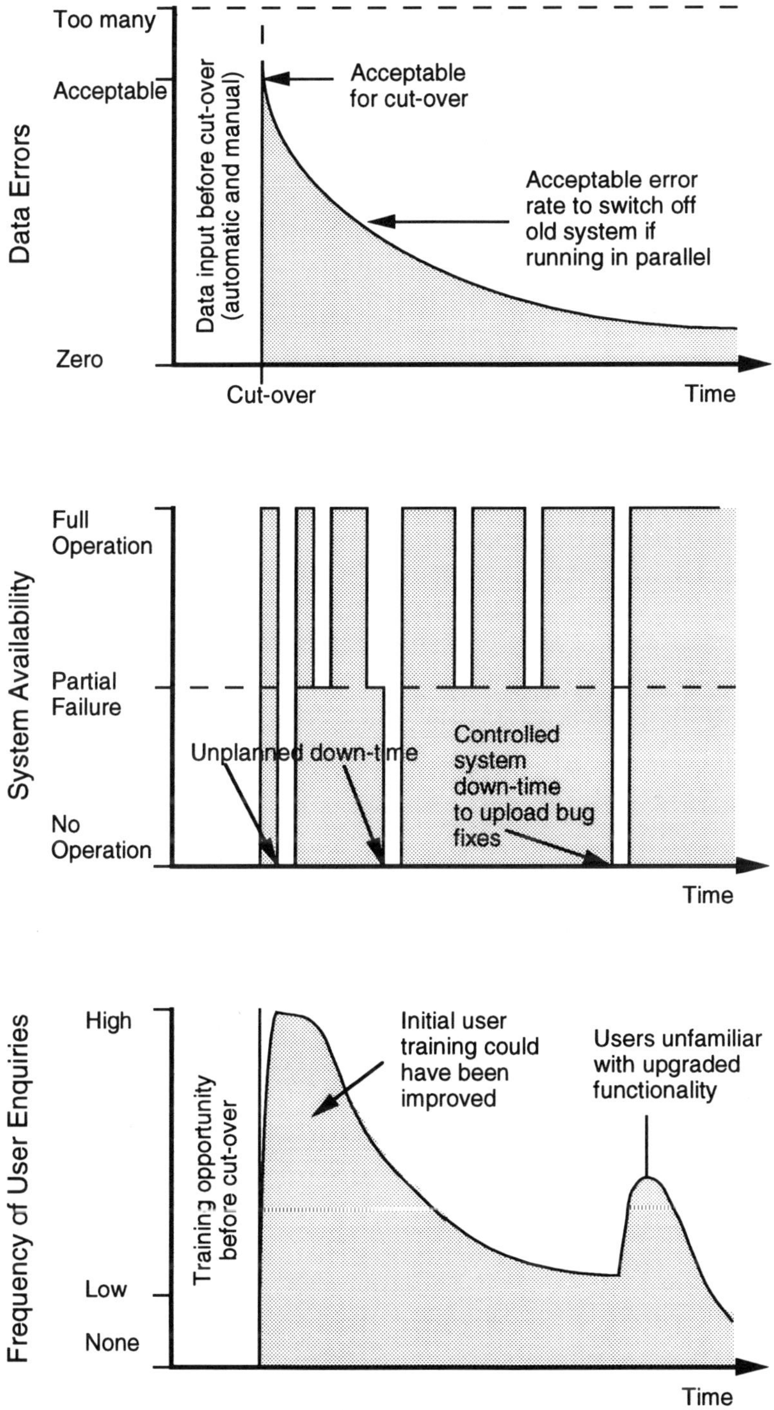

cutover when the system is supporting live manufacturing. The number of licenced users and percentage database occupancy are both likely to increased significantly after cutover. The number of users, for instance, may rise from the tens used for prototyping to hundreds for actual use. Consequently, even though some loading simulations may have been possible prior to cutover, the hardware platform may need to be upgraded to cope with the extra operational demands. Any changes in the hardware should be included as a revision to the IQ.

Contingency plans should exist for the host computer system and the various system users who are often distributed amongst departments at different localities on the pharmaceutical manufacturer's site. Users should be trained with regular refresher courses on how to implement these plans.

Change control must be maintained in the live production environment. Changes will include upgrades to system hardware platform, new releases of software packages, and any temporary program fixes undertaken by or on behalf of the pharmaceutical manufacturer. It is often tempting not to go through a formal change control procedure for temporary program fixes because the system will be returned to its original state and no one would be the wiser if it was not recorded that any change took place. It is for this reason, however, that such fixes must be recorded so that if GMP is compromised, it can be identified, corrective actions can be initiated, and any root cause can be traced and addressed. Quite often it is useful to establish a User Group to support and authorise changes and modifications to the system. The User Group is also a useful mechanism to collect reports of poor or faulty system operation. Training could also be organised via the User Group.

Electronic Document Management Systems

Automation systems used to support document control of project documents, data sheets, drawings, operating procedures, and so on must be validated. Examples include document management systems, EBRSs, and CAD systems. These systems can vary greatly in size and complexity from PC–based systems, to mainframe systems, to networked client-server systems connecting several sites together. The approach to validation will be similar to that outlined for business systems, but with specific attention given to

- Version control
- Access security
- Change control
- Archive and retrieval
- Change history
- Master records

The system design should always provide for the retention of full audit trails to show all changes to the records without obscuring the original records [8]. EDMSs often employ a WORM philosophy (Write Once, Read Many), whereby each change to a record is documented in its own right and associated to the original record. It should be possible to reconstruct a record by applying, in order, each change made to the original record. It should be possible to associate all changes to records with the persons making those changes. All changes should be accompanied by timed and dated signatures and the reasons for the changes. The master document can be paper or electronic, as discussed in Chapter 5 under document control. Whichever media is used for the master, it must be retained in a secure location. The use of any databases to reference or store records needs testing.

Electronic master documents will have electronic signatures accompanied by electronic time stamps. It must not be possible to "cut and paste" signatures. Security to prevent accidental or unauthorised changes and signatures is crucial, especially in light of the FDA's Code of Federal Regulation on Electronic Records and Electronic Signatures [9]. Similarly, the automation systems clock that is used to time stamp any signature must be tested for its accuracy and accessibility. It is often quite a simple task to modify the system clock, and security features should be established to prevent this from occurring.

An important function of an EDMS is the provision of copies to users. Some systems might have printers distributed around the site or facility so that copies can be printed near their point of use. In such situations, the supporting network configuration and print quality must be checked. Printed documents should have a limited lifetime, otherwise they might have been unknowingly superseded. The front page of documents should, therefore, include an expiry date a week or two after the date the document is printed. Security access to any distributed terminals used to request or view records must also be tested. Other tests that may include challenging user procedures should include ensuring that the correct version of a record is used, and that records are correctly authorised before they are used.

SUPPORTING TECHNOLOGY

Databases (Including Spreadsheets)

Databases containing data items critical to GMP must be validated. It is often not practical to verify the integrity of an entire database, because it changes so frequently. Validation must, therefore, cover both database management software and checks on the critical data items it manages.

Database management software usually consists of a standard package, perhaps with some configuration. Supplier Audits should review Predelivery

Testing to determine how much supplementary On-Site Testing is required. Evidence of Predelivery Testing should include Software Inspections. Some software may be resident on firmware and, as such, should be included within the Software Inspection. On-Site Testing will normally be restricted to verifying the basic operational capability of the database management software. Spreadsheet macros are considered as bespoke programming by the GMP regulatory authorities and must be fully specified and tested. If a distributed database is being used, then the effect of a system crash, making a portion of the database unavailable, should be carefully studied for its impact on GMP. Careful consideration should be given to any possible contention by multiple concurrent accesses wanting to change the same data. The management of small databases, likely to be based on a spreadsheet of data, is much simpler than that for larger databases that employ relational or object-oriented architectures. Practitioners should also be vigilant in case the number of database users exceeds the number of licenced users, because this could affect response times and data access contentions. Any modifications or upgrades to the software by the pharmaceutical manufacturer or the database supplier must be made under change control.

As mentioned earlier, the integrity of critical data items should be regularly checked. Critical data include batch records, loop specifications, calibration records, and labelling details. The mission criticality of on-line data will be a key factor in deciding the frequency of data checks. For instance, it has been recommended that LIMS databases have daily data integrity checks [10].

Contingency Plans should be established. If the database becomes unavailable, for instance, as the result of a system crash, and a manual paper system is employed to continue drug manufacturing, then procedures managing this changeover must be in place and include how to update the database when it becomes available again. Manual updates of the database will be prone to typographical errors and checks should be established to verify the integrity of updated data items. Alternative databases temporarily used instead of manual paper records to collect data in the absence of the intended database must also have the transfer of data back to the original database verified.

Networks

All communication links are potential sources of error and may result in the loss or corruption of data. Appropriate controls to ensure data integrity must be implemented. Network controls should be implemented on three levels:

1. Network hardware
2. Network software
3. Networked applications

Hardware controls should include ensuring that all the correct network cards are used, that shielding against electrical interference is provided, and that error correcting codes to restore degraded service are configured. Software controls should, meanwhile, include the configuration of network access points, the consistent use of user identifications, and checking that users are implementing passwords, and data access authorities (usually by User Group) are assigned. Finally, network applications must be checked to ensure they are correctly configured for the network. The overall network traffic flow should be checked; network bridges and routers should be reconfigured to remove bottlenecks and improve performance. It may be possible to reserve portions of the network bandwidth for particular applications, or to prioritise network traffic. Usually, the network is configured for disconnection by fault, but fault-tolerant features, such as standby hardware and resending data by different network routes, may have been made available in the network design. Consideration must be given as to whether and how automation systems can operate in isolation if the network fails. Fault diagnosis tools and manuals should be made available to personnel responsible for managing the network. If standard network products are used, then testing must confirm version details.

The FDA summed up the following aspects of network operation that require management and testing [11]:

- Control of records, such as batch records distributed over networks
- Remote control of computer systems across network
- Identity of those with access rights from remote sites (including suppliers)
- Nature and extent of management control over network (including security)

These topics are equally applicable for LANs and WANs.

If batch records are stored on the network, then they must be accessible from the network at the site where manufacturing took place [9]. Partially complete batch records that are under construction by a current production run should also be retrievable, but access should not hinder their final stages of compilation. Security implications, including the use of read-only access, should be considered for retrieved records.

VALIDATING EXISTING SYSTEMS (RETROSPECTIVE VALIDATION)

The following checklist is based on work by the German APV for practitioners validating existing automation systems (known as retrospective validation) that were not, or were only partially, developed in accordance with validation requirements [12]:

- Freeze the automation system to stop any changes.
- Prepare a Validation Plan.
- Conduct a GMP Assessment to determine the GMP–relevant components and functions of the system with reference to the past operational experience.
- Assess the completeness of documentation against a life cycle and evaluate the quality of documentation (a Supplier Audit may be required).
- Create/revise the documentation describing the automation system.
- Conduct a Design Qualification and a Hazard Study.
- Inspect critical application software, conduct an IQ, conduct an OQ with emphasis on GMP component and functions of the system, and conduct a PQ.
- Prepare a Validation Report.
- Release the automation system for use, if necessary implementing system modifications and/or additional organisational measures under change control.

Validating existing systems can be five times more expensive than if that same system had been validated when it was new. Practitioners should, therefore, consider whether it is cheaper to implement a replacement system rather than conduct retrospective validation.

Documentation

The basic documentary requirements for existing automation systems are the same as for new systems. The exception is that of a URS and Predelivery Testing which are not needed because the system already exists and is installed at the pharmaceutical manufacturer's site.

The content and structure of Validation Plans; specification and design documentation; GMP Assessments; Supplier Audits; Hazard Studies; and IQ, OQ, PQ, and Validation Reports should fulfil the recommendations outlined in Chapter 3. Validation Plans usually have an additional section giving a brief history of the system from its original procurement, through any developments, to the current system configuration. The Validation Plan should also indicate the new and existing documentation that will be used to support validation of the automation system. The intent of the current system may have changed from the original design intent documented in existing documentation. It may not be necessary to totally rewrite a System Specification. Instead it may be possible to write a short frontispiece to existing documents, defining the changes and their impact on the original design. Software Inspections are required if original Predelivery Testing records are incomplete, insufficient, or not available. Some practitioners also conduct a DQ before testing begins to review how the system's design intent is fulfilled. Testing will comprise IQ, OQ, and PQ. The IQ and OQ may both be conducted whilst the system is making pharmaceutical grade products for later sale. This often means that safety-related, disaster recovery, as well as other tests, cannot be tested. In such situations, some portions of testing may have to be delayed until a planned facility shutdown takes place. Some facilities may not have a planned shutdown for more than a year, in which case consideration should be given to especially planning one for the validation project. The final phase of qualification, the PQ, can use, but must not rely solely upon, historical evidence of dependable operation.

Supplier Audits

When auditing suppliers of automation systems that were procured without a validation requirement, it is important to determine the operational support for the current system, including any ongoing support services provided by the supplier. Remember that the original supplier may have been a function within the pharmaceutical manufacturer's organisation. In such instances, the Supplier Audit becomes an internal audit and document search.

The U.S. Pharmaceutical Research Manufacturers of America (PhRMA) Computer Systems Validation Committee [13] has recommended that pharmaceutical manufacturers target the following topics:

- *Documents:* A supplier may have discarded original project documents, or they may have become obsolete. Change control practices that do not ensure up-to-date system documents are risky for the operational phases of the life cycle because effective maintenance programs rely on these documents for the preservation of validation.
- *Testing:* Outdated module and integration testing documents, including Software Inspections, may be unusable for regression testing of the current system configuration. The audit should review test protocols to ensure that they reflect the current operating environment.
- *Manuals:* Maintenance to and enhancements of the system (including system upgrades) throughout years of operation may have resulted in changes to how the system is operated. A supplier may have outdated user manuals, or no manuals, with users relying on typed or handwritten instructions to supplement or replace old manuals. Audits should note if technical personnel review changes and edits for accuracy before releasing manuals to system users.

- *Operating Procedures:* Procedures for operating the automation system should be inspected for conformance to current company policies, regulatory requirements, and industry practices. Nonconformities should be noted as part of a list of follow-up actions to the inspection.
- *Maintenance:* Any support agreements should be reviewed with respect to current Contingency Plan expectations. It is common for contact addresses to change and for backup versions of the software to have been upgraded. Amendments should be made as required.

Note that the lack of specifications, test records, manuals, and operating procedures necessitates the pharmaceutical manufacturer to re-engineer the documentation, as far a reasonably practical. How difficult this task will be depends on the quality of available documentation, the assistance the original supplier can provide, and the experience of staff that the pharmaceutical manufacturer can assign to the validation. Many pharmaceutical manufacturers ask third-party validation specialists for assistance in such work because of the experience and knowledge they can provide. The cost of this exercise, of course, may make it cheaper to replace the system rather than retrospectively validate it.

Software Reuse and Portability

The reuse of components from existing automation systems (hardware and software) offers suppliers the opportunity to reduce the conventional development cost of new systems. Components may need to be generalised before they can be reused; others may have been designed for immediate reuse. Many suppliers reuse elements of software from previous versions as they progressively develop their software.

The implications of reuse must be understood before this approach is adopted. Systematic reuse requires a properly catalogued and documented record of reusable components. Libraries of available components can then be built. Documentation fully describing each component must exist and any problems with the components must be logged and corrected. The correct operation of a component in one system does not necessarily guarantee its successful application in another system. Reusable components should be scrutinised to assess any potential hazards before they are used. Components may need additional work to make them robust. This work is vital because, without detection, deficient components will be carried forward into new applications. The Therac-25™ radiation therapy computer system that was responsible for several deaths suffered common-cause failures from reused software [14]. Unfortunately, managers are often reluctant to cover any additional validation costs associated with making software components robust for reuse because of the difficulty in quantifying the long-term advantage of a library of proven reusable components [15].

Pharmaceutical manufacturers and suppliers are faced with the task of balancing increased programming efficiency offered by reuse and the potential hazards reuse may incur. It has been suggested that the reuse of small amounts of software can actually introduce more problems than writing the whole application from scratch because the new software must fit around the reused software. To reap the dividend of reuse, it has been recommended that at least 70 percent of a program must consist of reused software components of proven functionality [16]. Furthermore, it must be understood that, whilst reused software may be configured, any customisation will negate its proven component functionality and the software must be considered as bespoke for the purpose of validation.

Recent examination of some tableting PLC software revealed the original code to have been written in Spanish, with subsequent functional revisions in German and English before a final modification for a French application. It is important to realise with software such as this that older portions of the software may not have been developed to current validation requirements, and features from earlier versions that are no longer needed may still remain. This situation occurs quite regularly to suppliers who are asked by pharmaceutical manufacturers to provide standard software with a few additional features. Pharmaceutical manufacturers should be aware that such developments increase the validation requirements because the software can no longer be considered "standard".

A special case of reuse involves the portability of software across a range of operating platforms. Standard programming languages, communication protocols, and application environments should significantly reduce the modifications required to adapt software for different computers and operating systems. Practitioners sometimes use the term *open systems* to describe standard software capable of running on a variety of system architectures. As noted above, however, it is important to distinguish between customised and configured software when considering the validation implications of reuse. Practitioners should not underestimate the problems they may experience with portability.

Attention should also be applied to software downloaded from the Internet because the history and quality of such software and any supporting documentation is likely to be unknown. Without an audit trail to its original development, such software cannot be treated as standard software and should be subject to the more rigorous validation requirements of bespoke software.

Migration and Parallel Operation

Manufacturers should set and review a migration strategy that addresses both near-term and long-term corporate needs for individual automation systems.

When migrating from manual to computerised systems or upgrading automation technology, the following implications should be considered:

- Configuration flexibility and capacity for expansion
- Financial cost
- Installation impact on manufacturing
- Integration capability
- Performance improvement
- Personnel requirements
- Technology risk
- Validation requirements
- Vendor capability

Systems, manual or automated, being replaced by computerised systems should be run in parallel for a time to validate the migration [17,18,19]. It is unacceptable to rely on parallel operation as the sole basis of validation [20]. The replacement system must be validated in its own right. Automation systems employed should meet or exceed the validation requirements for the manual functions they replace [7]. The new automation system must be at least as reliable as the automation system it replaces. When it is obvious that the new system is better than the old one, the old one should be decommissioned. Practitioners should not necessarily run the system in parallel until their are no "bugs"; the real question is whether the bugs can be managed. Parallel operation, of course, may not always be possible or desired. The personnel requirements to run two systems together may be considered too high, or perhaps would require two production facilities.

Once an automation system has been implemented, the pharmaceutical manufacturer must appreciate that automation technology is continually advancing. The next generation of microprocessor technology and software (half the price or double the functionality) has been arriving on average every two to three years, and there seems to be no reason to suspect that this trend will not continue. The next generation may consist of an upgrade to the automation system or its replacement. The various migration options are shown in Figure 4.7 [21]. Not every option to upgrade may be taken, but care must be taken not to slip unknowingly into obsolescence when older versions are no longer supported by their suppliers. There may alternatively be reasons for ceasing all updates and establishing a legacy system.

Regular upgrades following an evolutionary migration are associated with low technology risks, but the combined validation effort for every upgrade can be considerable. One aspect of automation systems that can be overlooked is the upgrading of hardware components (such as printers, monitors, instruments) and system software (such as operating systems and

Figure 4.7. Migration Routes

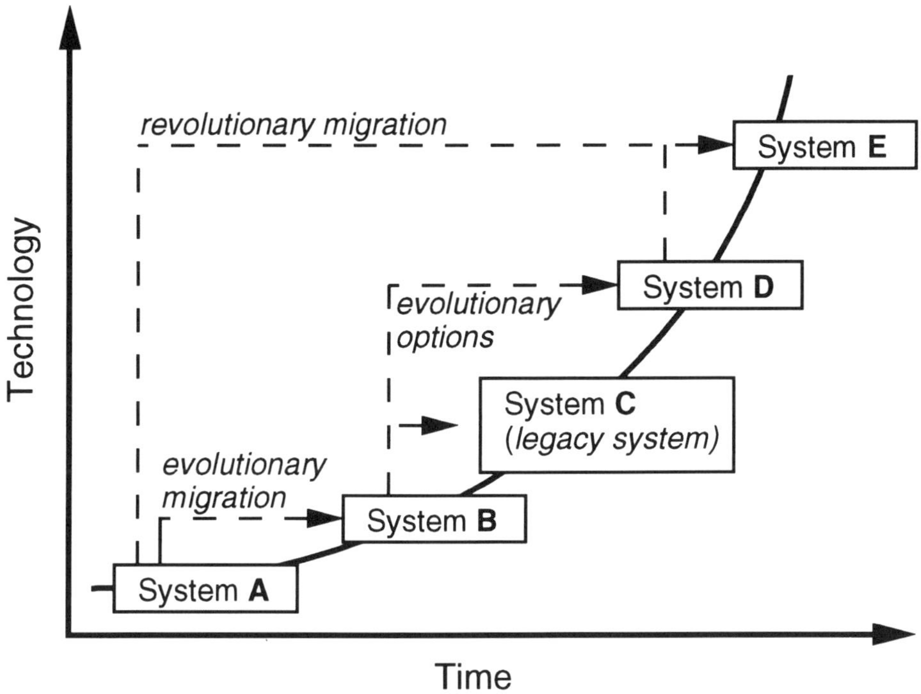

standard packages). In particular, system software is continually being upgraded, and whilst upward compatibility may be claimed on the initial release of an upgrade, confidence without supporting evidence should be limited. In this situation, it is recommended that installation of the upgrade is delayed until the new release is market tested.

Major step changes in technology across several generation upgrades (a revolutionary approach) will reduce the overall validation effort, but the technology risk can be high. Examples of step changes include the cutover of large systems, such as MRP IIs, where parallel operation may not be practical because of the large volume of data and user interaction. In order to reduce the risk, larger systems are usually implemented in stages with a progression of phased cutovers for main functional elements. Within an MRP II system, cutovers might include financials, customer services, and manufacturing.

Legacy Systems

Automation systems that do not implement software and hardware upgrades are called legacy systems. Updated software and hardware is usually only installed if they include bug fixes or if support for the old version is being removed. New versions of products, however, do not always bring operational benefits. Early adopters may find bugs yet undiscovered by the supplier (e.g., Pentium® processor). Equally, new product versions may actually degrade overall system performance (e.g., the original system memory is insufficient for the new data processing requirements of Windows 95®). In these circumstances, it is advisable to retain and operate the original system, wait a period (perhaps six months) for a favourable track record to be established by other industry practitioners with the updated products, and only then install the revisions.

Other legacy systems exist because suppliers are no longer supporting their software or hardware products. A decline in the number of users of a product may lead a supplier to question the financial viability of their continued support of the product. Pharmaceutical manufacturers must discuss this topic with their suppliers so that a suitable validation strategy can be planned.

Legacy systems are quite acceptable, providing the original system has been validated to current GMP requirements and that its validation status is being maintained. Validation activities will include the following:

- Establishing version and change control.
- Collating documentary evidence that the software and hardware provided by a supplier has been developed and maintained under a quality assurance regime supporting validation.
- Reviewing documentation and preparing any supplementary information required to make the documentation complete.
- Investigating the supply chain of any secondhand software and hardware used to maintain the system to establish whether it came from the original supplier and that it has not suffered any damage.
- Testing critical features with additional tests to supplement, where necessary, supplier testing.

If validation is not practical, pharmaceutical manufacturers should consider selecting and replacing legacy software and hardware with equivalent products or to replace the entire automation system. This may involve using alternative suppliers. New software or hardware in a legacy system will require validation to confirm that its functionality operates as required, and that it does not affect what remains of the original system.

REFERENCES

1. Freeman, M., Leng, M., Morrison, D., and Munden, R.P. (1995), Position Paper on the Qualification of Analytical Equipment, *Pharmaceutical Technology Europe*, November.

2. Huber, L. (1995), *Validation of Computerized Analytical Systems,* Buffalo Grove, IL: Interpharm Press, Inc.

3. Trill, A.J. (1994), A Regulatory Perspective, *Good Computer Validation Practices: Common Sense Implementation,* edited by T. Stokes, R.C. Branning, K.G. Chapman, H. Hambloch, and A.J. Trill, Buffalo Grove, IL: Interpharm Press, Inc.

4. Motise, P. (1996), *Inspection of Computerized Manufacturing Systems,* ISPE European Computer Systems Validation Conference, 24–25 September, Zurich, Switzerland.

5. Automation Research Group (1996), *Automation Straegies,* Special Issue (April).

6. ISPE (1995), Bulk Pharmaceutical Chemicals, *Baseline: Pharmaceutical Engineering Guide for New Facilities,* Volume 1 (First Draft), Tampa, Florida: International Society for Pharmaceutical Engineering.

7. UK Department of Health (1989), *Good Laboratory Practice: The Application of GLP Principles to Computer Systems,* London: United Kingdom Compliance Programme, Department of Health.

8. OECD (1995), *The Application of the Principles of GLP to Computerised Systems,* No. 10 OECD Series on Principles of Good Laboratory Practice and Compliance Monitoring, GLP Consensus Document, Environmental Monograph No. 116, Paris: Organisation for Economic Co-operation and Development, Environmental Directorate.

9. Final Rule for 21 CFR Part 11 (1997), Electronic Signatures and Electronic Records, *Federal Register,* 65(54).

10. U.S. EPA (1995), *Good Automated Laboratory Practices: Principles and Guidance to Regulations for Ensuring Data Integrity in Automated Laboratory Operations with Implementation Guidance,* Document Reference 2185, Washington, DC: Environmental Protection Agency.

11. FDA (1983), *Guide to Inspection of Computerized Systems in Drug Processing,* Technical Report, Reference Materials and Training Aids for Investigators, Rockville, MD: Food and Drug Administration.

12. APV (1996), The APV Guideline on Computerised Systems, Appendix U of the UK GAMP Forum's *Supplier Guide for Validation of Automation Systems in Pharmaceutical Manufacture,* Version 2, The Hague: International Society for Pharmaceutical Engineering.

13. Grigonis, G.J., Jr. and Wyrick, M.L. (1994), Computer System Validation: Auditing Computer Systems for Quality, Article on behalf of the PhRMA Computer Systems Validation Committee, *Pharmaceutical Technology Europe,* 18 (9): 32–39.

14. Leveson, N.G. and Turner, C.S. (1993), An Investigation of the Therac-25 Accidents, *IEEE Computer,* 26 (7): 18–41.

15. Sommerville, I. (1992), *Software Engineering,* 4th Edition, Reading, MA: Addison-Wesley.

16. Hatton, L. (1997), Unexpected (and Sometimes Unpleasant) Lessons from Data in Real Software Systems, *Safety and Reliability of Software Based Systems,* Springer-Verlag.

17. *Australian Code of Good Manufacturing for Therapeutical Goods* (1990), Medicinal Products—Part 1, Section 9, Woden, Australia: Therapeutic Goods Administration.

18. European Union Guide to Directive 91/356/EEC (1993), Computerised Systems, Annex 11 of *European Commission Directive Laying Down the Principles of Good Manufacturing Practice for Medicinal Products for Human Use.*

19. U.S. Code of Federal Regulations Title 21, Part 314 (last amended 1992), *Applications for FDA Approval to Market a New Drug or an Antibiotic Drug.*

20. Tetzlaff, R.F. (1992), GMP Documentation Requirements for Automated Systems: Parts 1, 2, and 3, *Pharmaceutical Technology,* 16 (3): 112–124, 16 (4): 60–72, 16 (5): 70–82.

21. Salazar, J.M., Gopal, C., and Mlodozeniec, A. (1991), Computer Migration and Validation: A Vendor's Perspective, *Pharmaceutical Technology,* June.

22. ICH Harmonised Tripartite Guideline for Good Clinical Practice (1996), IFPMA, May.

Chapter 5

Ongoing Support Programmes

Validation represents a business investment. It aims to ensure that automation systems consistently operate to their original design intent and that documentary evidence exists to demonstrate this to GMP regulatory authorities. This investment, however, will be wasted if the validated status is not maintained. Without support, the performance and operational regulatory compliance of automation systems will tend to decline. For instance, operators will inevitably forget about the repairs and improvements they made in the past if they have not updated system documentation. If a maintenance activity or modification was required, then whoever was conducting the work would either have to rely on their own memory of the system's history or spend time examining the system to establish how it works. This can often lead to operations staff feeling extremely frustrated.

This chapter discusses the ongoing support needed to maintain the validated status of automation systems. The ongoing support needed is the same irrespective of whether the automation system was validated as a new or existing system. Topics covered include the following:

- Operating procedures
- Repair and maintenance
- Document control
- Change control
- Security
- Contingency planning
- Training
- Performance monitoring

- Periodic review and revalidation
- Decommissioning

Ongoing support programmes will tend to fall into misuse, however, if they are not practical and efficient. Since between 30 percent and 80 percent of the overall cost of an automation system can be attributed to its operational phase, it is important to get ongoing support right.

Another important factor to bear in mind is that over the operational lifetime of the system, the minimum validation requirements are likely to rise, as indicated in Figure 5.1. If these minimum validation requirements exceed the original validation requirements, a decision will need to be made whether to conduct further validation or to replace the automation system.

OPERATING PROCEDURES

To deliver a product right the first time, every time, it has become common practice to conduct work in accordance with SOPs. The aim of the procedures is to institute a controlled and repeatable practice for the development,

Figure 5.1. Operational Lifetime Capabilities

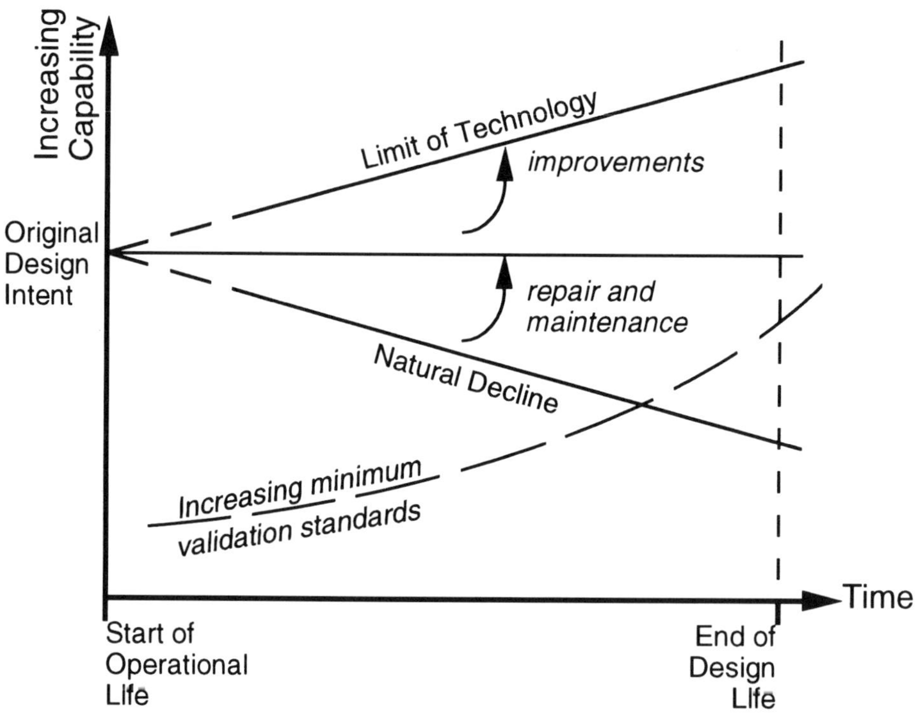

operation, and support of the automation system [1]. Procedures will include all those activities itemised above and any Service Level Agreements (SLA). Without SOPs, work cannot be conducted under management control. Effective management is essential for successful validation.

Wherever possible, SOPs should have a consistent format. A common style will help staff who are not familiar with the procedure to read and understand it much faster. Users should be encouraged to write their own procedures in an effort to ensure they are practical and do not miss important information or provide unnecessary detail. Some validation practitioners refer to this as SOP resilience—bias the procedures towards operator function rather than being too technically specific. This will allow the SOPs to be used with no or minimal modifications despite minor situation changes. All procedures will require review and approval by management who must check for consistency and compliance with other corporate procedures, standards, and regulatory requirements.

SOPs should be periodically reviewed at a frequency adequate to ensure they accurately describe the current working practices. They should be authorised before use and maintained under change control. A history of amendments and subsequent approvals of new versions should be kept; this is often appended at the end of their respective procedures. Some companies, however, prefer to keep a centralised library of amendments. In either case, it is vital that the current issue of an operating procedure is used. SOPs should be located near their point of use so that staff can easily access them. Old versions should be removed from circulation. There have been numerous incidents where staff have resorted to carrying uncontrolled photocopies, because access to controlled copies was not convenient. As soon as these uncontrolled copies became out of date, staff were unknowingly compromising validation.

The benefit of ISO 9000 certification for operating procedures has already been discussed in Chapter 2. Compliance with this standard is voluntary and provides a good basis for validation. However, ISO 9000 only certifies a consistent procedural approach; it does not certify the quality attributes of any particular piece of work.

DOCUMENT CONTROL

Documented manufacturing practice is vital for pharmaceutical companies because without it, they have no way of demonstrating validation to the various GMP regulatory authorities. This is not the only use for documentation though. Documentation also provides pharmaceutical companies with a corporate memory of how they implemented and used automation systems. Documentation can be used as an internal auditing aid, as training material, and as *aide memoirs* for operations personnel. It is also useful when setting up new facilities and processes, and setting up programmes of continuous improvement. Document control is essential especially during corporate mergers when documentation can be misplaced or lost, and during downsizing initiatives when support resources are reduced.

Documentation can be organised into a hierarchical structure consisting of policies, operating procedures, technical records, and operational data, as shown in Figure 5.2. Policies will include the Validation Policy and other corporate policies where they exist covering safety, environmental protection, and so on. Operational procedures were outlined in the previous section of this chapter and are usually referred to as SOPs; they include cleaning, calibration, and Quality Control analytical methods. Technical records include development and testing documentation for the automation system, whilst operational data include software listings, configuration details, and batch records. Once the hierarchical structure has been established, it is easier to ensure that the various levels of documentation have a consistent style, format, and amount of detail.

Figure 5.2. Documentation Pyramid

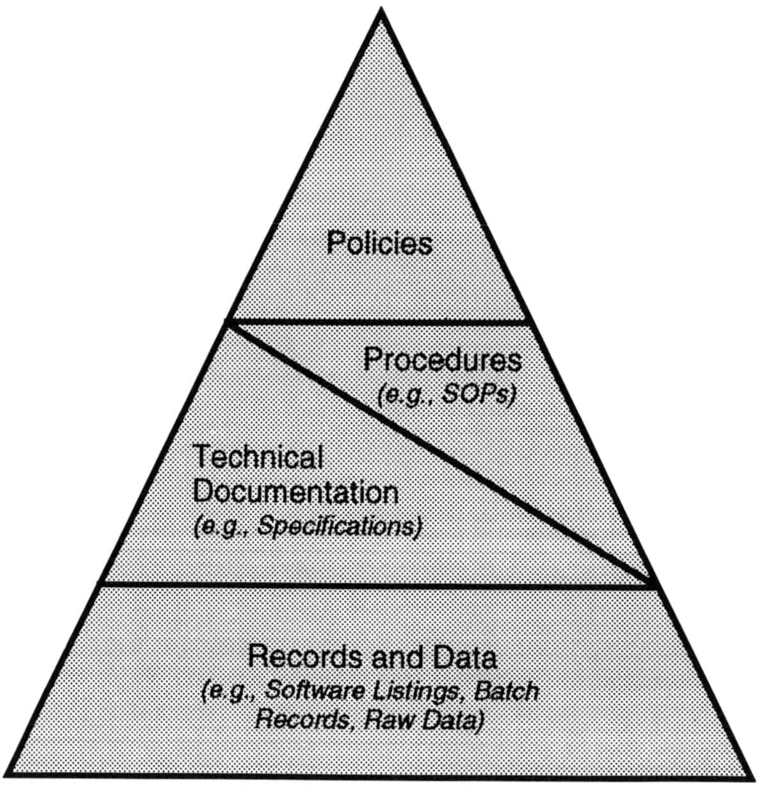

Quality

The quality of documentation must be assured. Poor documentation is usually characterised as rambling, with omissions in some areas and too much detail in others. This is hardly conducive to its use, let alone compliant with GMP. Those preparing documentation and records should, therefore, concentrate on ensuring that documents are

- Concise
- Complete
- Consistent
- Comprehensible
- Correct
- Controlled

Wherever possible, keep documents small, preferably less than 20 pages, and avoid the duplication of information. Minimise the number of copies, as this will make it easier to retrieve and update distributed documents. Some organisations print documents on coloured paper so that a black and white photocopy can be easily recognised as a copy of the master. Management must ensure personnel do not keep uncontrolled photocopies of documents, because they may be used when in fact they have been revised. Where paperless manufacturing systems distribute copies of documents, then they should be clearly marked as having a limited life so that if they are revised, old copies are not accidentally used. A life of one week is normally recommended. Keep the organisation and administration of documentation simple. Complex systems are much harder to manage successfully.

Individual documents should have the following controls:

- Document Title
- Document Number
- Version Number
- Page x of y
- Date of Issue
- Copy Number

Some organisations include a date for the next default review of the document. This review ensures that even if no changes have occurred, the document will still be examined to check that it is still current.

Centralised versus distributed administration of documentation has advantages and disadvantages. Centralised administration offers far fewer internal audits, economies of scale, opportunity to use sophisticated EDMSs, and easier control of master documents because they are in one place. Distributed administration meanwhile offers more "ownership" because it is closer to its users and it is easier to plan for busy periods. Most organisations tend to centralise administration by site, but either approach can be adopted as long as it is controlled.

Regulatory authorities will search documentation for keywords that in their experience are often associated with poor documentation [2]:

- Calculate—is the calculation specified?
- Automatic—is the degree of manual intervention specified?
- Typically, Usually—how often?
- Normally—what is normal, what is abnormal?
- Appropriate—what is appropriate, what is not appropriate?

A simple word search can be used on word processors when a document is being written to identify the use of these words. These words should then either be replaced with alternative phrases or clarified to remove any ambiguity.

Data collected directly from automation system equipment, and data or control signals transferred to the automation system, should be checked to confirm that they have been accurately and reliably transferred [3]. Live and master data should be distinguished.

Control

Documents must be reviewed and approved prior to issue. The review must be recorded using proformas or writing meeting minutes. The date of the review and the names of the reviewers must be recorded. Documents should be reviewed by a multidisciplinary team that includes technical and quality representatives. Each reviewer, however, does not necessarily have to be an authorising signature for the document as long as their comments are included in the review records. Reviewers should prepare for the review with copies of the document distributed prior to the review. The review must systematically cover each section of the document. If there are no comments regarding a section, then this should be indicated in the review records. Any corrective actions identified in the review must be assigned to personnel with a completion date. Care must be taken to ensure associated documents are also reviewed and updated.

At a recent conference, practitioners expressed the opinion that in their experience, 90 percent of the review comments concerned layout, spelling, and grammar [4]. The remaining review comments concerned content, omissions, and accuracy. Yet over 90 percent of the problems arising from poor documentation can be attributed to omissions [5]. Reviewers should bear this in mind and make the best use of their time.

A revision history should be created, if one does not already exist for the document, and updated with a reference to the review records. Many documents have their revision history appended at the end. Reviews that only involve a change to a few pages of an existing document offer the opportunity to reissue just those few pages. Less paper to distribute usually means faster implementation of the change. However, if the whole document is reissued, then the current document has only one set of authorising signatures and it is easier to track the current version of the document. Care must be taken to make sure that documentation does not become confused by too many individual page updates; reissue the whole document when there is a danger of this occurring.

Authorising signatures should be kept to a minimum and include a technical representative and a quality representative. Too many signatories will slow down the issue of documentation. The names and dates of signatories must be clearly indicated, together with the reason why they are signing. Signatures should be in black or blue pen because they are generally more resistant to fading. Where a document is circulated for review, then it may be necessary to pass the revised document around again to ensure that all signatories see the final document before signing. A copy of a document's surpassed version should then be retained and clearly marked as withdrawn.

Archives: Retention and Retrieval

Documentation should be stored at a separate and secure location [6]. Critical documentation, records, and data should be kept in a fireproof safe. Some documentation may be archived electronically, but advice should be sought from GMP regulatory authorities on which documents they would expect to inspect as paper. It is generally acceptable to store version histories on electronic media, as long as the current master copy is paper. Clinical trial data are often stored on microfiche or other electronic medium. It should not be possible to alter such electronic copies such that they could be interpreted as master records [7]. Valid record changes must also not obscure previous record changes. Paper archives should be established where there is a risk that the technology for restoring electronic copies on paper may become obsolete during the time that the documentation is required to be archived.

Record retention requirements are the same regardless of the medium [8]. The retention time for validation documentation relating to a drug product's manufacture is as at least one year after the product's expiry date. The retention time for validation documentation relating to a drug product exempted from expiry dates varies depending on whether it is supplied to the United States or to Europe. For the United States, it is at least three years after the last batch has been distributed [2,8], whilst for Europe documents must be retained for at least five years from its certification [6]. The UK's IQA

Pharmaceutical Quality Group suggests that all documents be retained for a period of at least five years from the last date of supply [9]. An effective solution for many organisations has been to store their documents for a period of seven years after the effective expiry date of a drug product or as long as the automation system is used, whichever is longer.

Where system obsolescence forces a need to transfer electronic documentation from one system or format to another, the process must be recorded step by step and its integrity verified [10]. An exact copy must be verified prior to any destruction of the original media. The obsolete system could alternatively be maintained as a legacy system, an approach that can be expensive and one that might still require transfer to a new system or format at a later date when maintenance become impractical.

Documentation required by regulators, including those stored electronically, must be accessible at the drug manufacturing site during an authorised inspection. It should be possible to give GMP inspectors, if requested, a true paper copy (accurate and complete) of master documentation regardless of whether the original's medium was magnetic, electronic, optical, or paper. True copies must be legible and properly registered, with two dated, independent signatures.

Retrieving documents from the archive after company mergers can be a problem—it is easy to lose track of which documents exist and where they are stored. Retrieval during a GMP inspection is usually required within about 20 minutes. Some documentation, however, may be held off-site at a supplier's premises (see Figure 5.3). The division of documentation between a pharmaceutical manufacturer and its suppliers should be defined in the Validation Plan or Validation Report. The drug manufacturer will be expected in most cases to retain a report reviewing documentation held by suppliers. These reports may stand-alone or be part of a Supplier Audit. Access to supplier documentation (normally within 24 hours) may be via a visit to the supplier's premises, courier or postal service, or via electronic links (subject to the FDA's new regulation on electronic records) and, as such, should be subject to a formally agreed-on access agreement. Some pharmaceutical manufacturers establish escrow accounts with their suppliers.

REPAIR AND MAINTENANCE

Routine repair and maintenance activities should be embodied in approved SOPs and cover instrumentation, computer hardware elements, and communication network components. The frequency of maintenance should be defined in these SOPs and, unless otherwise justified, comply with the OEM's recommendations. Maintenance frequencies may be determined by recalibration requirements and reliability-centred preventive maintenance calculations. Advice can be sought from supplier organisations, but it should not be

Figure 5.3. Custody of Documentation

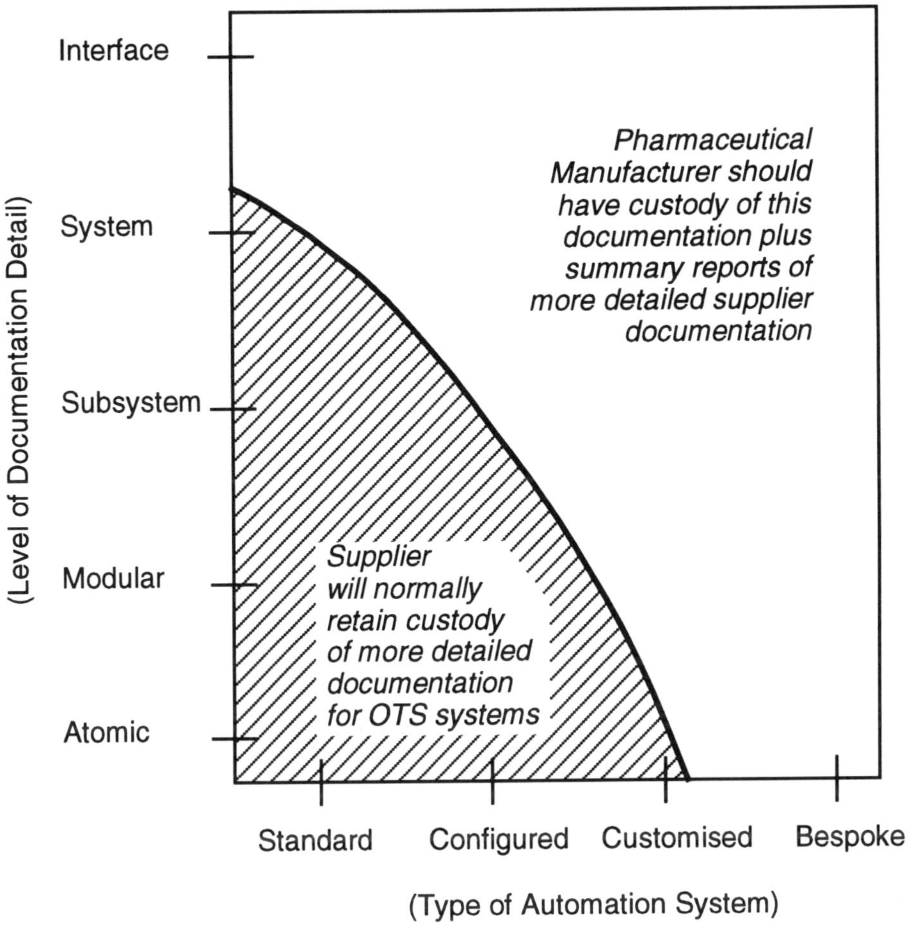

solely relied on because it is highly unlikely that they do not fully understand the precise nature of the pharmaceutical application [11]. Justifications for periodic inspection intervals should be recorded, remembering that they can be modified in the light of operational experience. Any change to recalibration periods or preventive maintenance intervals, however, must be controlled.

Repair and maintenance operations should not present any hazard to the manufactured product [6]. Defective elements of automation systems (including instrumentation and analytical laboratory equipment) should, if possible, be removed from their place of use (production area or laboratory bench), or at least be clearly labelled as defective. It is unlikely, unfortunately, that the precise time of failure will be known. This often leaves operations staff with a dilemma of what to do with the drug products that might or might not have been manufactured when the automation system was defective. Indeed, was there an initial partial failure and a period of degraded operation before any fault was recognised? No specific guidance can be given except to consider the merits of each situation, case by case, and ensure that a quality check is performed on product batches manufactured during the period when the automation system is suspected of malfunction or failure. It is best to play safe when considering the number of product batches that are potentially substandard and assume worst-case scenarios.

Calibrated equipment should be labelled at the time of each calibration with the date of the calibration and next calibration due date. This label facilitates a visual inspection of equipment to check whether it is approaching its next calibration date or is overdue. The label should also include as a minimum the initials of the engineer who conducted the calibration. Some companies also include space for a full signature and printed name, but this should not prove necessary if initials are legible and can be traced to the appropriate engineer. Where labels are used, however, care must be taken to apply them to a clean dry area so that they do not fall off. Labels should be considered as an aide memoir, with the master record being kept elsewhere (perhaps handwritten in a plant logbook or a calibration certificate in an engineering management system) in case the labels become detached. Calibration procedures must be agreed on and wherever appropriate refer to national calibration standards.

Maintenance and repair documentation may be requested during an inspection by a GMP regulator. Documentation for maintenance activities must include a description of the operations performed, who conducted the maintenance and when, and the results confirming that the maintenance work was completed satisfactorily. Calibration certificates should be retained. Repair records, meanwhile, should include a description of the problem, corrective action taken, acceptance testing criteria, and the results confirming that the repair work has restored the automation system to an operational state. Repair logbooks can be used to record nonroutine repair and maintenance work.

The GMP regulations require pharmaceutical manufacturers to maintain backups of software programs, data entered, and operational data to establish the proper performance of automation systems. Backup and restoration procedures are, therefore, needed. Each backup should be verified before it is stored in a secure location, preferably a fireproof safe. There have been several instances where backups have been incorrectly made and a restoration of the automation system was not possible. It is generally recommended that three backup copies are kept, one for each of the last three backups. This system is sometimes referred to as grandfather-father-son backups. Many organisations performs backups at least once a week, although the frequency will vary depending on the criticality and change of the automation system. The appropriate backup media can vary; examples include diskettes, cartridge tapes, removable disk cartridges, or remote-networked host computers. Any change to the backup procedure must be carefully considered and any necessary reciprocal modification to the restoration procedures made. Stored backups should be checked for accessibility, durability, and accuracy at a frequency appropriate for the storage medium [6,8]. The retention responsibilities for backups are the same as for other documentation and records.

Records should be kept regardless of whether or not the work was conducted by a contracted service supplier. If such engineering support is provided by an external agency using their own procedures, then those procedures must be subject to approval by the pharmaceutical manufacturer before they are used. Repair logbooks should note visits from external staff, recording their names, the date, and the summary work conducted so that additional information held by the supplier can be traced in the future if necessary. It is important that service arrangements defining when suppliers are used by pharmaceutical manufacturers to conduct maintenance and repair work are formally agreed. Such agreements are often embedded in contracts called Service Level Agreements (SLAs). The UK GAMP Forum promotes the development of a Maintenance Plan to define roles and responsibilities [12]. It is unacceptable to the GMP regulatory authorities not to have documentary evidence demonstrating management control of these activities.

CHANGE CONTROL

It has been suggested that one in five changes to automation systems may introduce new defects [2], which is why practitioners sometimes refer to a death rather than life cycle. Pressures to implement a quick and cheap fix have been blamed as a contributory factor. Beware of cosmetic, minor, and major changes—they all change the system. Minor decisions become significant when they go wrong. Understanding the impact of a local change does not necessarily imply understanding whether a ripple effect exists that will impact the system elsewhere. Even like-for-like changes can be dangerous, for instance, the documentation accompanying so-called "standard" products often reads subject to alteration without prior notification. Pharmaceutical manufacturers have accordingly implemented change control to demonstrate the management of all changes.

Change control includes document control and is associated with the following sequence of activities:

- Identify and specify change.
- Preview impact of change.
- Assess risk and impact if change is incorrectly implemented.
- Specify testing requirements and acceptance criteria.

- Implement change after authorisation.
- Test change with any retesting of the overall system.
- Accept change with independent review.
- Update documentation to reflect change.

Change control forms should be designed to demonstrate the management control of changes. These forms must be practical and their use coordinated by an assigned individual. The details of the proposed change must be clearly defined. It is often useful to identify the originator of the change so that points can be quickly clarified. The impact of the change on drug product quality, operator safety, and the environment is usually specified by specialist staff. A decision is then made to accept or reject the change; cost may be factor. High costs, however, are not an acceptable excuse to avoid or delay implementation of a change needed to achieve or maintain the standard of a drug product.

Testing should be implemented to test any modifications and the impact of these modifications on the system's overall operation. Repeated testing on the complete system is sometimes called *regression testing*. In principle, all system tests should be repeated after every change. In practice, however, this is too expensive. Dependencies between parts of the system should, therefore, be identified. A subset of original tests covering these dependencies should then be used to check that the change has not adversely affected other parts of the automation system. Some new specific tests may be needed to check modifications to the system, but it is likely that these can also be based on existing test specifications from the IQ, OQ, and PQ. In this manner, a high degree of confidence can be placed on changes to an automation system within a reasonable cost.

The availability of staff to authorise the progressions and acceptance of work must be taken into account and, if necessary, deputies assigned. At a minimum, three sets of signatories should be established: authorisation to implement change, acceptance of implemented change, and completion of all associated documentary requirements. The signatories for these stages represent the system owner (e.g., facility manager), the system user (e.g., senior operations engineer), and the system owner, respectively, with counter signatures by quality assurance personnel.

If there is more than one change awaiting implementation at any time, then the changes should be prioritised. There must be no interference between changes that are concurrently implemented. Changes to software may be bundled for collective release in a new version of the software. Major changes should follow the validation life cycle described in Chapter 3.

Special arrangements should be made for emergency situations where the authorisations of changes may be altered because of the availability of staff. The documentary requirements for emergency changes are the same as for nonemergency changes. Dates to remove temporary modifications should be adhered to, otherwise there is a tendency for them to become permanent by default. Software incorporating emergency or temporary changes must still be identifiable by a unique version reference. Without version control, it is all too easy to forget about changes and think that a modified version of software is unchanged.

Dependence on change control records supplementing original documents after system release hampers quality maintenance because maintenance personnel have no single set of updated documentation that describes the current system. Configuration management practices aligned with formal change control principles are one way to manage information and maintenance work activities.

SECURITY

System security covers physical security mechanisms and management procedures aimed at preventing the loss and corruption of system data, inadvertent or unauthorised changes, and restricted access [3,6]. Security practice should, therefore, address both operational and storage/archive facilities. Security controls must take account of whether the system is open or closed.

- *Closed Systems:* An environment in which access is controlled by persons who are responsible for the content of electronic records which are on the system.
- *Open Systems:* An environment in which access is *not* controlled by persons who are responsible for the content of electronic records which are on the system.

Single user-point systems are generally regarded as more secure than multiple user-point systems, because physical access is easier to control. A recent report investigated the vulnerability of open systems, suggesting that 1 in 3 unauthorised access attempts are successful, but that only 1 in 150 are typically detected [13]. Detected unauthorised access attempts must be recorded and investigated. If a significant security breach occurs, then senior management should be alerted immediately. There should be a defined procedure for the issue, cancellation, and alteration of authorisation for security access [6]. Security practice should be subject to periodic review.

Physical Access Controls

Wherever practical, automation systems should be located in rooms that can be securely locked when the systems are not being used. If this is not practical, then the systems should be placed away from easily accessible areas and chained. Do not place systems where they cannot be easily used or where objects could fall or interfere with their operation. Personnel should not be allowed to eat, drink, or smoke in the immediate vicinity of the system because of the likelihood that particles or liquid will be dropped inside the system's keyboard and equipment air vents.

Other physical security mechanisms may be incorporated into the automation system. Examples include the key operation of computer consoles and instrument calibration front plates, and biometric tests, such as retina scans, to access system functionality.

Some pharmaceutical organisations have introduced tamper evident labels on automation equipment to complement protection mechanisms. Such a management strategy does not directly protect the security of a system, but seeks to ensure that all access breaches are detected. Any security breaches, intentional or unintentional, benign or malicious, can then be investigated and corrective actions put in place.

All portable security equipment associated with an automation system (including keys and detachable programming devices) should be stored in a secure location, such as a locked cabinet or room, when it is not being used. An individual should be assigned responsibility for monitoring the correct use of logging procedures to record the release and return of equipment to authorised personnel. It should be possible to track who, why, and when portable equipment was used.

Logical Access Controls

Access requirements for single-user and multiple-user automation systems are described by the UK Department of Health [14]. Password access rights should be dependent on unique identification, usually a user identification accompanied by a user password. Access controls identifying users by group are not considered as secure as if they identified individual users because of the need to share passwords. Passwords should be subject to periodic checks, revision, and recall. Procedures should be established for the issue, control, and revocation of access rights that may consist of a hierarchy of access permissions. Access rights should be periodically challenged to ensure that security integrity is maintained. Records with time stamps should be kept of record changes and access attempts by unauthorised personnel. It is recommended that some common security passwords, such as names and birthdays, are prohibited [3].

An important feature of logical access control which should be incorporated wherever possible is that of an automatic log out of a user's account when it has not been used for some specified "time-out" period (e.g., 5 minutes). This will help ensure that a user's account, with its particular access rights, is not inadvertently left open for other potentially unauthorised users.

Systems with group access controls often time-out to a default operational level, only using passwords for access to special functions.

Software should be protected by backing up at regular intervals. Software backups will include each version upgrade of computer programs and interim copies of associated data files at intervals corresponding to the nature of change in the data. The backup and restoration of automation software should be specified in a procedure.

There has been much discussion about the security of dial-in access via modems (modular-demodulator units) to open systems. Unauthorised access must be prevented. Specific points for consideration include the following:

- Use a dedicated or restricted telephone line.
- Verify originating phone number.
- Record all unauthorised access attempts.
- Use a call-back system.
- Disconnect modem when not in use.

Some companies have restricted the use of the Internet and other open intercompany communication facilities (e.g., Intranet) to stand-alone automation systems that do not run GMP–related applications. This may be judged by some to be overkill, but these companies prefer to be safe rather than sorry.

Virus Controls

Computer viruses are small pieces of computer code that corrupt and destroy files and programs in a computer by embedding themselves within the computer's software. They copy themselves from one program to another, transferring from machine to machine without users realising it until it is too late. Advanced viruses change their characteristics each time they infect new software. Many viruses are little more than electronic graffiti, merely displaying messages on the user's computer screen to demonstrate infiltration. Other viruses, however, overwrite a computer's system software, rendering it useless.

In November 1995, Britain made its first conviction for computer misuse [15]. The individual concerned created two advanced viruses. Like most virus writers, his motive was malice rather than trying to blackmail firms. The first virus, called Pathogen, displayed the message *Smoke me a kipper, I'll be back for breakfast, unfortunately some of your data won't* and disabled the computer between 5 P.M. and 6 P.M. on Mondays if programs infected by the virus had been opened at least 32 times. The second virus, called Queeg, attacked computer systems in the same manner but with a different message and on Sundays between noon and 1 P.M. The virus writer spread the viruses by hiding them in computer games and antivirus software. The viruses together are thought to have caused many millions of dollars of damage. It is good practice to check all software to be used on automation systems for known viruses before the software is installed.

A German pharmaceutical manufacturer recently had a company-wide alert across its international operations because of a virus. The virus was introduced onto a PC with an upgrade of a standard instrument calibration software package. The PC was networked to local site and international operations. Luckily, the pharmaceutical manufacturer had the foresight to institute a virus checking facility as part of its security practice, and the virus was identified and removed before any damage was incurred. Virus-checking software, however, only checks for known viruses. Where such software is used, it should be regularly updated to include checks for the latest viruses. Some drug manufacturers insist that all computer systems and electronic storage media used on their premises are virus checked, including those used by visiting personnel.

Computer viruses can also be introduced when users load unauthorised computer games on automation systems. This often happens out of normal working hours when there is relatively little to keep operations staff occupied and is sometimes referred to as "midnight madness". A recent incident of this type affected an embedded PLC controlling an autoclave. The virus concerned was called "Jack the Ripper", one of the top 10 viruses reported in the United Kingdom in 1996, which produces slow irreversible corruption of data on disk [16]. The virus is believed to have been introduced via a game loaded on the PC–based SCADA system controlling the PLC. Management should ensure their staff are aware of the dangers viruses pose to GMP as a result of degraded functionality and compromised data integrity. Games should not be allowed. Staff must understand that disciplinary action, which could include losing their job, will be taken against those found responsible for loading unauthorised software.

Pharmaceutical manufacturers and suppliers alike must maintain vigilance against the introduction of viruses. However, organisations must also beware of hoax virus alerts. Checking automation systems for nonexistent viruses is a waste of effort. Management should, therefore, assess any alert on a case-by-case basis: verify the origin of the alert, evaluate the hazard posed by the virus, consider the ease of any action to mitigate the potential threat, and weigh the option of taking no action. The use of special antivirus procedures can help an organisation react quickly.

CONTINGENCY PLANNING

Contingency Plans must be formalised and cover remedial action for process automation system breakdowns, partial failures, and catastrophic failures [6]. The plans will detail fall-back action, including replacing equipment and repair, and documentary and authorisation procedures. A check should be made periodically that all support resources necessary to restore the system will be available in the event of implementing the contingency plan [3]. Failures and remedial activities must be recorded [6]. It is important that emergency protocols are defined and understood by the operating staff.

Personnel must be nominated either by name or job title with their responsibilities for implementing the Contingency Plan. It should be recognised that in emergencies or unplanned situations, normal job roles may not be applicable. It is important that lines of communication, both within the pharmaceutical manufacturing organisation and suppliers, are specified with names, addresses, and telephone numbers. Agreed on potential sources for temporary or permanent replacement of equipment, including software, should be detailed. Individuals and organisations nominated in the Contingency Plan must be competent to fulfil their duties. Reference should be made to any procedures required to enact this plan, such as procedures for security or restoring backups. If production can continue manually (paper-based) upon failure of an automation system, then the Contingency Plan must specify procedures for production records, such as batch records.

The Contingency Plan and any supporting standby systems and procedures must be tested periodically to ensure they are adequate. The plan should be reviewed and refined with growing operational experience. This includes the use of mobile automation systems built into lorries or trucks that can be driven onto the drug manufacturer's site and "plugged" in to replace local systems that for whatever reason have become unavailable. Standby automation systems must, however, be validated before they are used.

STAFF TRAINING

All personnel responsible for validation must be competent to fulfil their duties—having suitable experience and training or access to appropriate technical expertise and management skills [6,8]. Roles and responsibilities should be clearly specified and assigned [3] in the Validation Plans, Quality Plans, and job descriptions assigned to personnel. Résumés demonstrating the suitability of personnel should be stored and maintained in accordance with other GMP documentation and records. Pharmaceutical manufacturers must, therefore, ensure suppliers provide them with current résumés.

Initial training requirements should be outlined in the Validation Plan, and the timely provision of these requirements should receive full management support. Training courses should be prepared and presented by competent personnel. Many organisations collect feedback from course attendees to assess the quality of the training as well as measuring the how effectively the attendees have absorbed the course material. Questions to attendees might include the following:

- What does GMP, the FDA, and the MCA stand for?
- Why do we validate?

- What do we validate? (Where do you fit in it?)
- How do we validate? (Where can you get advice?)
- Who validates? (What are your particular responsibilities?)
- Recall your organisation's golden rules of validation.

Training requirements and records must be periodically reviewed. Training should be a continuous activity, with refresher courses for existing staff and induction courses for new personnel. Some organisations use job performance evaluations to help identify emerging training needs. Training records for all personnel should be kept up-to-date. GMP regulatory authorities may ask to inspect these records.

PERFORMANCE MONITORING

The performance of an automation system is monitored through operations, staff observations, and regular diagnostic tests. Operational observations are typically recorded in a facility (incident) logbook with time and date, comment, and the signature of person making the entry. Some logbooks also have entries noting the corrective action (perhaps the reference of a change request) against each originator comment.

Some organisations employ SPC to monitor the performance of their automation systems. SPC may be implemented directly by the automation system itself or by data collected from the automation system for evaluation elsewhere.

Many automation systems have automatic diagnostic facilities. Where such facilities exist, they should be used, and this may involve enabling them via a logical or physical switch. It is important that any diagnostic results are understood. The requirement to run and evaluate a diagnostic as acceptable may be defined in an SOP. If a diagnostic result identifies a deficiency, then this must be recorded in a predefined place that (as suggested above) may be the facility logbook. Some of the deficiencies may require immediate attention, such as alerts identifying the loss of availability of I/O cards or peripheral devices. Other deficiencies such as the above recommended disc utilisation will gather information to be used by periodic reviews. All problems should be diagnosed and any corrective action progressed through change control.

PERIODIC REVIEW AND REVALIDATION

Automation systems should be periodically reviewed [8] to confirm that its validated status has been sustained. Organisations often establish a review panel to conduct such periodic reviews. Before the panel meets, the chairman should estimate the time needed to undertake the review and determine the size and composition of the review panel. Members on the review panel should include operations staff and management, system support staff, and quality assurance personnel. User communities of networked applications should be represented by their departmental functions.

The review meeting must be recorded either by minutes or a formal report. It will normally begin by reviewing progress on actions assigned at last meeting and close by assigning a new list of actions which should be assigned to individuals with target dates for completion. The date for the next meeting should be agreed on. Many companies conduct periodic reviews every 12 months, or within shorter periods depending on:

- The system's potential impact on the quality of manufactured drug products.
- How easily unauthorised changes can be made against the system's access controls.
- Any recent problems experienced with the system's operation.

Topics for consideration in the periodic review should include, but are not limited to, the following:

- *Operating and Maintenance:* Check they are still current, including maintenance and calibration schedules, Contingency Plans, and backup and restoration procedures.
- *Documentation, Records, and Data:* Inspect for noncompliances and trends.
- *Change Control:* Check what has changed with automation system instrumentation, computer hardware, and computer software. Have the change control procedures been correctly adopted? Conduct spot checks to compare running systems with documentation. Have they been updated as changes have been implemented? Ensure any clock changes, such as the change between summer and winter time, have been correctly implemented. Review any outstanding change requests.
- *Security:* Review physical access; use of passwords, including frequency of change and list of active users; and unauthorised access attempts.
- *Contingency Plans:* Check software copyrights and licences. Some software applications cease to function upon expiry of a licence. Review any SLAs supporting the Contingency Plans and check that details are correct and still appropriate, and that the supplier is aware of its obligations.
- *Training:* Examine the need for refresher and induction courses.
- *Performance:* Check availability of automation systems and the level of utilisation of their databases and networks. If there were

any incidents, were corrective actions identified and have they been completed? How often was any help desk facility used? Exercise UPS batteries and check ongoing records monitoring the operating environment (e.g., humidity and temperature).

- *Revalidation:* Examine the need to revalidate if a lot of changes have been made or if regulatory requirements have altered. Check whether any unauthorised changes have been made.

The review panel meeting should take only a few hours if all the necessary information for the periodic review is collated before the meeting. Anecdotal evidence can be presented to the meeting.

If a periodic review identifies the need to reestablish or test the confidence in the validated status, the automation system should be revalidated. Revalidation does not necessarily imply a full repeat of the validation life cycle; partial requalification is acceptable when justified [11,17].

Periodic reviews and revalidation are shown in Figure 5.4's spiral validation life cycle for process automation systems. The spiral concept aims to capture evidence of revalidation as addenda to existing validation documents. If development has progressed to a point where the system cannot readily be assessed by reading the control and development documents together, a new control document incorporating all the amendments should be prepared and the original retained [3].

DECOMMISSIONING AUTOMATION SYSTEMS

Automation systems are decommissioned either when they have become technologically obsolete, they have become too unreliable, or the process they are controlling becomes obsolete. This activity is often called retirement in relation to laboratory management and analytical systems [10]. The automation system may still be needed at a later date to support a new or rejuvenated process. The validation requirements of decommissioning must be carefully considered. There are validation issues if its documentation is needed in relation to a future recall of a drug product or if the automation system is used again in the future.

Decommissioning will normally be based on an established shutdown procedure. There may, however, be special decommission operations that have not be used on the live system. Operations management must ensure that decommissioning hazards are identified and that procedures are defined to avoid any accidents.

If there is a possibility of the automation system being used again, then it should be disassembled and tagged, carefully packaged and labelled, and stored in a secure location. Documentary evidence supporting its validation must be archived. System Specifications, Predelivery Testing, IQ, OQ, PQ, and ongoing support procedures could prove very useful if the automation

Figure 5.4. Ongoing Validation Spiral

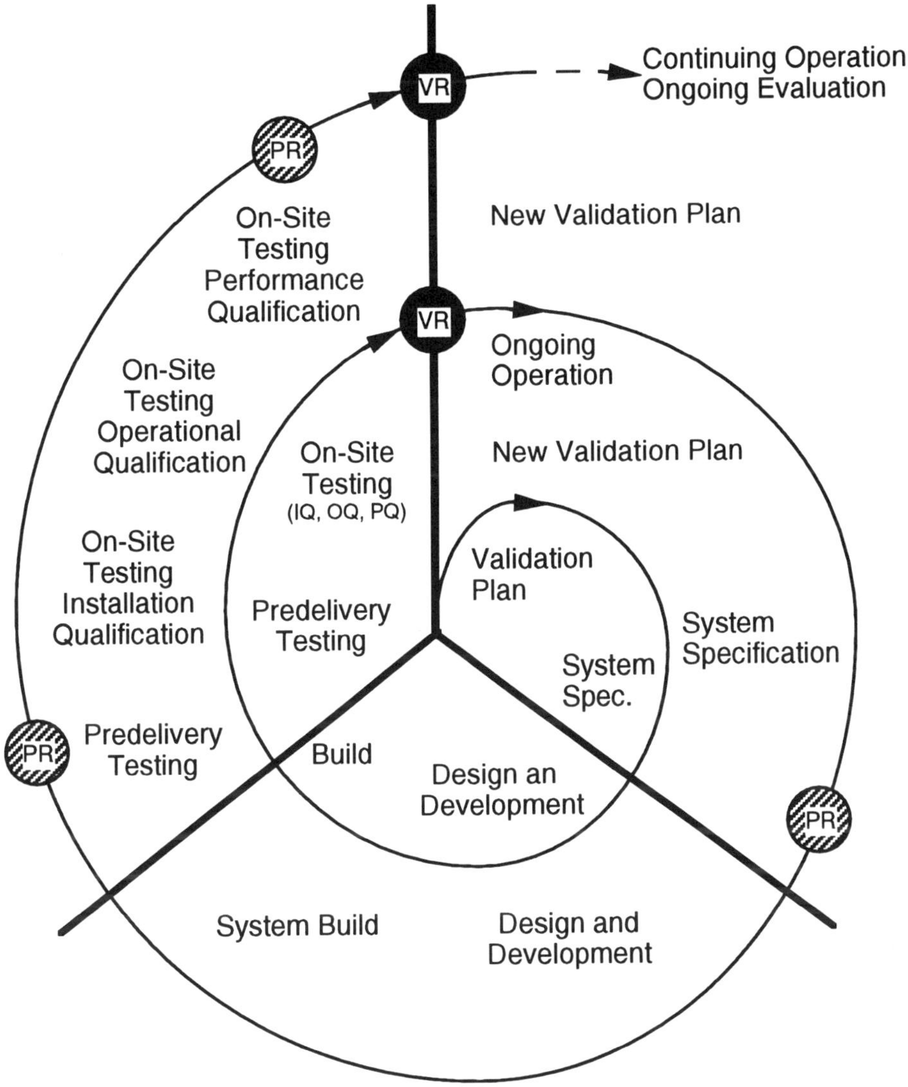

'VR' - Summary Validation Report (activity dependent), and 'PR' - Periodic Review (time dependent).

system is reused. Validation costs for the new system could be halved if it is similar to the original application. Documentary evidence of the automation system's validation should also be archived in case this information is required by an investigation into the recall of a drug product. Recalls can occur many years after decommissioning. The retention requirements for validation documentation have already been outlined earlier in this chapter.

When decommissioning is complete, a short report on the validation of the automation system should be composed to pass on any learning points. Only when this report has been issued and any archiving completed can operations managers relinquish their responsibility for the system.

REFERENCES

1. FDA (1987), *Software Development Activities,* Technical Report, Reference Materials and Training Aids for Investigators, Rockville, MD: Food and Drug Administration.
2. Clark, A.S. (1995), Inspection of Software Systems, ISPE European Computer System Validation, Zurich, 20–21 September, Zurich, Switzerland.
3. TGA (1990), *Australian Code of Good Manufacturing for Therapeutical Goods,* Medicinal Products—Part 1, Woden, Australia: Therapeutic Goods Administration.
4. Olsen, P. (1995), ISPE European Computer System Validation, 20–21 September, Zurich, Switzerland.
5. Wingate, G.A.S. (1996), Management for Operations Dependability, in *Life-Cycle Management for Systems Dependability,* edited by F. Redmill and C. Dale, Springer-Verlag.
6. European Union Guide to Directive 91/356/EEC (1993), Computerised Systems, Annex 11 of *Guide to Good Manufacturing Practice for Medicinal Products.*
7. FDA (1995), A Memo on Current Good Manufacturing Practice Issues on Human Use Pharmaceuticals, *Human Drugs Notes,* 3(3).
8. U.S. Code of Federal Regulations Title 21, Part 210 (last amended 1994), *Current Good Manufacturing Practice in Manufacturing, Processing, Packaging, or Holding of Drugs;* Part 211 (last amended 1995), *Current Good Manufacturing Practice for Finished Pharmaceuticals.*
9. UK IQA (1994), *Pharmaceutical Supplier Code of Practice covering the Manufacture of Pharmaceutical Raw Materials, Active Ingredients and Excipients,* Document Reference No. P00020, Issue 2, Institute of Quality Assurance, Pharmaceutical Quality Group.
10. U.S. EPA (1995), *Good Automated Laboratory Practices: Principles and Guidance to Regulations for Ensuring Data Integrity in Automated Laboratory Operations with Implementation Guidance,* Document Reference 2185, 1995 Edition, Washington, DC: Environmental Protection Agency.
11. FDA (1987), *General Principles of Process Validation,* Rockville, MD: Food and Drug Administration, Center for Drug Evaluation and Research.
12. UK GAMP Forum, *Supplier Guide for Validation of Automation Systems in Pharmaceutical Manufacture,* Second Version, The Hague: International Society for Pharmaceutical Engineering.

13. Kehoe, L. (1996), Behind the Net, Technology Section, *Financial Times,* London, 18 June.

14. UK Department of Health (1989), *Good Laboratory Practice: The Application of GLP Principles to Computer Systems,* London: United Kingdom Compliance Programme, Department of Health.

15. Uhlig, R. (1995), Black Baron Jailed Over Computer Virus That Caused Chaos, *Daily Telegraph,* London, 16 November.

16. Uhlig, R. (1996), Don't Let a Virus Eat Your Work, *Daily Telegraph,* London, 13 August.

17. Clark, A.S. (1988), Computer Systems Validation: An Investigator's View, *Pharmaceutical Technology,* 12 (1): 60–66.

Chapter 6

Working Relationships

GMP regulatory authorities require confidence that the automation systems used by pharmaceutical manufacturers consistently perform as intended by their specifications. To this end, pharmaceutical manufacturers who do not have a core competency in automation systems will often need the support of their suppliers (vendors, integrators, and consultants). This chapter explores these working relationships, the mutual expectations, and how successful partnerships can be established.

THE PHARMACEUTICAL MANUFACTURER'S PERSPECTIVE

The involvement of pharmaceutical manufacturers with automation systems can be viewed as consisting of four distinct activities:

1. The organisational preparation for validation
2. The project work to integrate the system in readiness for the manufacture of drug products
3. The operational use of the system to manufacture drug products
4. Inspection by GMP regulatory authorities

Organisation

Pharmaceutical manufacturers should carefully consider how they will establish a validation culture in their organisations. Work will include developing policies and procedures, as described in Chapter 2. Proactive companies will have the luxury of planning how to most cost-effectively institute organisational change. However, most companies see validation as a "grudge-spend" and will hang on as long as possible before committing any funds or preparing any preliminary plans. Such reactive companies are often forced to make speedy changes when a GMP inspection looms, or after corrective actions have been mandated by a GMP regulatory authority following complacent or substandard inspection preparations by the pharmaceutical manufacturer. Unplanned changes are often costly and inefficient, perhaps twice as expensive as planned changes.

It is advantageous when establishing a validation culture to tap into the experience of practitioners who have already instituted such changes in an organisation. A pharmaceutical manufacturer could seek advice from contacts in other pharmaceutical companies. The likelihood is, however, that the time and effort such contacts can give will be limited. Whilst many pharmaceutical companies are happy to discuss the general principles of validation, the detailed implementation of validation is seen by many companies as a competitive edge and, therefore, will not be disclosed. Where a pharmaceutical manufacturer has a sister company who is experienced with validation, then a secondment of key personnel may be possible. Most pharmaceutical companies, however, opt to recruit validation specialists or employ experienced consultants to supplement their management team. This approach offers the company a resource that can be effectively dedicated full time to planning and implementing the organisational change for validation. It is important to recognise that the effectiveness of the management team will be compromised if they do not have sufficient authority to institute change or if members are distracted by other unconnected duties. The most effective management teams are usually found within quality departments because of their historic authority to prevent the release of drug products that are deemed not to be GMP compliant.

Projects

Most projects are supported by suppliers, even if the supplier role is taken by an internal group within the pharmaceutical manufacturer's organisation. The validation responsibilities for projects have already been discussed in Chapter 3, but as yet, the respective viewpoints of the supplier and the pharmaceutical manufacturer have not been presented.

The pharmaceutical manufacturer, generally, has the most influence at the beginning of a project when the URS is being established. Suppliers have little involvement at this stage and, hence, their influence is limited. Pharmaceutical manufacturers must resist the temptation to continually tinker with their URS, as this can have a significant impact on the supplier's work. Emphasis should be placed on establishing the core functional requirements and operator interface. Modifications should always be discussed with the supplier. Too often, unnecessary work is passed onto the supplier, with slippage to the project. It is worth spending time getting the URS as complete as possible before the supplier starts work. Some pharmaceutical manufacturers ask consultants or equipment vendors to help them derive the URS in an attempt to improve its quality.

As the project progresses, the influence of the pharmaceutical manufacturer decreases. The automation system is being built in accordance with the URS and as work progresses, the cost in changes to these requirements rises steadily (see Figure 3.2).

Validation should comply with the pharmaceutical manufacturer's Validation Plan. Many pharmaceutical manufacturers, however, experience a nasty surprise when their supplier fails to deliver a validation package that meets their expectations. A retrospective exercise for validation then becomes necessary. This is usually very expensive and the supplier is likely to ask for extra funds. If the contract value cannot be exceeded, this work usually falls back to the pharmaceutical manufacturer to complete. To add to the problem, there are nearly always production pressures to get the automation system running in accordance with the original delivery date. It is important, however, that the pharmaceutical manufacturer does not use the automation system until sufficient documentary evidence has been collated to consider the system validated; otherwise, GMP regulatory authorities will consider manufactured drugs to be GMP noncompliant.

Pharmaceutical manufacturers should carefully select their suppliers not only on technical ability but also on validation capability. It is all too easy for a supplier's sales representative to indicate an understanding of validation; what matters is that the supplier's personnel assigned to the project understand validation.

Beware of suppliers claiming their products or services are GMP regulator approved; there is no such generic approval [1]. The only claim that can be made is that a particular application of a product or service passed an inspection at a particular point in time. The same product or service may not pass a repeat inspection by the same GMP regulator at a later date. Equally, there is no guarantee that same product or service implemented elsewhere will pass a GMP regulator's inspection. Buyer beware; follow up on supplier's cited satisfied customers.

The supplier's progress on a project should be monitored and documentation should be reviewed as it becomes available. It may be necessary for the pharmaceutical manufacturer to spend some time with the supplier to help them develop the validation capability of their project team. Alternatively, the pharmaceutical manufacturer could employ, or ask the supplier to employ, an independent validation consultant to assist the supplier and, thereby, reduce the demands on the manufacturer's own personnel. If the supplier does not have a proven validation track record, it is advisable not to enter into fixed-price contracts. Inexperienced suppliers who underestimate their validation costs may be tempted to compromise on quality rather than introduce project slippage and exceed their budgets.

Operations

Operational dependability is a vital element of GMP compliance. An insight into the operational problems experienced with automation systems is given by an analysis of Eutech Engineering's database of over 350 automation system malfunctions experienced by a number of international chemical and pharmaceutical manufacturing companies in the 1990s [2]. The results are presented in Figure 6.1.

- Poor application design and programming errors accounted for 29 percent of malfunctions, indicating the importance of a supplier's project capability. Some of these problems were due to poor change control of the installed automation system by the pharmaceutical manufacturer and the lack of documentation provided by servicing engineers. It is all to easy for operations staff to make changes on quiet shifts and forget to record what they did; it then

Figure 6.1. Automation System Malfunctions

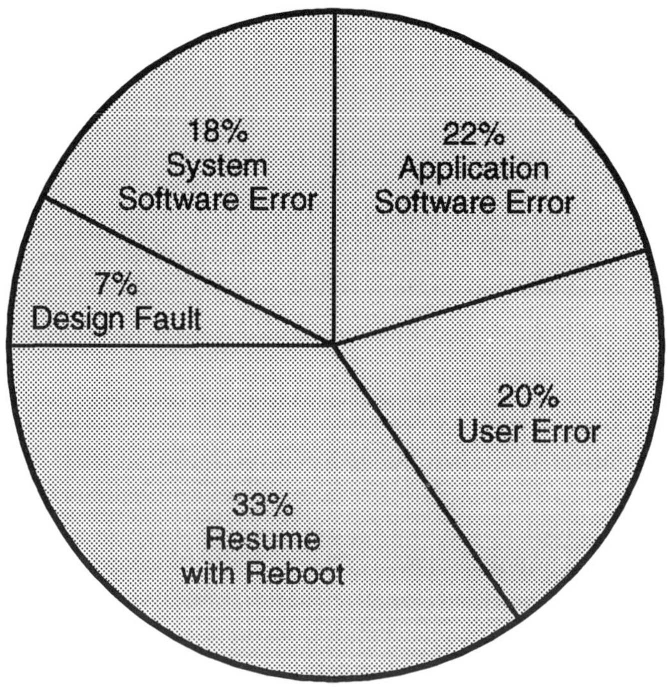

comes as a great surprise to the responsible managers that the documentation describing their system is out of date.

- The importance of conducting Supplier Audits for commercial off-the-shelf (COTS) software is highlighted by the 18 percent of malfunctions attributed to standard software.
- The importance of training system operators is demonstrated by the 20 percent of malfunctions attributed to human error. Pharmaceutical manufacturers must ensure training is given with approved SOPs before operators are required to use the automation system.

Unfortunately, the remaining malfunctions could not be diagnosed because a simple reboot of the software resumed normal operation and subsequent investigation could not identify any reasons for the malfunction.

A selection of operational lessons gathered from a book considering management issues for systems dependability are listed below [3]. Whilst there are undoubtedly others lessons relevant to pharmaceutical systems, these would seem to convey the key points of learning:

- Management should be commensurate with the criticality of the system.
- Ensure competency of operations staff as individuals and teams.
- Control access to the system, including keys and passwords.
- Control the use of system overrides.
- Communicate learning from incidents.
- Ensure essential records are kept and maintained.
- Monitor changes and maintenance to the system.
- Ensure manufacturer's recommended operating instructions are followed.
- Ensure appropriate national and international standards are adopted.
- Audit and follow-up outstanding issues with suppliers and sub-contractors.
- Ensure contingency plans are practical.
- Maintain a positive attitude amongst operations staff.
- Regularly audit systems to verify their specifications are still current and that they perform as intended.

It is evident that organisations must be ever vigilant of their GMP automation systems and continually develop their management capability for validation.

Regulatory GMP Inspections

GMP regulatory authorities hold pharmaceutical manufacturers accountable for validation. Manufacturers cannot pass on this responsibility to their suppliers. Pharmaceutical manufacturers cannot claim budgetary constraints as an excuse for insufficient personnel or unvalidated systems. The pharmaceutical manufacturer must, therefore, ensure that their validation work is properly funded and that suitable personnel and suppliers are assigned.

Most inspections by GMP regulatory authorities skip automation systems because few investigators are suitably qualified. When occasionally nonexpert investigators attempt such inspections, the results are often unpredictable [4]. Inspections conducted by automation system experts often uncover significant instances of noncompliant GMP practice. Whether or not an automation system expert will be conducting the inspection will only be known a few weeks or days before the inspection. Not surprisingly, the inspection of automation systems is often compared to Russian roulette. The best way to be prepared is not to take the risk of noncompliance and validate all automation systems that might be subject to inspection.

THE SUPPLIER'S PERSPECTIVE

Suppliers fall into three main categories: equipment vendors, service providers, and consultants. Equipment vendors are considered here to supply and integrate automation systems. Service providers provide ongoing operational services, such as calibration and maintenance. This supplier role may be fulfilled by an internal department within the pharmaceutical manufacturer's organisation.

Pharmaceutical manufacturers expect suppliers to provide solutions satisfying their needs and to demonstrate control of the work assigned to them. It sounds simple. In practice, however, suppliers sometimes fail to satisfy the manufacturer's expectations. This may not be solely the fault of the supplier. There must be a timely flow of information both ways between the supplier and the pharmaceutical manufacturer. Good project management skills are vital.

Equipment Vendors

Equipment vendors (including system integrators) should be employed under a contract that includes a statement of responsibilities [5]. This position is mandatory for companies operating under ISO 9000. The contract should include a Supplier Quality Plan that will outline working procedures and key personnel. Suppliers often face complex resourcing problems as projects start and finish, but they should, nevertheless, be expected to make every effort to keep these key individuals on the project. Any changes in the Supplier Quality Plan should be agreed on with the pharmaceutical manufacturer in advance of any change.

The supplier's influence on the design of the automation system rapidly increases as more and more money is committed to the progressing project. The cumulative earned income follows as S-curve throughout the project life cycle, as shown in Figure 6.2. At first, there is little income generated, and the scope of supply is being refined; then work begins in earnest until the bulk of the work has been completed, at which point relatively little new earned income is generated as the project closes. In many instances, at the end of a project, changes can be prohibitively expensive. It is at this point that if a change is implemented that system integrators and equipment vendors generally have a resource planning problem as some project staff will have been moved onto new projects. Any changes in personnel should be agreed to with the manufacturer to ensure that the capability of the personnel fulfilling the contract is not compromised.

Many suppliers have sought accreditation with ISO 9000, which has necessitated the establishment and maintenance of a documented quality system. The quality system should be an integrated process throughout the entire life cycle, thus ensuring that quality is being built into the automation system as development progresses, rather than being discovered at the end of the process. This sentiment is echoed by GMP regulatory authorities. In the past, equipment suppliers kept very little data that could be used by

Figure 6.2. Supplier Perspective

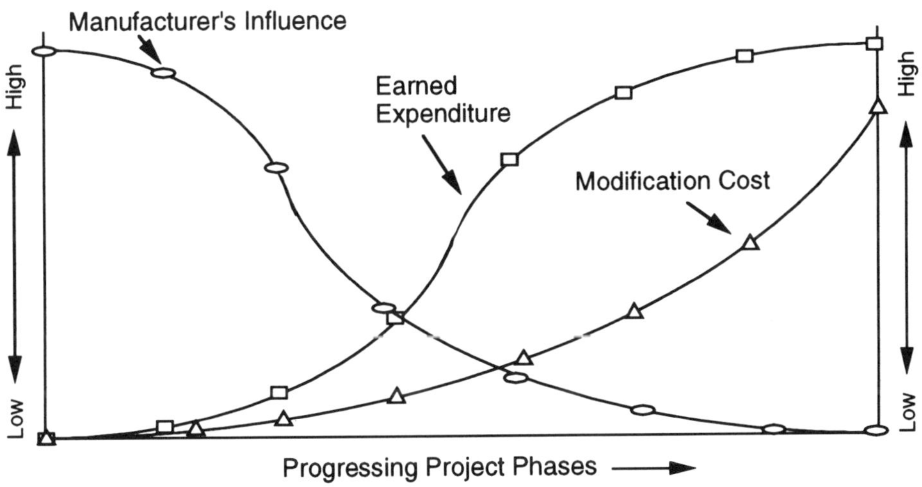

pharmaceutical manufacturers as supporting evidence for validation. Now things are getting better. However, existing products that entirely or partially consist of older components will be supplied for many years to come. Suppliers must not hide this fact from their customers.

Service Providers

Service providers contract resources to pharmaceutical manufacturers for work other than project work, usually under Service Level Agreements (SLAs). Work will include calibration, maintenance, and modifications. The comments made for equipment vendors apply equally to service providers. A particularly important factor is, however, that the supplier's records complement those of the pharmaceutical manufacturer. There have been numerous instances of service engineers not documenting their work. There must be a complete audit trail of evidence supporting validation. Agreement should be reached on who holds key documentary evidence and any retention facilities required by the supplier.

Consultants

The use of validation consultancy offers pharmaceutical manufacturers and suppliers quick access to GMP expertise. Consultants may be employed to advise on GMP requirements for automation systems, rather than to conduct validation, although the two roles may be combined. Consultants bring knowledge of their own experience and an independent view on industry practice (including a detailed understanding of current and emerging GMP standards and guides) to complement the pharmaceutical manufacturer's or supplier's in-depth knowledge of their working practices. This partnership approach to consultancy is illustrated in Figure 6.3. It must be appreciated, however, that whilst consultants bring an insight into what works and what does not work, they must respect confidentiality agreements with previous clients and establish agreements with new clients.

Consultants should endeavour to help their clients achieve GMP compliance whilst minimising the change to the client's established working practices. Consultants, therefore, should be sympathetic to a client's GMP history and any organisational pressures affecting the implementation of validation. The aim should be to deliver a smooth transition to GMP compliance, and this may necessitate a phased introduction of new and revised working practices. Existing procedures should be adapted wherever possible, rather than introduce entirely new procedures. Consultancy generally requires much more than just technical expertise!

The U.S. GMPs state that consultants must have sufficient education, training, and experience to advise on the subject for which they are retained [6]. Consultants may belong to an external contracting organisation or a

Figure 6.3. Using Consultants

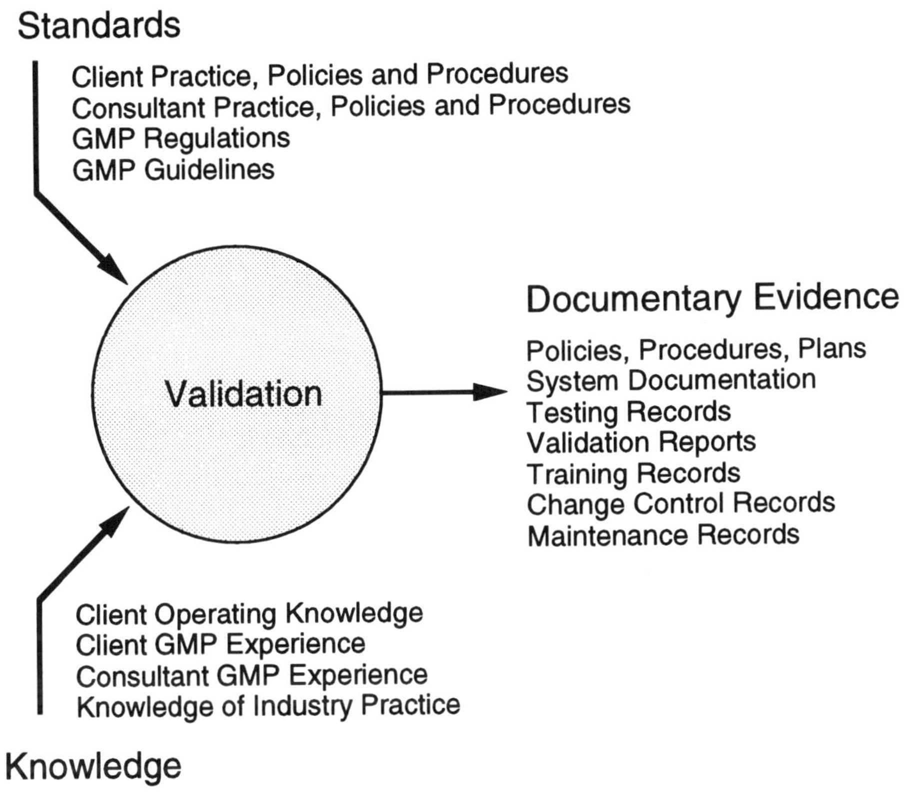

support organisation internal to the pharmaceutical manufacturing company. Consultants should be used only where they can demonstrate

- Technical competency (competent staff)
- Extensive experience (proven track record)
- Recognition of their expertise (nationally or internationally)
- Cost-effectiveness (customer commendations)

Pharmaceutical manufacturers must maintain records stating the name, address, and qualifications of any consultants used and the type of service they provided. Suppliers should inform pharmaceutical manufacturers where they employ a consultant on a specific project in case the manufacturer considers it prudent to keep a record of that consultancy in respect to the delivered validation by the supplier.

THE GMP REGULATOR'S PERSPECTIVE

Whilst there are no obvious differences in the basic principles of validation expected by the various GMP regulatory authorities (see Table 6.1), different regulators will not necessarily accept each other's findings. It is important, therefore, to understand the different operating philosophies held by GMP regulators. There is, nevertheless, one common attribute of the GMP regulatory authorities and that is their need for documentary evidence of validation or, as members of the FDA often put it, "In God we trust, everyone else needs documentation". This stringent approach has largely come about as a result of the "Generic Drug Scandal" in the late 1980s when the FDA uncovered instances of fraud by pharmaceutical manufacturers.

Inspection Practice

Inspections determine if processes are adequately validated with documented evidence that provides a high degree of assurance that a specific

Table 6.1. Regulatory Requirements of Automation Systems

Australian Code of GMP Medicinal Products—Part 1, Section 9	European Union Directive (GMP) 91/356/EEC Annex 11	United States Code of Federal Regulations, Title 21, Part 211 (GMP) Clause 68
Competent personnel	Competent personnel	Calibrated, inspected and checked to assure proper performance
Validation life cycle	Validation life cycle	Maintain written records
Maintain written records	Contracted out services	Authorised changes
Detailed description	Detailed description	Verify accuracy of inputs and outputs
Processing checks	Processing checks	Security
Software quality	Software quality	Backup data files
Testing	Siting of equipment	Hard-copy records (or alternative)
Operating procedures	Testing	
Operator training	Change control	
Change control	Record and analyse errors with corrective actions	
Security	Security	
Contingency plan	Contingency plan	
Data storage	Data storage	
Ongoing evaluation		

process will consistently produce a product meeting its predetermined specifications and quality characteristics [7]. Inspections are conducted before a new drug can be approved, to verify production method and technology changes, and periodically verify every two or three years that validation is being maintained. Increasing scrutiny is being applied to constituent automation systems [8].

The majority of inspectors working for regulatory agencies do not have specialised knowledge of computer systems and technology. Should the assigned regulatory agents responsible for an inspection be particularly anxious about the validation of automation, then advice and assistance can be requested from a specialist inspector within the agency.

The preparation for inspections includes a risk assessment based on the product, process, and technology mix including the use of automation systems, and a review of the company's inspection history. The assessment of automation systems forms only part of an inspection exercise for a manufacturing facility [9].

Once on-site, inspections by GMP regulators usually adopt a survey approach similar to the four-level review process promoted by the FDA [10]:

Level 1: Recognise how the automation system interacts with manufacturing.

Level 2: Evaluate the quality procedures used by pharmaceutical manufacturers to control their operations.

Level 3: Examine documentation in the validation package supporting an automation system.

Level 4: Review software source code as appropriate (Software Inspection).

The first review level is necessary to confirm the inspector's understanding of the criticality of automation systems and set the inspection priorities. This will involve discussions with the pharmaceutical manufacturer's senior technical management and a tour of the manufacturing facility. The second review level should identify poorly defined or missing procedures. This will affect the expectations of the third review level and the scope and detail of validation documentation. Particular automation systems subjected to inspection will have been identified in the first review level. During the tour, the GMP inspector may have noted component details of the automation system and any associated systems (computer hardware, software, and instrumentation) using a portable computer and checked that evidence of validation exists for these items [8]. The fourth review level is usually only invoked by specially trained GMP inspectors for software configurations and customisations, but may be extended to standard OTS packages where deficiencies are identified. Throughout the review process where customary or reasonable validation evidence is lacking or incomplete, inspection scrutiny may be increased [8]. Conversely, if the preliminary review of the validation evidence does not raise apparent or suspect problems [11], then scrutiny may be reduced.

The Validation Plan and Validation Report are typically amongst the first documents to be inspected. Inspections of automation systems are predicated on the assumption that pharmaceutical manufacturers have effective record retention systems [12]. Significant problems may arise during inspections where record storage or retrieval systems are inefficient or ineffective [8]. Sometimes GMP inspectors will ask for supplementary information to be sent to them once their site visit is finished.

Paul Humphreys of the Australian Therapeutic Goods Administration (TGA) recently gave the following insight into their inspection practice for validation documentation [13]:

Item 1: Computer System (including logic flow diagram or schematics, hardware layout and interaction, and functional requirements—GMP impact areas)

Item 2: System Control Documentation and Change Control

Item 3: Software Quality Assurance

Item 4: System Security (including backup)

Item 5: Data Changes (including audit trails, and critical data entry)

Item 6: System Validation (including operator training)

Auditing practices are widely discussed between regulatory authorities and a common approach is emerging. Opportunities for harmonising U.S. and European auditing practices are being investigated by the International Conference on Harmonisation (ICH) [14]. European and Australian auditing practices are harmonised through the Pharmaceutical Inspection Convention (PIC) [15].

ISO 9000 and Validation

Questions are often raised concerning the acceptability of ISO 9000 accreditation of pharmaceutical manufacturers and their suppliers in lieu of validation. GMP regulators do not accept this position. ISO 9000 and other software development processes do provide a foundation for validation, but they do not replace the specific needs of GMP validation. This perspective is supported by recent research which suggests that ISO 9000 and other software development processes help improve bad practices rather than improve good practices, although good practices may improve a little (see Figure 6.4) [16]. Those who are familiar with ISO 9000 will also know that the annual follow-up audits supporting an organisation's ongoing certification by an

Figure 6.4. Improving Quality of Programming

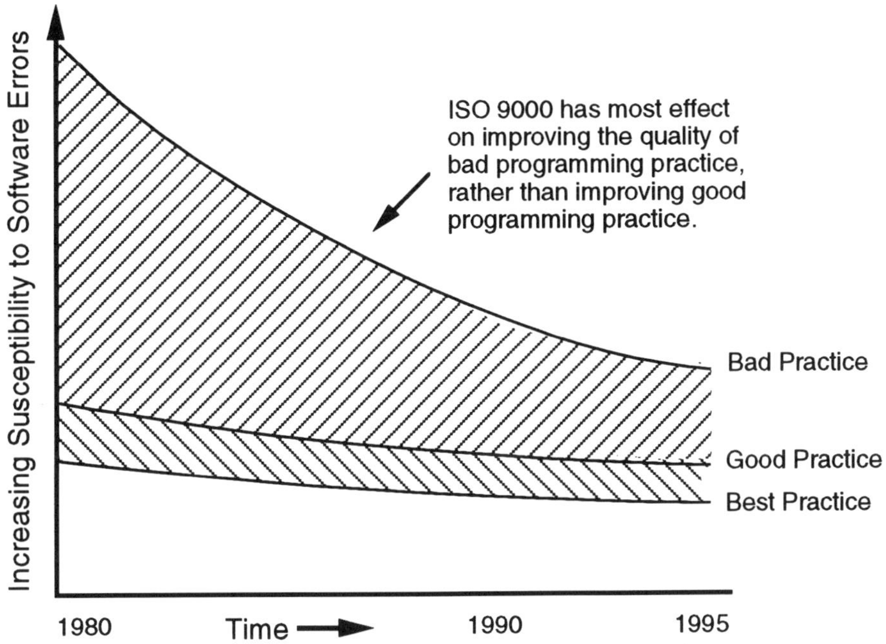

accredited body almost always uncover problems with management procedures and their application, even though some of these audits are very brief—perhaps only a day long. Holding an ISO 9000 certificate does not guarantee high quality work; it is just an indicator of capability. GMP regulators would seem to be right in their cautious attitude towards ISO 9000.

Constructive Relationships

Most GMP regulatory authorities have a very positive perspective toward the validation of automation systems and wish to develop constructive relationships with the pharmaceutical industry. Inspectors frequently attend conferences to present papers and participate in discussion panels. Indeed, recently, several European conferences have used live video links with the FDA. Inspectors will also take the opportunity to meet industry organisations, individual pharmaceutical manufacturers, suppliers, and consultants in specially arranged meetings to discuss validation issues. Such meetings cannot go into the specifics of particular automation system applications, but emerging issues and concerns can be raised and provide valuable information to validation practitioners. Discussions are often a two-way process, with the regulators not only giving clarification on their expectations but also seeking advice on what is practical and sensible. In addition, the EMEA and the U.S. FDA can both be contacted through the Internet on http://www.eudra.org/home.html and http://www.fda.gov, respectively. The result has been a pyramid of GMP assistance, as illustrated in Figure 6.5. The regulator's open attitude has been one of the primary factors for the success of validation in the pharmaceutical industry and, in particular, how to deal with emerging technologies and the novel application of automation systems.

Access to Inspection Findings

A citation of noncompliance, known as a "483", is drafted by the FDA at the close of the on-site inspection with a pharmaceutical manufacturer. An opportunity to clarify issues is given before the close of the inspection and the formal issue of the citation. Similar reports are written by the EU agencies and the Australian TGA, but unlike the FDA citations that are available to the public in accordance with the U.S. Freedom of Information Act, these reports are confidential to the inspected manufacturer and the regulatory authority.

GMP inspection reports are unlikely to have sections dedicated to the validation of automation systems. It is far more usual to note issues affecting automation systems with the production facility or service utility that was

Figure 6.5. Hierarchy of GMP Assistance

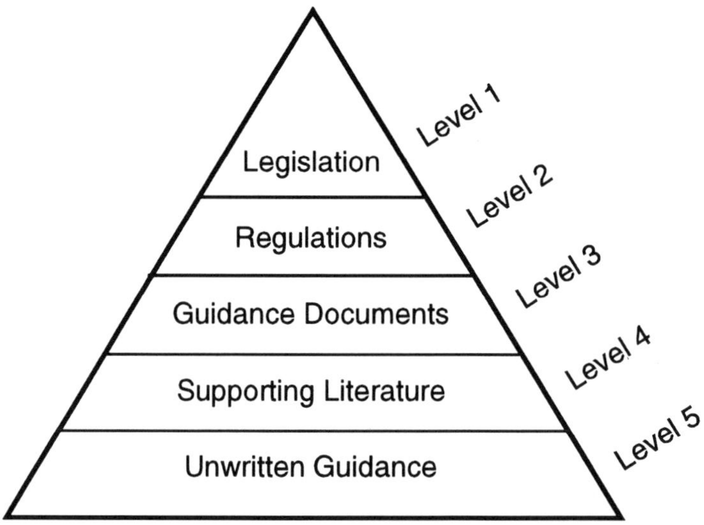

found GMP noncompliant. In summary, the GMP regulatory authorities require assurance regarding

- Life cycle approach adopted
- Risks to product identified
- Risks to product assessed
- Demonstrate risks controlled
- Validation management
- Independent auditing

If all these topics have been adequately instituted, then there should be no citations of GMP noncompliance affecting automation systems.

Poor Excuses

Many excuses have been given to GMP regulatory authorities when inspections have found validation to be deficient. Sam Clark, a former FDA investigator now working for Kempers-Masterson, recently listed some of the excuses offered to him when he was inspecting automation systems [17]. Clark listed these excuses under two categories. Firstly, some responses were from pharmaceutical manufacturers who simply did not validate an automation system that was inspected. The excuses offered included the following:

- We do not have the resources.
- We have used the system for years.
- We do not have anyone who can do that.
- It was done, just not documented.
- We got the system from a reputable supplier.

None of these excuses could be accepted. Pharmaceutical manufacturers should not release drug products whose manufacturing practice is not completely validated.

Secondly, other excuses were presented by pharmaceutical manufacturers for incomplete, inconsistent, or missing documentary evidence supporting validation:

- We do not need written procedures—all our people are professionals.
- We have excellent training programmes.
- We have done it this way for years and have not had any problems.
- It was done, just not documented.

Without documentation, there is no physical evidence that validation took place, regardless of whether it was sufficient. Hence, the saying "If it ain't written, it ain't done". GMP regulatory authorities may well believe on a personal level that a pharmaceutical manufacturer did conduct suitable validation, but there have been too many cases of fraud for the regulatory authorities to accept GMP compliance without documentary evidence. It is imperative that pharmaceutical manufacturers collate documentation supporting their validation as evidence to be presented to GMP regulators on inspection.

GMP AND FREE TRADE AGREEMENTS

As discussed in Chapter 1, GMP regulatory authorities, whilst government agencies, actually represent the interests of public health. It is occasionally suggested, nevertheless, that countries institute GMP as a means of protecting their domestic market for their national pharmaceutical manufacturers to supply. This issue is succinctly covered by the agreement on Technical Barriers to Trade (TBT) in the current General Agreement on Tariffs and Trade (GATT).

GATT is a global trade agreement instituted on 1 January 1948. It has been amended several times following international negotiations called "rounds". The most recent round, which dealt with TBT, was called the Uruguay Round and was formally ratified by 115 countries at Marrakech on 15 April 1994. The administration of GATT is the responsibility of the WHO. The Agreement necessitates GMP regulatory authorities to demonstrate that neither the intent nor the effect of their mandatory requirements on pharmaceutical manufacturers create unnecessary obstacles to international trade:

> *Members shall ensure that technical regulations are not prepared, adopted or applied with a view to or with the effect of creating unnecessary obstacles to international trade. For this purpose, technical regulations shall not be more trade-restrictive than necessary to fulfil a legitimate objective taking account of the risks of non-fulfilment would create. Such legitimate objectives are inter alia . . . . the prevention or deceptive practices [or] protection of human health or safety.*
> (Article 2.2)

There is no obligation to "harmonise down" to a common standard, providing Article 2.2 is not breached; there is, however, clear encouragement for harmonisation. Other free-trade agreements, such as the North America Free Trade Agreement (NAFTA) between Canada, Mexico, and the United States, are subordinate to GATT.

Embedded within GATT is a Code of Good Practice (CGP). The code has several important implications for the regulation of GMP:

- Foreign parties are to be given advance notice of developments in national GMP requirements and an opportunity to comment before they become mandatory.
- Mandatory GMP requirements are to be developed, wherever possible, from existing international standards. It is recognised that exemplary circumstances may exist, such as climatic or geographical factors or fundamental technological problems.
- Regulatory authorities are to establish, wherever possible, mutual recognition of other national GMP inspections.

The last two items above are embedded in the policy of the pharmaceutical industry's own Technical Requirements for Pharmaceuticals for Human Use as developed by the ICH. Western European GMP regulatory authorities have formed the PIC of GMP, which endeavours to assure uniform GMP compliance through the coordination and harmonisation of training for inspectors.

LEGISLATION COMPLEMENTING VALIDATION

Whilst the primary purpose of validation is to satisfy the GMP requirements of regulatory authorities representing the end consumer of drug products, it may also help meet other legislative obligations. Such legislation is usually based on the need for contracts to define agreed-on goods or services. Goods and services, including software-based systems [18], must correspond to their description and be of a merchantable quality (fit for purpose) [19,20,21]. Both GMP and contract law share the objective of fit for purpose and this should be achieved through good professional practice. Neither GMP requirements nor legislative obligations aim to be adversely restrictive, but rather to maintain standards and practices. There is, however, a difference in perspective. Whilst GMP holds the pharmaceutical manufacturer solely accountable, the other legislation obligations may allow liability to be shared with suppliers. In contract law, if the supplier knows the customer's application intent (regardless of the product's common usage), the goods or services must be fit for that intended purpose.

Contract Terms and Conditions

Contracts made in relation to validation work should make reference to the Validation Plan, any Supplier Quality Plans, and, where appropriate, the System Specification discussed in Chapter 3 to define the scope of work, goods, and services. The contract should include terms and conditions to define individual responsibilities, the assignment of responsibilities to third parties, confidentiality, intellectual property rights (IPR), and terms of payment. It is very important that infringements, liabilities, and insurance are also covered and how these are affected by circumstances outside the control of the pharmaceutical manufacturer and the supplier.

A "breach of contract" is established against noncompliance of a contract. Failure to supply an agreed product (goods or services) can result in a suite for damages. Product distributors are not normally liable unless they label products falsely or the original producer is unknown. GMP regulatory authorities hold pharmaceutical manufacturers accountable for ensuring contracted work is completed in compliance with GMP requirements, irrespective of whether any breaches of contract were attributable to suppliers. A manufacturer cannot pass on responsibility to their equipment suppliers.

Exclusion clauses are usually implemented as a defence against damages. However, within the United Kingdom, their use is limited, and negligence can never be the subject of such a clause [22]. Excessive and restrictive liabilities are often subject to a test of "reasonableness". Alternatively, indemnities can be used to pass damage responsibility to a third party who supplied the source of system noncompliance. There may, of course, be a joint responsibility between the primary subject of the breach of contract and the third party, in which case responsibility may be shared. In this way (depending on supply roles), a combination of system integrator, equipment hardware supplier, and software supplier may be held accountable for breach of contract between the customer and the primary supplier. Examples of accountability include software installed on an inappropriate hardware platform, system inappropriately used, or operational instructions not followed. Indemnity is strictly controlled through common law; there must be no doubt of accountability. Secondary contracts limiting the liability of the initial contract are legally permissible, but are unlikely to pass the "reasonableness" test. The EU Directive on Unfair Terms in Consumer Contracts (93/13/EEC) interprets all ambiguous contract clauses in favour of the customer, which in the case of validation is likely to be the pharmaceutical manufacturer [23].

Associated with the breach of contract is "misrepresentation". This is a misleading understanding given outside the contract, but that is integral to the contract agreement. Such an understanding might involve the qualification and experience of personnel implementing the contract. The pharmaceutical manufacturer or supplier may be allowed to rescind the contract, but only to recover costs where misrepresentation is fraudulent or negligent [24].

Duty and Standard of Care

Duty of care is based on avoiding reasonably foreseeable adverse consequences. The failure of "duty of care" implies negligence. It has been successfully applied to deficiencies in

- Design
- Construction
- Inspection
- User instructions
- Data security

and hence covers some basic attributes of GMP. In addition, there is the general expectation of safe operation [25,26,27]. Data security which includes access security is mandated in many counties by laws protecting individuals and organisations from the misuse of information [28].

Within the United Kingdom, a "standard of care" is imposed on the equipment producer who is liable to compensate the pharmaceutical manufacturer for personal loss but not for corporate damage [29]. The concept of "standard of care" is very similar to that of "duty of care".

Prosecution for negligence of care must usually be brought within some limited period from the date of supply. In the United Kingdom, this period is 3 years from loss or awareness of loss and cannot be brought after 10 years from the date of original supply. Other legislation may strengthen the regulation affecting some aspects of supply, such as supply chains [30].

Legal Defensive Positions

The overwhelming majority of contracts are brought to a successful close. If fulfilment of the contract is disputed, however, the prosecuted party has four basic defences:

1. Presentation of an ISO 9000–accredited quality system, adherence to established company and industry practices, and use of competent personnel.
2. Demonstrating the likelihood that the adverse consequence was introduced by the user subsequent to delivery by the supplier. Evidence of predelivery inspection and testing is required.
3. Presentation of a "development risk" whereby the bespoke nature of an application is presented as a source of acceptable risk. This argument, however, is usually self-defeating because in such circumstances it is "reasonable" to apply more rigorous development practices.

4. The goods or services supplied conform to the customer's formal requirements and it was these requirements that were deficient. In practice, user requirements are rarely precise enough to begin debating this defence.

These defences highlight the importance of mutual respect within a working supplier-customer relationship. It is in both parties interest to ensure contracts are fair and rigorous.

Liability of Personnel

Employees can, in theory, be sued for breach of contract if they are shown not to have taken reasonable care in their duties. In practice, this rarely happens due to the limited recoverable resources from the individual. Instead, the employee is subject to disciplinary action and the possibility of dismissal.

Negligent work by an employee under employer management or established employer practice is the responsibility of the employer. It is the employer's responsibility to demonstrate their management and practices were not negligent to defend against this position. Company directors representing the employer may be accountable for the employee's negligence if they have a duty covering the negligence and there is "gross negligence". Proving gross negligence in the absence of unambiguous evidence is extremely difficult.

Contractors under a "contract for services", like employees, can be sued for breach of contract where they are shown not to have taken reasonable care in their duties. In practice, however, because of their limited recoverable resources, it is far more likely that they will be dismissed. The position of contractors as "independent" for the purpose of prosecution for negligence is complex. Independence implies that the contractor worked outside employer management and employer practice. This is rarely the case and contractors are treated by the law as employees.

GMP regulatory authorities also have a "duty of care" to the pharmaceutical manufacturers inspected, but what constitutes their duties is not precisely defined. Few cases have been successfully brought by drug manufacturers against GMP regulators.

REFERENCES

1. Motise, P. (1996), *Inspection of Computerized Manufacturing Systems,* ISPE European Computer Systems Validation Conference, 24–25 September, Zurich, Switzerland.

2. Wingate, G.A.S., Smith, M., and Lucas, P.R. (1995), *Assuring Confidence in Pharmaceutical Software,* Safety and Reliability of Software Based Systems, First Annual ENCRESS Conference, September, Bruges, Belgium.

3. Wingate, G.A.S. (1996), Management for Operations Dependability, in *Life-Cycle Management for Systems Dependability*, edited by F. Redmill and C. Dale, Springer-Verlag.

4. Krankling, L. (1995), *Pharmaceutical Engineering* Interviews Ken Chapman, *Pharmaceutical Engineering,* 15(4): 46–49.

5. European Union Guide to Directive 91/356/EEC (1993), Computerised Systems, Annex 11, *Guide to Good Manufacturing Practice for Medicinal Products.*

6. U.S. Code of Federal Regulations Title 21, Part 210 (last amended 1994), *Current Good Manufacturing Practice in Manufacturing, Processing, Packaging, or Holding of Drugs;* Part 211 (last amended 1995), *Current Good Manufacturing Practice for Finished Pharmaceuticals.*

7. FDA (1987), *General Principles of Process Validation,* Rockville, MD: Food and Drug Administration, Center for Drug Evaluation and Research.

8. Tetzlaff, R.F. (1992), GMP Documentation Requirements for Automated Systems: Parts 1, 2, and 3, *Pharmaceutical Technology.*

9. Trill, A.J. (1993), Computerised Systems and GMP—A UK Perspective, Part 1: Background, Standards and Methods; Part 2: Inspection Findings; Part 3: Best Practices and Topical Issues, *Pharmaceutical Technology International.*

10. *The Gold Sheet* (1996), 30 (7), July.

11. Tetzlaff, R.F. (1993), Validation Issues for New Drug Development: Part 3, Systematic Audit Technique, *Pharmaceutical Technology.*

12. FDA (1992), Compliance Program Guideline Manual, 7346.832, Pre-Approval Inspection Investigations, Rockville, MD: Food and Drug Administration.

13. Humphreys, P. (1996), *Australian GMP Trends for Computer Systems,* ISPE/PDA Joint Conference on Computer-Related System Validation, 2–3 May, Basel.

14. Kessler, D.A. (1994), Harmonisation, *Pharmaceutical Engineering.*

15. PIC (1992), *Guide to Good Manufacturing Practice for Pharmaceutical Products,* Convention for the Mutual Recognition of Inspection in Respect of the Manufacture of Pharmaceutical Products (PIC), Document PH 5/92, Pharmaceutical Inspection Convention.

16. Hatton, L. (1997), Unexpected (and Sometimes Unpleasant) Lessons from Data in Real Software Systems, *Safety and Reliability of Software Based Systems,* Springer-Verlag.

17. Clark, A.S. (1995), Inspection of Software Systems, ISPE European Computer System Validation, 20–21 September, Zurich.

18. Lloyd, I.J. and Simpson, M.J. (1997), Computer Risks and Some Legal Consequences, *Safety and Reliability of Software Based Systems,* Springer-Verlag.

19. UK Sales of Goods Act (1974).

20. UK Supply of Goods and Services Act (1982).

21. U.S. Food, Drugs and Cosmetics Act.

22. UK Unfair Contract of Terms Act (1977).

23. Unfair Terms in Consumer Contracts, EU Directive 93/13/EEC (1993).
24. UK Misrepresentation Act (1967).
25. UK Supply of Machinery Regulations (1992).
26. UK Health and Safety at Work Act (1974).
27. UK Environmental Protection Act (1990).
28. UK Data Protection Act (1984).
29. UK Consumer Protection Act (1987).
30. UK Product Safety Regulations (1994).

APPENDIX 6A. DEFICIENT DOCUMENTARY EVIDENCE

Failure to use standardised document formats

Incomplete definitions

Constraints not cited

Formulae inconsistencies

Inappropriate or inconsistent "<" and ">"

Legends with inconsistent or misleading scales

Excessive changes

Different corrections not distinguished

Not reporting significant changes

Standard reports and forms not used (raw data recorded informally)

Illegible writing

Raw data records not available

Inconsistent dates

Inconsistent units of measure

Lack of double checking for accuracy

Not reporting all adverse reactions

Problems and deviations not fully reported

Unusual or unexpected recorded results

Records retained informally

Inappropriate procedures

Deficient procedures

Staff responsibilities not defined

Training records not up to date

Poorly organised documents and records

Hard-to-follow documents and records

Report conclusions that seem too good to be true

Reports with exaggerated claims

Reports with political half-truths

Reports with incorrect absolute terms (all, every, none, never, etc.)

Chapter 7

Validation Capability

Validation covers many activities that can be classified as responsible engineering rather than specific to GMP. When budgeting for validation, it is important to distinguish between responsible engineering and specific validation requirements. It is the experience and opinion of the author that validation implemented by competent and experienced practitioners should add no more than 5 percent to the project cost of a new automation system, and there is scope to reduce this percentage. This additional effort is usually associated with the system's qualification rather than its development. It is also suggested that the validation of existing automation systems can cost up to five times more than validating a new system. This will vary, however, depending on the use of competent and experienced validation practitioners and the suitability of existing documentation to support validation. If validation costs are greater than these, then it is probably either due to excessive validation work or attributing quality management support work to validation. It is very important when planning validation budgets to understand where the costs of a project are actually spent.

PERSONNEL

Personnel with general computer awareness and who are inexperienced with the requirements of validation will typically take twice as long to validate as experienced practitioners. Specific experience of the system under validation should reduce this to one and a half times longer than experienced validation practitioners. It is because of metrics like these that many pharmaceutical manufacturers have developed their own internal validation expertise or used experienced validation consultants to validate their automation systems.

The capability of personnel has, in the past, been dependent on their professionalism. This, however, is no longer enough. Pharmaceutical manufacturers must be able to demonstrate the capability of their personnel to GMP regulatory authorities and this necessitates documentary evidence. When selecting validation personnel, the following profiles should be considered:

Profile of a Validation Expert

- graduate or post-graduate in science discipline
- four or more years of GMP experience with computer systems
- very good communicator
- validation experience with more than 1 company
- journal publications or conference presentations

Experts should have experience in validation within more than one organisation. Practitioners must take care not to slip into a mind-set that there is only one way to validate. Instead they should be flexible in their approach so that when the inevitable problems arise, minds are not closed to exploring new solutions. Validation experts do not have to be leaders as long as they are supported by managers and they can eloquently express their views to those managers so that the appropriate direction can be given to the validation engineers.

Profile of a Validation Engineer

- technical background involving computer systems
- technical qualifications associated with computing systems
- two or more years of GMP experience, not necessarily involving computer systems

A validation engineer must have a certain tenacity to complete work and be able to progress work without constantly seeking advice. This is not to say, however, that they should be discouraged from seeking advice, but they should have sufficient judgement and validation knowledge to make some basic decisions themselves.

Management Style

Managers should not rely on the experience of individual personnel alone. When assembling validation teams, it should be remembered that less experienced personnel can be given additional training either through formal courses, attendance at industry seminars and conferences, or informally by working in teams containing seasoned practitioners. The personal motivation and commitment of each individual is also crucial. Many organisations recognise this and promote a positive attitude amongst staff:

- Aim for "how we can" rather than "why we can't".
- Do not be limited to (perceived) constraining perspectives.
- Avoid working in isolation and seek (but not to distraction) the opinion of colleagues.
- Give constructive feedback.
- Prepare for meetings and make a positive contribution.
- Make statements that add value and stick to the subject at hand.
- Explain reasons for disagreements and offer alternatives.
- Be specific when making commitments and honour their enactment.

Where staff have a negative attitude, management should consider ensuring their staff:

- Have a higher visibility of the development process.
- Be given a clear definition of product requirements.
- Be assigned clear job responsibilities.
- Be allowed to concentrate on design and not control.
- Give prompt feedback on project issues.

This will result, hopefully, in increased job satisfaction. It should be recognised, however, that some staff enjoy fire fighting and believe a structured approach restricts their initiative. The aim is to not to dictate but rather to give guidance within a validation framework.

Estimates of days' effort for validation activities presented in this chapter are based on the premise that experienced and motivated practitioners are used to conduct the validation. Planners should make allowances that, towards the end of a project, the effectiveness of personnel tends to reduce because of lost project momentum. Pharmaceutical manufacturers can compensate for this by giving the achievement of planned milestones a high profile in their organisations and duly praising staff and suppliers when work schedules are fulfilled. If there is a clear definition of work, then a fixed price should be negotiated with suppliers. Sometimes, however, the nature of the work cannot be fully specified, in which case phased projects are more appropriate. Either a fixed-price first phase can be offered to a supplier to plan and define the remaining work, which can then be conducted under a fixed-price arrangement, or a time-and-materials approach may be adopted until work has progressed to a point where a fixed price can be offered to complete the work. Both of these mechanisms should help work close out as planned without the final stages going on and on apparently out of control.

EFFORT TO VALIDATE NEW SYSTEMS (PROSPECTIVE VALIDATION)

Industry metrics for validating new systems (known as prospective validation) are given in Table 7.1 and assume that work is conducted by experienced validation practitioners and that established procedures for conducting validation are available. The estimates take account of some variable factors, as indicated in the right-hand column of the table, and are based on practical experience.

The metrics presented assume that the supplier's normal working practices are sufficient to satisfy ISO 9000. Suppliers will normally quote additional work for validation. The extra work normally covers documentation

Table 7.1. Metrics for Validating New Automation Systems

<table>
<tr><th rowspan="3">Validation Activity</th><th colspan="4">Days Effort Per Automation System</th><th rowspan="3">Notes/Factors for Consideration</th></tr>
<tr><th>Small</th><th>Medium</th><th>Large</th><th>Very Large</th></tr>
<tr><th>PLC, IPC</th><th>SCADA</th><th>DCS, MES</th><th>MRP II</th></tr>
<tr><td>GMP Assessment</td><td>3</td><td>5</td><td>7</td><td>10</td><td>Complexity of system
Poor supplier support +25%
Each MRP II site +25%</td></tr>
<tr><td>Supplier Audit</td><td>4</td><td>4</td><td>4</td><td>5</td><td>Per supplier</td></tr>
<tr><td>Validation Plan</td><td>3</td><td>4</td><td>4</td><td>5</td><td></td></tr>
<tr><td>System Specification</td><td colspan="4" rowspan="4">The supplier should be conducting this work, as it is not specifically supporting validation. The level of documentary evidence produced by the supplier's normal working practices, however, may not be sufficient to support validation. The additional requirements for validation should not normally exceed 3-5% of the cost of the automation system.</td><td rowspan="4">Complexity and degree of bespoke development:-
Configuration?
Macros?
Customisation?
Interfaces?
Other bespoke features?</td></tr>
<tr><td>Design & Development</td></tr>
<tr><td>Build</td></tr>
<tr><td>Predelivery Testing</td></tr>
<tr><td>On-Site Testing</td><td>10</td><td>15</td><td>25</td><td>40</td><td>Phased roll-out +50%
Each MRP II site +30%
Each comms link +10%</td></tr>
<tr><td>Validation Report</td><td>4</td><td>6</td><td>7</td><td>10</td><td>Include general review of validation document pack</td></tr>
<tr><td>TOTAL</td><td>24+</td><td>34+</td><td>47+</td><td>70+</td><td>Project Management?</td></tr>
</table>

practice rather than additional systems engineering. This additional amount should not normally exceed 3–5 percent of the cost of the automation system. The percentage should be nearer 3 percent for large systems such as MRP II, and not exceed 5 percent for smaller systems such as PLC applications. If the percentages are larger than this, then questions should be asked whether the supplier is charging too much—perhaps they do not understand what is required or how they can most efficiently conduct the extra work.

Suppliers of automation systems can reduce the cost of System Specification, Design & Development, System Build, and Predelivery Testing if they spread the cost over several similar systems. Pharmaceutical manufacturers can similarly reduce the cost of Supplier Audits, Validation Plans, and On-Site Testing, if they use similar automation systems elsewhere in their manufacturing operations. Validation Reports are specific to individual automation systems, and there is little opportunity for pharmaceutical manufacturers to reduce the cost of this activity other by ensuring the validation project has few issues requiring reporting. Pharmaceutical manufacturers may also reduce costs by sharing documentation or conducting joint Supplier Audits with other manufacturers.

The metrics given for an MRP II system's On-Site Testing should be read with caution because they are based on the GMP–specific testing required and do not take into account general application testing. It is assumed that non-GMP functionality has already been tested. The amount of GMP–specific testing required can vary considerably depending on whether the system is used at a single or multiple sites, and how the system (or variant) is used at each site. Supplementary testing may also be required to establish confidence in the GMP capability of the supplier's core MRP II product, if the Supplier Audit has uncovered deficiencies in the supplier's development practice.

EFFORT TO VALIDATE EXISTING SYSTEMS (RETROSPECTIVE VALIDATION)

Retrospective validation is conducted when an existing automation system must fulfil the requirements of GCP/GMP/GLP but has already been developed without validation. Factors that will affect the effort required to validate an existing system include the following:

- Staff stability during the system's original development
- Age of the original software and whether it was developed in accordance with a quality life-cycle methodology
- Hardware stability during the system's lifetime
- Programming languages used
- Programming style and formats used

- Level of documentation supporting the system's original development
- Implementation of change control throughout system's lifetime

Some of these factors have been taken into account for the estimates given in Table 7.2 (see the right-hand column). All of the industry metrics given in the table assume that work is conducted by experienced validation practitioners and that established procedures for conducting validation are available. Practitioners must not take these estimates as absolute and should themselves consider each retrospective validation project on a case-by-case basis to take account of the individual influences affecting the validation of existing automation systems. This is especially so for the testing metrics which are based on the assumption that the automation system in question is in a period (several years) of highly reliable operation, having had only a

Table 7.2. Metrics for Validating Existing Automation Systems

<table>
<tr><td rowspan="3">Validation Activity</td><td colspan="4">Days Effort Per Automation System</td><td rowspan="3">Notes/Factors for Consideration</td></tr>
<tr><td>Small</td><td>Medium</td><td>Large</td><td>Very Large</td></tr>
<tr><td>PLC, IPC</td><td>SCADA</td><td>DCS, MES</td><td>MRP II</td></tr>
<tr><td>GMP Assessment</td><td>3</td><td>5</td><td>7</td><td>10</td><td>Poor documentation +25%
Poor supplier support +25%
Each MRP II site +25%</td></tr>
<tr><td>Supplier Audit</td><td>4</td><td>4</td><td>4</td><td>5</td><td>Per supplier but audit not always necessary</td></tr>
<tr><td>Validation Plan</td><td>3</td><td>4</td><td>4</td><td>5</td><td></td></tr>
<tr><td rowspan="2">System Specification</td><td colspan="4">Collate and repackage existing documentation with supplements as necessary.</td><td rowspan="2">No documentation +200%
Poor documentation +100%
Each comms link +10%</td></tr>
<tr><td>10</td><td>15</td><td>20</td><td>50</td></tr>
<tr><td>Design & Development</td><td colspan="4" rowspan="3">Automation system has already been delivered without validation.
Conduct Design Qualification, Software Inspection and Hazard Study (3-5 days each) to verify system design as used.</td><td rowspan="4">Complexity and degree of bespoke development
Each MRP II site +30%
Large MES +50%</td></tr>
<tr><td>Build</td></tr>
<tr><td rowspan="2">Predelivery Testing</td></tr>
<tr><td>9</td><td>12</td><td>15</td><td>30</td></tr>
<tr><td rowspan="2">On-Site Testing</td><td colspan="4">On-Site Testing may need to repeat some Predelivery Testing to confirm core system functionality</td><td rowspan="2">No evidence of Predelivery Testing +200%
Poor evidence of Predelivery Testing +100%
Each MRP II site +30%
Each comms link +10%</td></tr>
<tr><td>15</td><td>25</td><td>35</td><td>50</td></tr>
<tr><td>Validation Report</td><td>4</td><td>6</td><td>7</td><td>10</td><td>Include general review of validation document pack</td></tr>
<tr><td>TOTAL</td><td>48+</td><td>71+</td><td>92+</td><td>160+</td><td>+ Project Management</td></tr>
</table>

few cosmetic changes during this period. Testing in such circumstances is often limited to include all critical GMP functionality, a check on all GMP–sensitive data, and some general tests (including challenge tests) to confirm the system's defined operation.

Suppliers and pharmaceutical manufacturers alike can reduce the cost of retrospectively validating automation systems by spreading the cost of GMP Audits, Supplier Audits, System Specification, and On-Site Testing over several similar systems. Pharmaceutical manufacturers may also reduce costs by sharing documentation or conducting joint Supplier Audits with other manufacturers. Conducting Design Qualification, Software Inspection, and Hazard Study will normally take between 3 and 5 days each to verify system design as used, depending on the complexity of the system. Validation Reports are specific to individual automation systems, and there is little opportunity for pharmaceutical manufacturers to reduce the cost of this activity other than by ensuring the validation project has few issues requiring reporting.

Suppliers leading retrospective validation will typically require an additional 20 percent days' effort in the form of support from the pharmaceutical manufacturer. The support will include understanding the automation system's development history, understanding the current intent of the automation system, and technical advice.

IMPROVING AN ORGANISATION'S CAPABILITY

Experience has shown the significant advantages for suppliers of automation systems (internally within pharmaceutical manufacturing organisations, systems' integrators, and equipment vendors) who improve their validation capability. In particular, the risk of noncompliant validation is reduced, and conducting validation itself becomes more cost effective and time efficient. Annual returns on investment for the quality improvement of computer-related systems in other industries have ranged from 4.5 [1] to 7.5 [2]. Similar dividends would be expected for the pharmaceutical industry.

ISO 9000 alone does not provide a suitable framework for improving validation capability. The standard focusses on improvement in processes and ignores due regard for the quality of the end product. As the Director of Corporate Quality at Motorola comments:

> *With ISO 9000 you can still have terrible processes and products, you can certify a manufacturer that makes life jackets from concrete, as long as those jackets are made according to documented procedures and the company provides the next of kin with instructions on how to complain about defects* [3].

The Quality Manager of Oracle UK also notes that ISO 9000 cannot be relied on as a statement that supplied products or services are fit for purpose [4].

Indeed, automation systems often carry a warranty similar to that shown below:

> *Although the software producer has tested the software and reviewed its associated documentation, the software producer makes no warranty or representation, either expressly or implied, with respect to the software or documentation, its quality, performance, merchantability, or fitness for a particular purpose. The licensee assumes the entire risk with regard to the use of the software and documentation.*

A framework recognising the symbiosis between both process and product was first proposed by the Software Engineering Institute (SEI) at Carnegie Mellon University and called the Capability Maturity Model (CMM). The CMM framework is based on five evolutionary levels of capability from ad hoc, chaotic processes to mature, disciplined processes [5]:

Level 1: The quality process is characterised as ad hoc and occasionally even chaotic. Few processes are defined, and success depends on individual efforts and heroics.

Level 2: Basic project management processes are established to track cost, schedule, and functionality. The necessary process discipline is in place to repeat earlier successes on projects with similar applications.

Level 3: The quality processes for both management and engineering activities is documented, standardised, and integrated into a standard quality process for the organisation. All projects use an approved, tailored version of the organisation's standard quality process for developing and maintaining systems.

Level 4: Detailed measures of the quality process and product quality are collected. Both the quality process and products are quantitatively understood and controlled.

Level 5: Continuous process improvement is enabled by quantitative feedback from the process and from piloting innovative ideas and technologies.

An assessment of capability generates a profile from which an organisation can identify necessary initiatives to support a general improvement in capability. In the same manner, the profile can help organisations prevent management oversight of crucial activities supporting a level of capability.

Brian Dodd of Searle Pharmaceuticals recently reported that most pharmaceutical manufacturers are at Level 3 or Level 4 and are content with their capability [6]. Surely as an industry, should we not aspire to Level 5 and endeavour to improve our capability? The continuous improvement of Level 5 should be accompanied by manufacturing performance improvement (MPI).

Whilst there is an inevitable cost associated with validation, this can be offset by tangible MPI benefits to the extent that they could equate to or even exceed the cost of validation.

The proliferation of process improvement models (ESPRIT's BOOTSTRAP, British Telecom's Software Assessment Method (SAM), Hewlett-Packard's Software Quality and Productivity Analysis (SQPA), Scottish Enterprise & Compita's Software Technology Diagnosis (STD), and Bell Canada's TRILLIUM) based on SEI's CMM framework and the current development of a proposed international standard (SPICE) substantiate the value of the CMM framework [7].

An adaptation of SEI's CMM framework for application to the validation of automation systems is shown in Figure 7.1. This is not a definitive capability framework, rather it aims to indicate how one might be developed. An additional sixth level (0) has been added to deal with organisations who have not yet embarked on any validation capability.

The validation capability framework can be used by pharmaceutical manufacturers for self-inspection or for Supplier Audits. The framework should be accompanied by a questionnaire to assess accurately the organisation's capability. Organisations will often have a capability profile that includes elements of capabilities from several levels. The assessed level of capability will be that with which an organisation is entirely compliant. Some validation capabilities and characteristics are shown alongside each of the capability levels in Figure 7.1, which should help organisations place themselves within the framework.

In the capability framework presented, it has proven quite difficult to align validation activities between Level 3 and Level 4. The divide suggested is based on an established project by project capability of Level 3 compared to the ongoing inherent organisational capability of Level 4. In the framework, Level 4 equates to a fully compliant regime of validation for GMP. A capability below this level will almost certainly be regarded by GMP regulatory authorities as insufficient for GMP. Noncompliance may not be identified on an initial or limited inspection. Pharmaceutical manufacturers must not become complacent and should prepare for further and detailed inspections. The regulator's position with individual cases of GMP noncompliance will vary with the severity of the deficiencies they find. Generally, however, they will give the pharmaceutical manufacturer a period of time to take corrective actions before they take the matter further.

Level 5 in the capability framework, meanwhile, signifies the opportunity for pharmaceutical manufacturers and their suppliers to reap the reward of tangible MPI benefits discussed earlier. Principal capabilities associated with Level 5 might include selecting preferred suppliers, conducting joint Supplier Audits with other organisations and sharing audit reports, developing in-house validation experts, conducting internal capability assessments to identify improvement opportunities, and planning for technology migration to exploit any new innovations.

Figure 7.1. Validation Capability Framework

Capability Level	Organisational Characteristics	Principle Capabilities	Validation Outcome
5 *Continuous Improvement*	Ongoing evaluation of validation experience -o- Pilot innovative ideas and technology	Preferred Suppliers Shared Audits Validation Experts Capability Assessments Technology Migration	*increasing cost-effectiveness & time efficiency*
4 *Managed*	Quantitative -o- Establish metrics for validation practice -o- Problem prevention	Validation Policy Supplier Audits Intergroup Coordination Contingency Plans Security & Access Practice Backup and Restoration Performance Monitoring Training Records Periodic Review	
3 *Standardised*	Qualitative -o- Validation practice is documented	Commitment of Senior Management Assigned Validation Staff Validation & Quality Plans Project Procedures Formal Peer Reviews Change Control Quality Assurance Document Control	
2 *Repeatable*	Validation is managed -o- Learning may be lost	User Requirements Project Plans Informal Internal Reviews Some End of Project Reports Quality Control Document Archive	
1 *Ad hoc*	No discernible management -o- Often chaotic	Commitment of Individuals	*increasing risk of validation noncompliance*
0 *Not Performed*	No requirement to validate, or do not yet understand how to apply validation		

Based on the experience of the author, most pharmaceutical manufacturers who have embarked on validation are at Level 3 or Level 4. The exception are those pharmaceutical manufacturers whose senior management are still not committed to the implementation of validation and rely on their subordinates to enact validation without the practical support they could offer. Such pharmaceutical manufacturers are usually at Level 2, having passed through a transitional period of the ad hoc approach characterised in Level 1.

A slightly different situation exists with suppliers of automation systems to the pharmaceutical industry. Suppliers generally understand the benefits of a quality approach, but unless the pharmaceutical industry forms a significant proportion of their sales, then it is unlikely they really understand how their quality approach relates to the requirements of validation, despite what the supplier's salesmen might say. For this reason, whilst a supplier might be Level 3 or 4 on the CMM, the same supplier is likely to be Level 2 on the validation capability framework. It is very important for pharmaceutical manufacturers to undertake a Supplier Audit to determine the actual capability of their suppliers, and, in particular, to assess the competence of personnel assigned to their project.

REDUCING COSTS

The cost of automation validation can appear prohibitive, and one option to reduce costs is to stop using automation systems. This option, however, means that the benefits of implementing automation systems, namely improved manufacturing performance and product quality, are lost.

Alternatively, investigating the efficiency of validation practices can lead to improved methods and reduced cost. For example, it may be cheaper to replace existing automation systems rather than validate existing systems, and managers should evaluate the relative costs before the start of a project. There are numerous other opportunities for reducing the cost of validation, including the following:

- Early definition and controlled maintenance of cost-effective working practices: improved working efficiency.
- Off-site contractor work packages: reduced infrastructure costs.
- Experienced validation staff: reduced learning curve.
- Reuse of validation experience between similar computer systems: improved working efficiency.
- Independent checks on coordination and consistency of working practices: reduce inefficiencies.
- Review validation practice, keep it simple: excessive paperwork and management is burdensome and an unnecessary cost.

- Joint Supplier Audits between pharmaceutical manufacturers: share the cost of audit activity.

This list of options is not exhaustive and not all will be appropriate to any one organisation. Nevertheless, no organisation can afford to ignore such opportunities in the current economic climate. Having said this, when making savings, it is important not to be too zealous such that the satisfactory GMP compliance is compromised. The cost of noncompliance (e.g., nonissue, delay, or revoking of a drug licence) can be significantly more expensive than, what in hindsight, might appear to be a marginal validation saving.

An analysis by management consultants KPMG of overbudget costs is presented in Table 7.3 and highlights some key areas for validation project manager to consider. The main problems are associated with project control, not the selection of particular software solutions or hardware platforms. The individual capability of project managers is vital, as is the ability of project team members to communicate effectively between themselves and end users. The consequences of early delays in a project, for whatever reason, must not be quietly forgotten under the belief that the project can catch up later. The ramifications of delays must be incorporated into revised project plans and their impact on overall project timings and cost reported to senior management at an early stage so that a way forward can be agreed on. There is nothing worse than shattering senior management expectations of full delivery, on time to budget, with delays and overspending just before the project's original date of completion. Further, project managers must ensure that a clear and unambiguous project definition exists which is understood by all parties concerned with the project. Validation Plans and User Requirements Specifications must be complete and approved before the project's implementation begins; suppliers must understand how they fit in. This is especially so for projects involving automation system technologies and/or new drug manufacturing applications with which the project team is not experienced. The lessons derived from Table 7.3 are not peculiar to validation projects; it's just common sense. Some organisations formally conduct risk analysis excerises to assess and manage perceived project risks.

Table 7.3. Reasons for Increased Project Costs

Problem	Percentage of Projects Affected
Inadequate Project Management	32%
Lack of Communication	20%
Poor Project Definition	17%
Unfamiliar with Application	17%
Inappropriate System Selection	9%

REFERENCES

1. Humphrey, W.S., Snyder, T., and Willis, R. (1991), Software Process Improvement at Hughes Aircraft, *IEEE Software*, (July): 11–24.
2. Dion, R. (1992), Elements of a Process Improvement Program, *IEEE Software,* 17(2): 39–42.
3. Henkoff, R. (1993), The Hot New Seal of Quality, *Fortune International,* (28 June): 62–65.
4. Coaster, A. (1992), *ISO 9002: The Good, the Bad, the Ugly,* Proceedings of the Third European Conference on Software Quality, November, Madrid.
5. Paulk, M.C. (1995), The Evolution of the SEI's Capability Maturity Model for Software, *Software Process—Improvement and Practice* (Pilot Issue): 3–15.
6. Dodd, B. (1996), *Why Harmonisation? Overview of Worldwide Regulatory Situation on Computer Systems*, PDA/ISPE Joint Conference on Computer-Related System Validation, 2–3 May, Basel, Switzerland.
7. Rout, T.P. (1995), SPICE: A Framework for Software Process Assessment, *Software Process—Improvement and Practice* (Pilot Issue): 57–66.

Chapter 8

Topical Issues

PENTIUM® PROCESSORS

Between 1983 and 1995, certain versions of Pentium® processors manufactured by Intel contained a defect in floating point divide operations. Automation systems based on this processor that are used in GMP applications must be identified and evaluated to determine whether any use of the erroneous operation is detrimental to the application. Several options exist if there is detrimental effect: replacement of the defective processor, software modification, or withdrawal of the system from its GMP application. Intel has undertaken to replace, without charge, defective Pentium® processors with an upgraded processor version that does not have the defect. The entire process of identification, evaluation, and corrective actions should be documented and any changes fully tested [1].

STANDARD SOFTWARE

Stating that a piece of software is "standard" is not sufficient in itself to relax the pharmaceutical manufacturer's responsibility for testing a software product. There is no magic number of applications that can be quoted to qualify a piece of software as "standard". Indeed, it has been suggested that 20 percent of the operational errors experienced by automation systems can be attributed to standard software, so the validation of such software would appear to be very important [2].

Standard software should not be used until it has been assessed to determine whether exact copies have been widely used for at least six months, and that the user community has not reported any problems that could affect its GMP application. Many so called "standard" products have many minor versions, each of which may only have a few users. Care must also be taken to establish that the product has been developed under a quality management system and is under version and change control. Recent press reports have passed surprise at the ad hoc software development used by some the world's best known software companies providing "standard" software products. Pharmaceutical manufacturers realising that they are early adopters should conduct additional testing and ensure they are kept informed of any problems as they are discovered in the user community.

Documentation accompanying standard software can be used to reduce significantly the amount of application documentation specifically produced by a pharmaceutical manufacturer for validation. Figure 8.1 illustrates how supplier documentation can complement a pharmaceutical manufacturer's validation package. The scope and detail of application-specific documentation will depend on how much configuration is needed to implement a supplier's OTS product. A Supplier Audit and GMP Assessment will be key to determining the quality of supplier documentation and the supplementary work required by the pharmaceutical manufacturer.

THE YEAR 2000 (Y2K)

Many problems will be experienced by automation systems when the year 2000 arrives. As recently reported in the press, a very large number of the automation systems developed before the 1990s have not made allowance for the year 2000 [3]. It must not be assumed that recently procured automation systems and software are immune to problems arising from the year 2000. IBM personal computers, for instance, have only been "millennium friendly" since 1995. Examples of potential "millennium bugs" are given in Table 8.1.

In addition to the problems listed in Table 8.1, there is also the issue of the ripple effect of errors within solutions integrating multiple software products or hardware platforms with coresident software, which is independent until a crash scenario occurs. Validation practitioners should take a "systems approach" and consider the collective impact of operating systems, network software, OTS software packages, and bespoke programs on the overall operability of an automation system. It should also be noted that whilst the original implementation of a system may be millenium friendly, subsequent modifications may not be.

The FDA has said that until the year 2000 arrives, it will not cite pharmaceutical manufacturers for not validating this aspect of their automation systems' operability unless the manufacturer has specified their systems to be

Figure 8.1. Validation Referencing Supplier's OTS Product Documentation

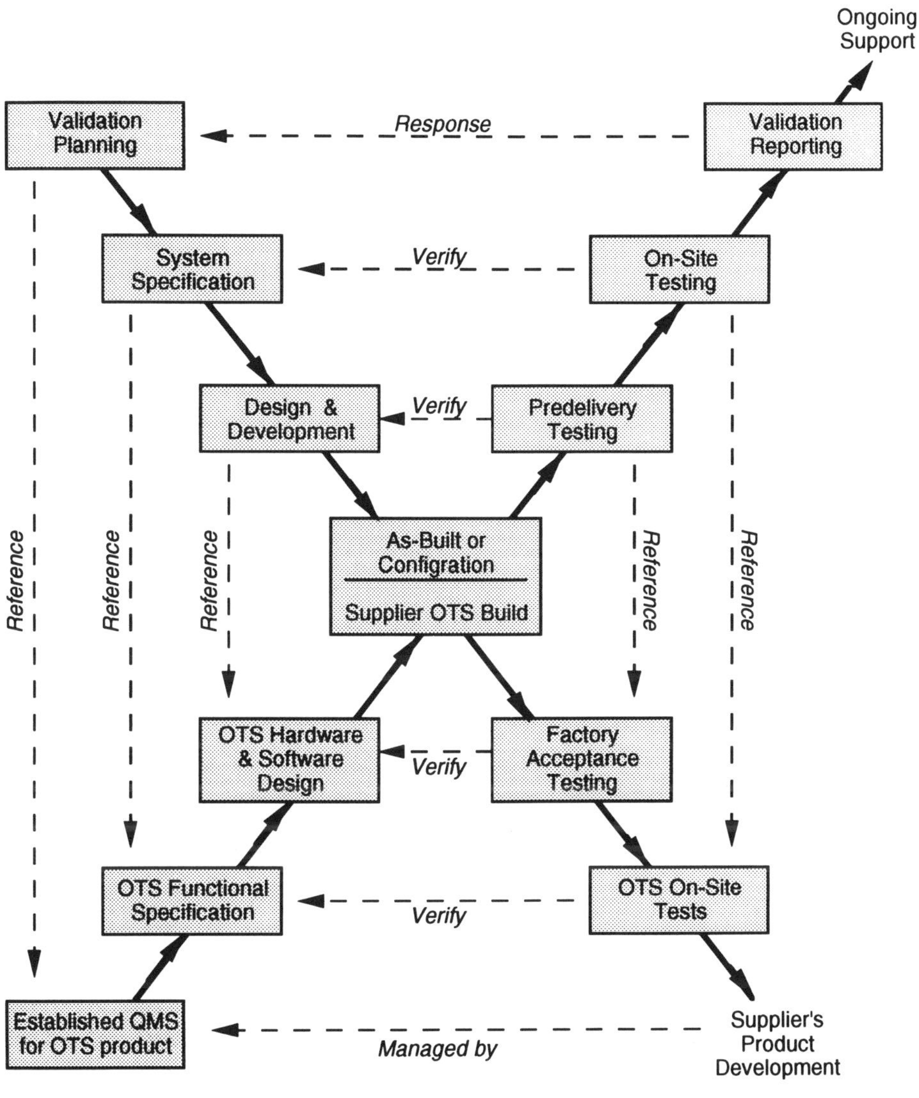

millennium friendly [3]. At the time this book went to press (June 1997), a policy statement on year 2000 inspection policy is awaited from other national GMP authorities. The MCA is already informally asking pharmaceutical manufacturers for Y2K assurance and have issued a guidance note [25].

There has been much speculation about the cost of removing millennium bugs and the potential high charges that might be made by suppliers

Table 8.1. Potential Y2K Problems

Stock Control	When the year 2000 arrives, those systems using the last two digits of the year for dates will overflow and the year will be interpreted as 1900. Stock control systems using the principle of first-in, first-out management control are, therefore, susceptible to malfunction. Stock received on or after 1 January 2000 will be viewed as being older than stock received before the year 2000. The result is that older stock will be left on the shelf—possibly leading to large stock write-offs when expiry dates are exceeded.
Quality Control	Some pharmaceutical manufacturers have already come across the date overflow problem with calculated shelf life and expiry dates for pharmaceutical products. Up to 1 January 2000, quality control dates which fall after 31 December 1999, will be viewed as expired because their "use by" year number is lower than the current year number.
Archive Management Systems	Databases and archive management software often have the facility to remove old items after a specified retention period. If the software has a date overflow problem, then it will delete items with retention dates beyond 31 December 1999, calculating that the retention period has passed.
Statistical Process Control	When sorting data into chronological sequence for analysis, possibly as part of a SCADA or LIMS system, the date overflow problem will manifest itself by placing data relating to the year 2000 before that of 1999. The problem may be readily diagnosable on simple trends, but it could generate hidden control problems which are not so easy to identify within complex Statistical Process Control (SPC) software calculations.
Batch Records	The year 2000 is a leap year, and it is an exception to the more widely known rule that century years are not leap years. Any batch record systems or systems that do not take account of this leap year will not include 29 February 2000 in their sequence of time stamps and will lead to audit trail problems.
Special Values	Some programmers have used 00 and 99 as a special values, possibly to signify a null input or end-of-file. The consequences of interpreting valid data with these special meanings has lead some practitioners to suggest that considerable amounts of GMP data could vanish at the turn of the century.

as the year 2000 approaches. Pharmaceutical manufacturers should start checking their automation systems, software licences, firmware, and Service Level Agreements (SLAs) now. Millennium bugs could cause catastrophic crashes, degraded system functionality, as well as corrupted or deleted manufacturing records. Millennium bugs are worth fixing before they are activated. Validation practitioners should be extremely wary of software packages that do not explicitly cite they are "millennium friendly". Many packages are likely to have been developed a number of years ago, or incorporate software that has evolved from earlier versions; therefore, they are unlikely to have considered the potential effect of the year 2000. In some instances, it may be more economic to replace an automation system or software package than make it millennium friendly, but such decisions should be made only by pharmaceutical manufacturers on a case-by-case basis. A list of millennium friendly software products is being collated by Taskforce 2000 on the Internet (http://www.weblaw.co.uk).

WINDOWS ENVIRONMENTS

Some Windows environments do not provide a pre-emptive multitasking environment with processing management provided through system calls within software. The following comments are related to Windows environments up to and including version 3.11. Windows 95® should alleviate many of these problems.

All Windows 3.11® applications share the same address space. This means that one Windows application can unintentionally corrupt the system resource (programming code or data) of another Windows application. Such faults are extremely difficult to track down. For example, an incorrectly loaded pointer in a program written in "C" may not directly affect that program, but rather affect an entirely unrelated application. The problem does not occur in Windows 95® because each application runs in a separate address space. It is important to note, however, that Windows 3.11® applications running under Windows 95® will still share a single address space, so the above hazard will still exist. There is no point in buying Windows 95® and using your original Windows 3.11® applications.

A similar issue exists with applications that crash. These applications can be reopened, but their originally allocated system resources will not be recovered. The system may be able to continue to run without any immediately noticeable effect on system performance. In the long term, however, as more Windows applications crash, the system's performance is likely to degrade and affect automation system control. To recover the system resources belonging to crashed Windows applications, the system's execution must be returned to DOS with the loss of all applications, and the environment must be established once more with its applications. It is important that these situations are covered by management and operator procedures.

Another concern with environments has been the propagation of software viruses. Whilst Windows 95® has proved less susceptible than DOS or version 3, viruses still pose a real threat to automation systems [4]. The cost of utilities to combat virus infections varies and does not necessarily reflect their effectiveness. Whichever utility is used, it should be frequently updated because new varieties of viruses continue to appear regularly.

Screensavers provide yet another hazard. Many are available without charge (freeware), are copied and distributed without controls, and, as such, may contain software viruses. Some screensavers have also been known to demand so much processing power from the host automation system that the primary application has insufficient resource to run at full speed. If this occurs with real-time systems, then the performance of the primary application could be seriously degraded and perhaps compromise GMP.

ELECTRONIC RECORDS AND ELECTRONIC SIGNATURES

The topic of electronic records and signatures has been much debated in recent years. The main issue is the authenticity of personnel identification that must be equivalent to handwritten signatures. The misuse of the electronic signatures must be deterred.

There has been considerable discussion in the pharmaceutical industry regarding electronic records and electronic signatures, and Paul Motise of the FDA recently gave some feedback on their current thoughts [5]. Since then, a new Code of Federal Regulations for accepting electronic records and electronic signatures has been issued, and the FDA is enforcing it beginning 20 August 1997 [6].

Electronic records must conform to the requirements of Document Control described in chapter 5. These requirements include

- Being able to discern between invalid and valid records
- Ensuring the correct sequence of changes and their respective authorisations
- Ensuring that changes to records do not obscure earlier modifications
- Ensuring it is not possible to alter in any way the audit trail of changes made to an electronic record

Examples of electronic records include computer files and scanned images, such as microfiche or microfilm. If these records are presented as master data to GMP regulatory authorities, they must be true copies and electronically signed. The term *true copies* implies that electronic records are

- Accurate in their content to the original record entry
- Complete, no missing content
- Retrievable from their storage media
- Reproducible in a printed form if necessary

Electronic signatures must be under the control of an administration procedure that ensures the signatures are [5]

- Unique to an individual
- Time stamped and consistent across time zones

- Associated to their meaning (e.g., review, approval, authorship)
- Bound to their master document with protection against unauthorised copying or alteration
- Appear in full on printed copies of electronic records

Electronic signatures can consist of either two elements that, combined uniquely, identify an individual (e.g., identifier and password) or a single biometric element. The use and management of passwords has already been discussed in Chapter 5. Organisations must verify the identity of individuals before assigning them electronic signatures. Signatures must be trustworthy and legally equivalent to handwritten signatures.

DATA INTEGRITY

Associated with the security issues affecting electronic signatures is data integrity. The FDA has been particularly sensitive to this topic, since the Generic Drug Scandal in the late 1980s indicated that corrupted data was a widespread problem in that sector of the pharmaceutical industry. Continuing concerns regarding data integrity were highlighted by the FDA's Joseph Philps at the University of Georgia's GMP Conference in 1996 [8].

Data integrity affects all data supporting GMP and, therefore, includes purchasing records, inventory control records, batch recipes, production records, QC laboratory data, training records, and so on. Data may be held in databases, spreadsheets, as parameters within an application, as optical records, electronic records, or paper records. Many pharmaceutical manufactures have not considered any form of control for maintaining data integrity. The GMP regulators will assume all data amendments and deletions to be unauthorised unless there are documented instructions specifying the activity as authorised. Security measures, such as those outlined in Chapter 5, should be implemented and include the following:

- Change control with full audit trail
- Backup and recovery procedures
- Checks for software viruses
- Limited accessibility
- Checks for unknown changes

Original records should be checked to verify their authenticity and that their quality has not degraded. Copies of data must be complete and accurate. Any loss in data integrity must be fully investigated and reported. The GMP regulators will expect any resulting recommendations to be implemented as soon as reasonably practical.

SIMULATION PACKAGES

Simulation packages can be used to support the pharmaceutical manufacturing process (for instance, exploring/optimising the performance envelope of a manufacturing process, or reproducing/investigating manufacturing incidents) or to assist the testing of an automation system and thereby reduce On-Site Testing. In either case, the simulator itself must be validated in accordance with the principles laid out in Chapter 3. This is because we must place assurance in the correct and reliable operation of the simulator itself before we can place confidence in its results. Potential users should conduct a Supplier Audit on the organisation supplying the simulation package to verify that it is fit for its intended application.

Validation must establish that the simulator (software and hardware):

- has been developed under a quality regime
- is suitably documented (e.g., specifications, design, user manuals)
- has been demonstrably tested against acceptance criteria
- has been widely and successfully used in industry

Many simulators use a model (sometimes referred to as an engine) of the manufacturing process or automation system architecture. Such models can be extremely complex, based on new technologies, such as fuzzy logic or neural nets, and linked to databases. Configuration details for the intended application must be validated. Databases containing details of the simulated automation system, live manufacturing process data, and any derived values should be checked to verify data integrity.

Many simulators have been developed by small companies and have a very small user community. This cost to validate simulators by such suppliers can, therefore, be very high, and this should be taken into account by pharmaceutical manufacturers when they decide whether or not to use such packages. It is also important to note that the FDA and other GMP regulators have highlighted the need for comprehensive On-Site Testing (IQ, OQ, PQ), of the actual system installed. Simulators would, therefore, appear to have a role in Predelivery Testing and as a general development/investigation tool, but not as a mechanism by which On-Site Testing can be dramatically reduced.

AUTOMATIC TESTING

Testing requires a significant proportion of the total validation effort. Automatic testing offers the opportunity to reduce the time required by personnel to test an automation system. Automated testing tools can

- Automate test data-set generation
- Automate running of tests from test specifications
- Provide test coverage statistics

Automatic testing is suitable for modular testing, integration testing, and OQ. Some modular testing, however, may be more efficiently achieved through isolated manual tests. Automatic testing utilities are expensive and a payback on the investment will be achieved only if they are used for large systems or a number of similar smaller systems. Automatic testing does not deplete the need for Software Inspections.

An overview of an automatic testing tool is given in Figure 8.2. Tests to be executed by an automatic testing utility can be produced manually or automatically. Manually written tests are specified using a programming language that can be later executed by the automatic test utility. Alternatively, the automatic test utility may record user keystrokes as they use the application to be tested and convert these recordings into readable, editable test methods that can be rerun against the application whenever required. Similarly, realistic data sets can be generated. Test methods are played back against the application to be tested, either on the system under test or a test environment.

Thousands of combinations of tests can be generated, more than could ever be tried manually. These tests can be run in batches, perhaps overnight to relieve demands on working office hours. This is especially useful when dealing with a large number of tests or tests that take a long time to run. A history file of test outcomes is generated by the automatic test utility. The history file logs the progression of tests and reports which tests succeeded and which failed. The history file may also include diagnostic information identifying which aspect of the failed tests deviated from the intended successful outcome. Programmers then correct the software errors. The entire test set can then be rerun automatically to eliminate the risk of introducing new errors when the application is modified.

The GMP issues raised by automatic testing include the following:

- Validation of the automatic test utility
- Version and change control of tests and associated data sets
- Reconciling the need for master paper test records

Pharmaceutical companies should audit the suppliers of any automatic testing tools used to help qualify their automation systems. Supplier Audits have already been discussed in Chapter 2. The design, development, testing and operation of automatic testing tools should be documented and subject to change and version control. As a minimum, there should be three detailed test scenarios where the automatic testing facilities are manually checked.

Figure 8.2. Automatic Testing Tool

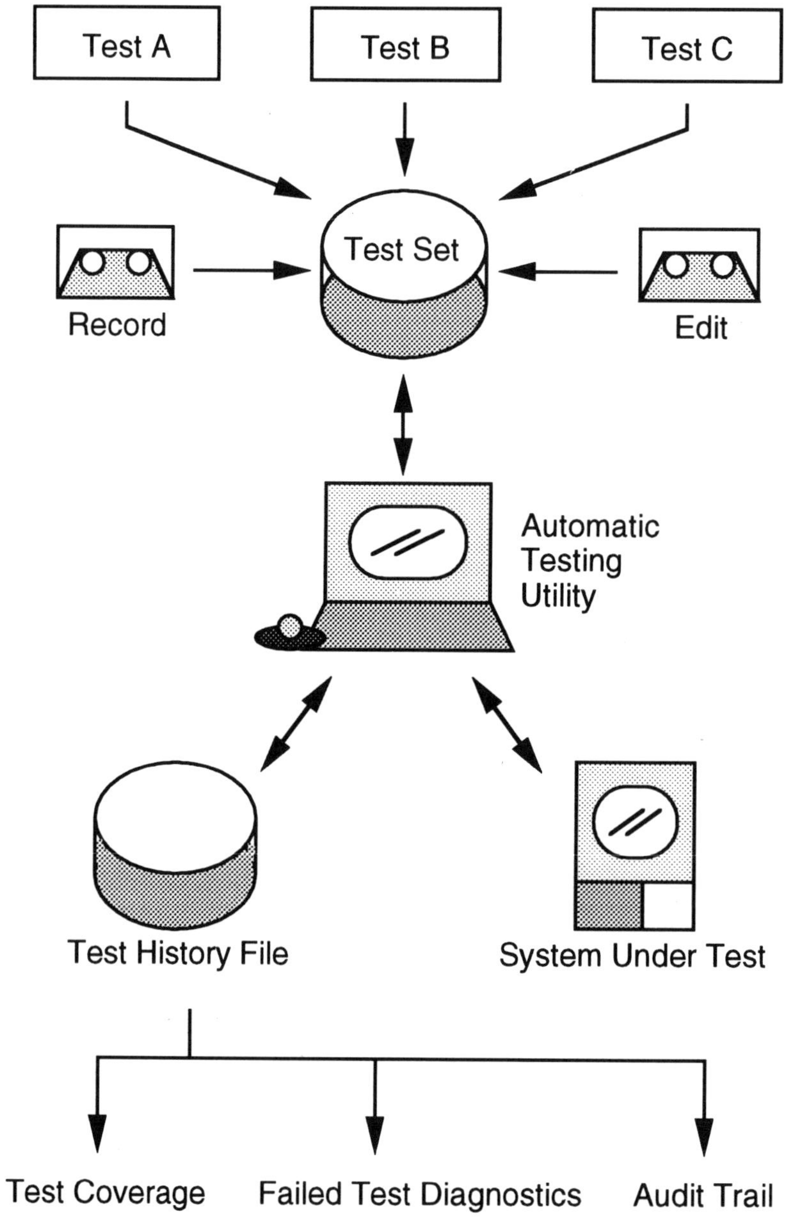

The number of detailed test scenarios will be commensurate with the criticality of the associated GMP application whose qualification the testing tool supports.

JOINT SUPPLIER AUDITS

A new development in Supplier Audits is the notion of a joint audit scheme whereby a number of pharmaceutical manufacturers cooperate in conducting a single audit on an individual supplier and share the audit report. Initial results are encouraging; by supplying a largely common report that satisfied the varying requirements of the participants, the costs to each participant have been cut by over 60 percent compared to one-off audits.

The cost savings by pharmaceutical manufacturers in one-off audits can be extended to follow-up audits conducted by the same or revised members of the original joint audit. User groups may be instituted informally by individual pharmaceutical manufacturers or more formally by the suppliers themselves. Not all members need attend every audit; membership of the audit team can rotate, ensuring continuity by retaining some members between successive audits.

Joint audits can also reduce the cost and disruption experienced by the supplier. Michael Wyrick, of Eli Lilly, recently reported that a joint audit by a large user group on an a particular MRP II supplier reduced the number of annual audits received by that supplier by about 80 percent [7]. The supplier may be given permission by the users participating in the joint audit to use the information from the audit with prospective customers and to disseminate it to user groups. Some of these prospective customers may wish to use the joint audit report in lieu or to supplement their own Supplier Audit. The agreement of the original joint audit participants should be sought before the report is handed over to any new pharmaceutical manufacturers in case there are any confidentiality issues. A small charge may be levied to cover the administration costs of duplicating and dispatching a copy of the report.

Three main concerns have been raised during joint audit by pharmaceutical manufacturers, the supplier, and the auditor [8]. Pharmaceutical manufacturers have been concerned about losing their personal insights and opinion of the supplier. The audited suppliers have been concerned about the risk of damaging audit reports being made available to other pharmaceutical manufacturers. The auditors have been concerned about the liability associated with distributed audit reports. These issues of sanitised audits, confidentiality, and liability must be addressed within the management of joint audits. The success of joint audits to date, however, would suggest that they will become common in the future. It must be recognised, however, that the role of User Groups in freely sharing information and experiences and providing advice on validation to the supplier is key to their continued success.

THIRD-PARTY CERTIFICATION OF VALIDATION

Interest has been expressed by both pharmaceutical manufacturers and suppliers in third-party certification of validation work [9]. Certification would relieve much validation work currently required by pharmaceutical manufacturers. Similarly, the rigour of inspections by GMP regulatory authorities could be relaxed because they could place confidence in the accredited inspection of a third-party agency. GMP regulatory authorities are interested in this opportunity but do not yet accept certification as a substitute for validation.

Suitable certification could be based on a ISO 9000-3 (TickIt) for software, or some other independent conformity assessment scheme, such as that proposed by Lloyd's Register or the UK Department of Trade and Industry's Framework for Safety-Critical Objects (FRESCO). The FRESCO project is independently investigating accreditation and certification of automation systems based on the emerging IEC 1508 standard for safety-related systems and includes a study of the certification opportunities for validation in the pharmaceutical industry [10]. It has suggested three levels of certification:

1. Application Independent Certification
2. Application Dependent Certification
3. Operations, Maintenance, and Modification Certificate

Pertinent issues considered by FRESCO include potential liabilities, the cost to users of the assessment and certification, and the benefits to other users and regulators. All of these issues are very important if a third-party accreditation scheme is to be successfully established for validation. The results of the FRESCO project were published at the end of 1996.

NEW VALIDATION GUIDES AND REGULATIONS

Between 1994 and 1996, various pharmaceutical industry initiatives around the world produced eight significant validation guides:

1. The German APV guide to Annex 11 (Computerised Systems) of the European Union GMP Directive [11]
2. The German GMA-NAMUR working party's recommendations for computer validation [12]
3. The ISPE/FDA guide for instrumentation and controls [13]
4. The OECD's computer validation guide for laboratory systems [14]
5. The UK GAMP Forum's automation validation guide for suppliers [15]

6. The UK IQA's guide on applying ISO 9000 to the pharmaceutical industry [16]
7. The U.S. EPA's computer validation guide for laboratory systems [17]
8. The U.S. PDA's computer validation guide for pharmaceutical manufacturers [18]

Further developments are expected in 1997/8. The German GMA-NAMUR is publishing three new guides:

1. NE 68: Validation for Process Control—Retrospective Validation of Existing Plants
2. NE 71: Standard Operating Procedures (SOPs)
3. NE 72: Validation Support for DCS

The UK GAMP Forum is likely to extend its guide with two short guidance notes on validating process computer systems and EDMSs as additional appendicies to the guide, and the U.S. PDA is publishing a significant development of its computer validation guide.

The intent of the German APV, the German GMA-NAMUR, the UK GAMP Forum, and U.S. PDA initiatives to coordinate their respective guides was announced at the ISPE's European computer validation meeting in Amsterdam in March 1995. It is vital that all of the various initiatives develop a consistent international approach and a standard lexicon for validating automation systems. Inconsistencies will at best prevent standardisation and at worst breed confusion between practitioners and GMP regulatory authorities. It is too early to comment on the success of this harmonisation, but at the time of publication of this book, the guides appear to be highly complementary.

In addition to the industry guides listed above, a proposal has recently been made by the FDA to update the U.S. GMP regulations, which include a strengthening (or as the FDA put it, a "clarification") of the validation requirements placed on the use of automation systems [19]. The preamble to the proposed amendment discusses the need to cope with advances in technology, that suppliers cannot validate but rather support a pharmaceutical manufacturers validation, and the need to demonstrate the preservation of a validated status. Particular expectations concerning automation systems are listed below and have been incorporated into the guidance presented in this book.

- Change control and revalidation
- Equipment (and software) suitability
- Software backups and performance data
- Document retention requirements

The FDA stresses that these amendments are part of an ongoing process of continuous improvement and that further amendments are likely in the future. Industry comment on the proposed amendment has been collected by the end of 1996, ready for issue of the revised GMP regulations in 1997.

The FDA is also in the process of revising its computer validation guides [8]: the inspection guide published in 1983 and known as the "Blue Book" [20], and the technical reference on software development [21]. Both should be ready for publication in 1997/1998 and copies will be made available over the Internet. A glossary of terminology designed for use by FDA staff is already available [22]. Paul D'Eramo is revising the Blue Book. The average FDA investigator has very general background training, and the revised Blue Book aims to gives these investigators a foundation in what they should expect in the way of validation for automation systems. Investigators will be directed to bias inspections towards the most critical automation systems associated with a manufacturing process. Specific assistance will be given on how to deal with modern technology, risk analysis, the role of suppliers supporting validation of automation systems conducted by pharmaceutical manufacturers, and retrospective validation of existing automation systems. Meanwhile, David Bergeson is revising the technical reference on software development. This revised document will have the same basic format as its original version, promoting the waterfall development life cycle, but will have new sections addressing software engineering, configuration management, and a discussion on software metrics.

Practitioners may also be interested to know that the FDA has also compiled an internal training course (No. 545) on the topic of computer system validation for its investigators. The course (based on overhead slides) includes the application of GMP regulations to automation systems, pharmaceutical manufacturer's policies and procedures, life cycle development and support of automation systems, problems associated with poor systems, how to inspect automation systems and their users, and an inspection exercise.

In addition to these FDA developments, a working party representing GMP regulatory authorities has been established to draft an "umbrella" document to harmonise international guidelines, GMP requirements, and standards for automation systems in the pharmaceutical industry. The working party was formed following a seminar held at Sydney (Australia) in September 1996 and organised by the Pharmaceutical Inspection Cooperation Scheme (PIC/S), formerly known as the Pharmaceutical Inspection Convention (PIC). Members of the PIC/S working party include the original European Union membership of PIC plus Switzerland's OICM, the TGA, and, it is hoped, the FDA. At the moment, a target date for the issue of the draft umbrella document has not been set.

VALIDATING EMERGING TECHNOLOGIES

Last but by no means least of the topical issues covered in this chapter is the validation of emerging technologies. This topic nearly always raises debate when discussing the particular requirements of different technologies. In such debates, it is necessary to determine whether the technology can be validated. Useful guidance in this respect is given by Ken Chapman [23], who recounts a meeting of the PMA's Computer System Validation Committee in 1992 that considered the validation of systems based on new technologies. The PMA considered two categories of systems:

1. Those in which the rules and related databases can change without human intervention, as experience grows
2. Those in which such changes can be made only with human intervention

The first category cannot be validated because the unpredictability of "correct" test results renders functional testing impossible. Automation systems based on these technologies must not, therefore, be implemented in support of drug manufacturing. Examples of systems in this category might include neural nets, fuzzy logic, and expert systems.

The second category can be validated because their functionality can be predicted and, therefore, tested against predetermined acceptance criteria. Systems in this category include those based on object orientation and formal methods.

The use of object orientation and formal methods would appear to be set to grow in popularity over the coming years. Recent research, however, suggests these techniques do not in themselves yield higher quality systems [24]. Formal methods, nevertheless, do facilitate more comprehensive testing and hence more errors are likely to be detected before release of the software system for use.

Whichever automation technology is used, the validation approach to be adopted should be based on the life cycle presented in Chapters 3 and 5, placing emphasis on GMP critical aspects of the automation system. If there is any doubt in the most appropriate validation approach, then pharmaceutical manufacturers and suppliers alike should discuss their application with GMP regulatory authorities. The regulators have a vested interest in understanding new technologies because they must understand them and the associated validation implications when inspecting their application elsewhere.

REFERENCES

1. FDA (1995), A Memo on Current Good Manufacturing Practice Issues on Human Use Pharmaceuticals, *Human Drug Notes,* 3(2).
2. Wingate, G.A.S., Smith, M., and Lucas, P.R. (1995), *Assuring Confidence in Pharmaceutical Software, Safety and Reliability of Software Based Systems,* First Annual ENCRESS Conference, 12–15 September, Bruges, Belgium.
3. Motise, P.J. (1996), Toward the Electronic Government: Year 2000, a Potential CGMP Problem? *Human Drug CGMP Notes,* FDA, December.

4. Uhlig, R. (1996), Don't Let a Virus Eat Your Work, *Daily Telegraph*, London, 13 August.

5. Motise, P. (1996), *An Update on Electronic Records and Electronic Signatures,* Process and Computer Validation '96, Spring Innovations, 22–23 April, UMIST Conference Centre, Manchester University, England.

6. Final Rule for 21 CFR Part 11 (1997), Electronic Signatures and Electronic Records, *Federal Register*, 62 (54).

7. *The Gold Sheet* (1996), 30 (7), July.

8. Bratt, A., Gladders, M.J., and West, A. (1995), Experiences in Audit Sharing, *Pharmaceutical Engineering,* (15) 4.

9. Selby, D. (1994), *The Objectives of the FORUM,* Good Automated Manufacturing Practice in the Pharmaceutical Industry, Management Forum Conference, 1 March, London.

10. Hunt, J.R., Lucas, P.R. and Wingate, G.A.S. (1995), FRESCO, *Achieving Safety in Control Systems,* (Edited by T. Anderson and F. Redmill), Springer-Verlag.

11. APV (1996), The APV Guideline on Computerised Systems based on Annex 11 of the EU-GMP Guideline, in *Supplier Guide for Validation of Automation Systems in Pharmaceutical Manufacture,* Version 2, The Hague, Netherlands: International Society of Pharmaceutical Engineers.

12. NE 58: Abwicklung von qualifizierungspflichtigen PLT-Projekten (version 04.06.96); [including . . .] Dannapel, B., Hensel, H., Mockel, B., Muhlenkamp, J., Muller-Heinzerling, T., Otto, A., and Teuchert, V. (1995), Qualifizierung von Leitsystemen: Ein Gemeinschaftsprojekt von GMA und NAMUR zur Validierung, *ATP—Automatisierungstechnische Praxis,* 37 (10): 64–76.

13. ISPE (1996), *Baseline Pharmaceutical Engineering Guide: A Guide for New Facilities,* Volume 1: Bulk Pharmaceutical Chemicals, Developed in Partnership by International Society of Pharmaceutical Engineering and U.S. Food and Drug Administration. Incorporates chapter on Instrumentation and Controls, Tampa, FL: International Society of Pharmaceutical Engineering.

14. OECD (1995), *The Application of the Principles of GLP to Computerised Systems,* No. 10 OECD Series on Principles of Good Laboratory Practice and Compliance Monitoring, GLP Consensus Document—Environmental Monograph No. 116, OECD Environmental Directorate, Paris: Organisation for Economic Cooperation and Development.

15. UK GAMP Forum (1996), *Supplier Guide for Validation of Automation Systems in Pharmaceutical Manufacture,* Version 2, The Hague, Netherlands: International Society of Pharmaceutical Engineers.

16. IQA (1994), *Pharmaceutical Supplier Code of Practice Covering the Manufacture of Pharmaceutical Raw Materials, Active Ingredients and Excipients,* Document Reference No. P00020, Issue 2, Institute of Quality Assurance, Pharmaceutical Quality Group.

17. EPA (1995), *Good Automated Laboratory Practices: Principles and Guidance to Regulations for Ensuring Data Integrity in Automated Laboratory Operations with Implementation Guidance,* Document Reference 2185, 1995 Edition, Washington, DC: Environmental Protection Agency.

18. PDA (1995), Validation of Computer Related Systems, *PDA Journal of Pharmaceutical Science and Technology,* Technical Report No. 18.

19. Hubbard, W. (1996), *Current Good Manufacturing Practice: Amendment of Certain Requirements for Finished Pharmaceuticals; Proposed Rule* (U.S. Code of Federal Regulation Title 21, Parts 210 and 211), Rockville, MD: Food and Drug Administration.

20. FDA (1983), *Guide to Inspection of Computerized Systems in Drug Processing,* Technical Report, Reference Materials and Training Aids for Investigators, Rockville, MD: Food and Drug Administration.

21. FDA (1987), *Software Development Activities,* Technical Report, Reference Materials and Training Aids for Investigators, Rockville, MD: Food and Drug Administration.

22. FDA (1995), *Glossary of Computerized and Software Development Terminology,* Issued August, Rockville, MD: Food and Drug Administration.

23. Chapman, K.G. (1994), Validation Concepts and Key Terminology, in *Good Computer Validation Practices: Common Sense Implementation,* edited by T. Stokes, R.C. Branning, K.G. Chapman, H. Hambloch, and A.J. Trill, Buffalo Grove, IL: Interpharm Press.

24. Hatton, L. (1997), Unexpected (and Sometimes Unpleasant) Lessons from Data in Real Software Systems, *Safety and Reliability of Software Based Systems,* Springer-Verlag.

25. MCA (1997), *Computer Systems and Year 2000 Conformity Requirements,* MCA Guidance Note No. 1 (Version 1.00), February–May.

Chapter 9

Conclusion

Validation practices have been reviewed in line with current expectations of GMP regulatory authorities and industry practice. This chapter concludes the review with some insights into the world of validation, some survival hints for practitioners, and some golden rules. The remainder of this book collates some case studies that discuss the practicalities of validating a range of different automation systems.

VALIDATION INSIGHTS

The various GMP regulations used around the world are based on three fundamental concepts of quality assurance [1]:

1. Quality, safety, and effectiveness must be designed and built into a product.
2. Quality cannot be inspected or tested into a finished product.
3. Each step of the manufacturing process must be controlled to maximise the likelihood that the finished product will be acceptable.

The implementation of these concepts requires validation. This includes validating the use of automation systems supporting the manufacture of drug products. Only pharmaceutical manufacturers, however, can conduct validation; suppliers cannot validate. Pharmaceutical manufacturers can, nevertheless, use information provided by suppliers to support their validation.

A common approach to validating automation systems has emerged during the late 1980s and early 1990s and is now maturing. The aim of this book has been to present this maturing approach and, with case studies, bridge the gap that has existed between the theory and practice of validation. A glossary of terms listing a selection of definitions from various regulatory and industry sources has been included as Appendix 2 to this book. Unfortunately, a universal set of validation definitions has not yet been established, although it is dearly needed.

The benefits of a widely adopted industry framework for validating automation have been recently extolled by Tony Trill of the MCA. The benefits include the following [2]:

- Establishing a common management practice
- Defining customer and supplier responsibilities
- Stabilising standards and their interpretation at a realistic level
- Linking validation to existing standards (e.g., ISO 9000)
- Reducing the costs of validation
- Shortening the time required for validation
- Ensuring appropriate documentation is produced for validation projects
- Improving the quality and reliability of delivered systems

This all makes good business sense and should eliminate the need for corrective work because the original validation was deficient. Both pharmaceutical manufacturers and their suppliers should know what is required and where points of clarification with GMP regulatory authorities are required. An established industry approach may also provide the basis for the international acceptance of validation work by various GMP regulatory authorities. The acceptance by GMP regulatory authorities of each other's inspection findings, however, is not expected in the near future.

VALIDATION SURVIVAL GUIDE

A positive attitude is essential when beating the validation blues! This does not, however, mean that managers and practitioners will not come across problems when validating automation systems. In such situations, it is often useful to focus on why validation is needed and reflect on the following advice:

- Do not assume validation has an intrinsic value—it has none. But your core product or service does. Can you quantify the benefits of validation for your business?
- Aim to build the principles of validation into the culture of your organisation. It was never intended to be a separate function.

Mould the principles of validation to suit your own working practices. It is often more cost-effective to use the services of an outside consultant than your own in-house staff.

- Err on the side of caution when estimating the cost of validation. During projects, do not be complacent: challenge any overspend or project slippage. Resist making changes to project requirements that are not really necessary, as these could considerably increase costs.
- Avoid validation for GMP becoming validation for Great Mounds of Paper. Documentation for its own sake will not ensure GMP compliance. If documentation is not useful, it is not likely to be needed for validation.
- Training is critical, but it must be the right training. Most training courses do not consider the practical application of validation and are a complete waste of time.
- You will not get your validation practices perfect the first time—they will need to be refined, so expect and plan for continuous improvement.

A proactive management style will minimise any problems experienced. The motivation and commitment of practitioners must be maintained. They must feel that they have management support in their work.

TEN COMMANDMENTS FOR VALIDATING AUTOMATION

Many light-hearted publications have published lists of 10 commandments for validation practitioners. None of these lists, however, is carved in stone, and there is some flexibility in deciding what should be included in the way of guidance. The checklist given below should help practitioners concentrate on the key issues affecting validation:

- Thou shalt plan validation of thy automation systems.
- Thou shalt validate with competent personnel.
- Thou shalt implement a regime of change control.
- Thou shalt specify procedures for thy validation.
- Thou shalt document thy automation systems.
- Thou shalt write and approve qualification protocols.
- Thou shalt execute thy qualification protocols and record thy test outcomes.
- Thou shalt write and approve summary validation reports.

- Thou shalt operate and maintain thy automation system in a state of control.
- Thou shalt periodically review thy automation systems' validation.

Remember that the GMP requirements for software are the same as for manufacturing records and documentation. Similarly, automation hardware (including computers and instrumentation) should fulfil the GMP requirements of manufacturing equipment.

Specific guidance on the validation of different types of automation system can be found in the case studies collated in part two of this book. The authors of these case studies are themselves experienced practitioners, and they have been encouraged to focus their papers on the key issues affecting their particular type of automation system.

GOOD BUSINESS SENSE

Validation should bring benefits to pharmaceutical manufacturers, their suppliers, and the end users of drug products. Pharmaceutical manufacturers should be able to rely on implementing automation systems correctly the first time, every time. Meanwhile suppliers should, by building in quality, be able to reduce predelivery costs for the same reason. A quality approach should also improve time and budget management. Finally, there should be savings because of fewer postdelivery problems:

- Product recalls
- Product returns
- Customer complaints
- Maintenance
- Customer queries

All of the above should be reduced. Customer satisfaction would tend to lead to further orders and promotion within the industry as a highly competent supplier.

To avoid insufficient and excessive standards of work, and to avoid duplicating tasks in their entirety or in part, pharmaceutical manufacturers and suppliers should work together in partnership. They must be able to work as a team and, as such, must be able to communicate effectively. The parallel mutual benefits of cooperation between customers and suppliers are outlined in Table 9.1.

A further benefit is the reduced time and effort to audit the GMP compliance of an automation system. Such an attribute yields a distinct marketing advantage to suppliers and gives pharmaceutical manufacturers visibility of their own validation capability before a GMP regulatory inspection.

Table 9.1. The Benefits of Cooperation Between Customers and Suppliers

Customer	Supplier
Meet user needs	Satisfy customer
Be easier to set up	Be handed over sooner
Be in production sooner	Be paid sooner
Break down less often	Fewer warranty visits
Be easier to repair	Shorter warranty visits
Be easier to further develop	Be easier to modify or upgrade
Be used more efficiently	Good reference sites for new customers
Cheaper overall	Cheaper overall
Preferred supplier	Repeat business

TRENDS IN VALIDATION

The validation of automation systems has been a topical issue for over a decade, as discussed in Chapter 1, and still accounts for up to 10 percent of citations for GMP noncompliance by regulatory inspectors [3]. The importance of validating automation systems is set to continue with GMP regulators' interest in the role of existing and new automation technology throughout the supply chain of drug manufacturing from R&D establishments, through the supply of BPCs and finished drug product processing, to distribution [4]. Indeed, as discussed in Chapter 8, the FDA is updating U.S. GMP legislation and guidance in a proposed amendment to the U.S. GMP regulations [1]. This will emphasise the need to validate automation systems used to monitor and/or control the manufacturing process.

Technology

In the 1980s, the use of automation systems was largely limited to PLCs and SCADA systems. More recently, a greater variety of automation systems has been used and integrated. Figure 9.1 illustrates how automation systems can support various aspects of pharmaceutical manufacturing operations. Different selections of automation systems can provide similar collective "patchwork" coverage of manufacturing operations. Pharmaceutical manufacturers must choose their preferred solution with a selection of systems that are not only technically capable but also validation compliant.

Specialist intelligent instruments for measurement and analysis will become increasing important as novel control parameters become more common. Such instrumentation will reduce the variability and increase the

Figure 9.1. Automation System Patchwork Coverage of Manufacturing Operations

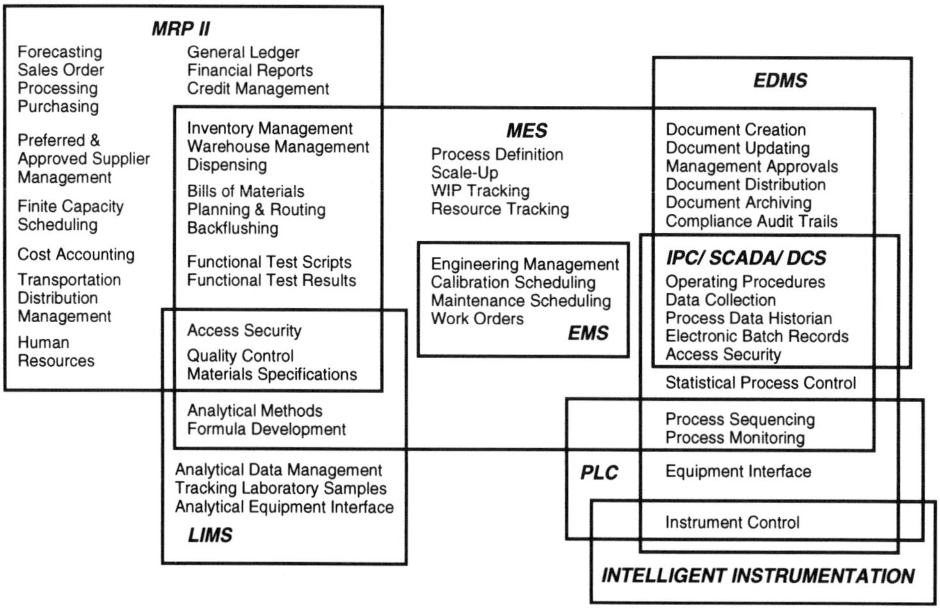

flexibility of manufacturing processes and is, therefore, of interest to the GMP regulatory authorities. Many companies are now also investigating the use of intelligent instrumentation for preventative maintenance, to increase reliability of instruments and process equipment, and to cut maintenance costs.

There is a growing trend towards decentralised process control and the interconnection (possibly with Fieldbus™) of automation systems including intelligent instrumentation, IPCs, PLCs, SCADA, and DCS under the umbrella of MES. IPC, PLC, SCADA, and DCS batch control solutions are subject to GMP because they implement manufacturing control on the production process. Although few IPCs are currently used in the pharmaceutical industry, recent functionality developments and their growing reputation in the chemicals sector would suggest that they will become a common pharmaceutical batch control solution in the future. Similarly, MES products have only recently become available and are subject to GMP scrutiny because they coordinate, supervise, and manage production.

Laboratory systems such as LIMS have also come under increased regulatory scrutiny as the complexity of the software they deploy has become more advanced.

Business systems such as MRP II have become regulatory concerns because they are no longer used solely for financial information and production forecasting but can now manage production materials, plant configuration, production routings, operating procedures, batch records, and distribution details—all of which are subject to GMP.

Looking further into the future, totally automated facilities loom that are truely paperless. Robotics and Automated Guided Vehicles (AGVs) will be commonplace, whilst conventional operator interaction will virtually disappear. Some pharmaceutical manufacturers claim to have paperless facilities now but in the experience of the author, they still employ a lot of paperwork (e.g., printed SOPs and printed work orders). Paperless facilities will bring their own set of problems, such as the use and control of electronic signatures, which is already beginning to be experienced by firms implementing EDMSs.

Regulation

The MCA has reported major inspection problems with automation systems during inspections of UK and oversees sites [4]. About half of the problems related to a complete absence of (or inadequate) validation data. This was closely followed by inadequate system descriptions (documentation) and a lack of documented alternative procedures to cover computer downtime. Problems were also highlighted with automated production lines, stock control, and system security. The MCA expects an increase in reported problems with automation systems validation over the coming years.

The results of a PMA survey have recently been presented. More than 152 citations were reviewed for GMP noncompliance by the FDA between 1984 and 1994, which included approximately 600 observations on various aspects of validating automation systems [5]. These data, together with a survey of 158 FDA observations covering all of 1995 and a large portion of 1996, have been used to produce Figure 9.2 and Table 9.2. Figure 9.2 shows a steady rise in problems identified with validating automation systems, and although there was a slight decrease in 1994, validation is still an important ongoing issue. Table 9.2 breaks down the FDA's observations into different categories. The five categories with the most observations, in descending order, cover testing and qualification, change control validation approach, specification and design, and quality assurance. An earlier survey in 1988 also identified system development and qualification as top issues [6].

The regulatory trends identified above represent significant industry deficiencies with automation system validation. The deficiencies contravene fundamental requirements in the GMP regulations. There is a continuing need to educate pharmaceutical manufacturers and their suppliers in practical validation compliance. One way in which GMP regulators can assist in this process is to harmonise their GMP requirements. The European Union's

Figure 9.2. Noncompliant GMP Inspections Referencing Automation Systems

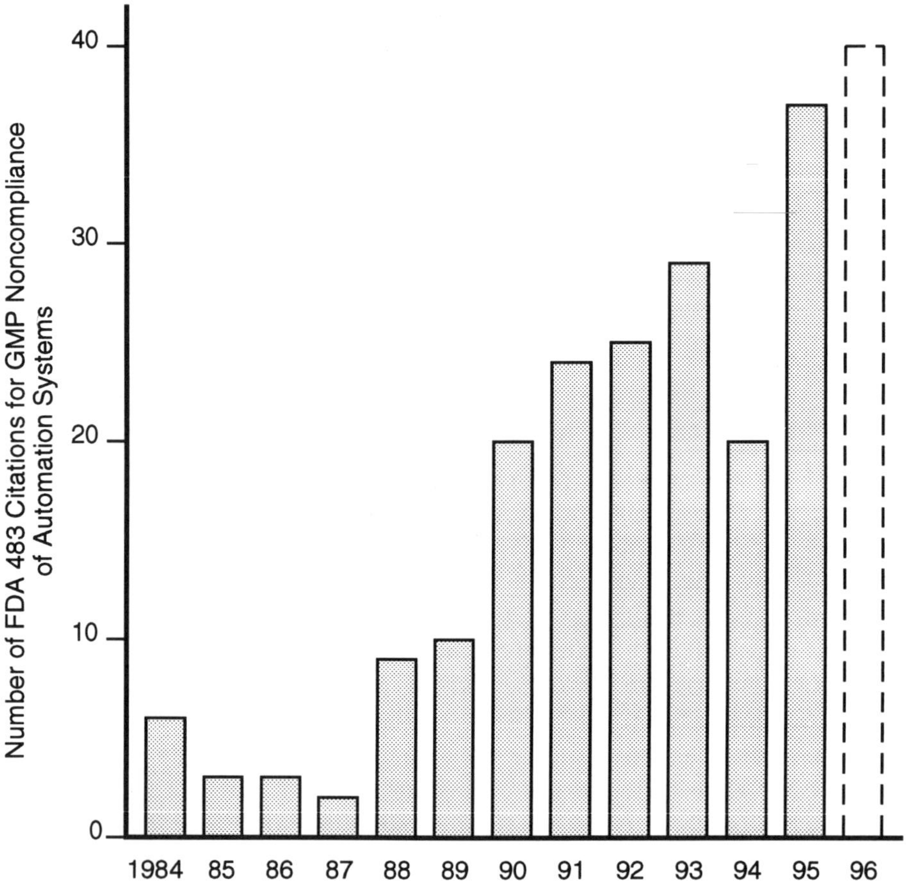

Note: Total number of FDA 483 citations for GMP noncompliance of automation is projected for 1996.

GMP Directive, which has already been adopted by countries outside the Union, has shown that harmonisation can work. The only outstanding issue appears to be that of consistent inspection standards between different national regulatory authorities and this, potentially, may be affected by national politics.

THE FINAL ANALYSIS

In the final analysis, pharmaceutical manufacturers have no choice but to validate their automation systems, otherwise their licence to market a drug

Table 9.2. GMP Observations Referencing Automation Systems (FDA: 1984–1996)

Deficiency Observed	Number	%
Testing and Qualification	154	20.3
Change Control	141	18.6
Validation Approach	109	14.0
Specification and Design	97	12.8
Quality Assurance and Auditing	95	12.5
Operating Procedures	53	7.0
Security Practice	31	4.1
Equipment Records and Maintenance	25	3.3
Training, Education, and Experience	15	2.0
Various Others	35	4.1

will be revoked or not issued in the first place. The cost of validation need not be excessively high if the exercise is focussed. Validation should be commensurate with the potential impact of the automation system on GMP. If there is no potential impact on GMP, then validation is not required. If there is a potential impact, then the whole system should be validated, with particular attention on the GMP aspects of the system's functionality. Impact analysis can be approached by considering BRAN:

- Benefits
- Risks
- Alternatives
- No action consequences

Benefits and risks should cover manufacturing performance, regulatory compliance, patient risk, corporate reputation, and so on. Alternatives cover the manufacturing process, manufacturing equipment, automation technology, and even the replacement of an automation system by a manual system. Finally, it is always worth considering the consequences of taking no action. There is a significant trend away from the idea that new systems are necessarily better systems. Unless a new system or upgrade is widely used, the number and severity of any bugs is unknown and will not be discovered until it is used. Meanwhile, operational experience with an existing or widely used system should have uncovered most of the operational problems. If measures can be or have been introduced to control or contain these known problems to an acceptable level, then it may be safer not to implement the new system or upgrade.

The validation life-cycle approach has proven itself as an effective method of ensuring the quality, safety, and efficacy of manufactured drug products. It should be no more than commonsense good practice and it should deliver tangible business benefits. Pharmaceutical manufacturers must not, however, confuse current industry practice with good practice. Standards are improving and drug manufacturers must get used to the increasing expectations of regulators. It is also important to realise that this does not necessarily mean more paperwork and bureaucracy. Validation is often misunderstood in this respect. GMP regulatory authorities are not enforcing validation for its own sake, but to protect the end users of drug products. Validation cannot be ignored; it is here to stay.

REFERENCES

1. Hubbard, W. (1996), *Current Good Manufacturing Practice: Amendment of Certain Requirements for Finished Pharmaceuticals; Proposed Rule* (U.S. Code of Federal Regulation Title 21, Parts 210 and 211), Rockville, MD: Food and Drug Administration.
2. Trill, A.J. (1996), *MCA View on the Presented Initiatives,* ISPE/PDA Joint Conference on Computer-Related System Validation, 2–3 May, Basel, Switzerland.
3. *The Gold Sheet* (1996), 30 (7), Chevy Chase, MD: F-D-C Reports Inc.
4. Trill, A.J. (1996), *Regulations and Computer Systems Validation in Context,* Management Forum Seminar, Computer Systems Validation: A Practical Approach, 6–7 November, London.
5. Dillinger, A. and Hambloch, H. (1996), *R/3 Validation at Pharmaceutical Companies,* Process Industry Workshop, SAPPHIRE '96, 12–14 June, Vienna, Austria.
6. DIA (1988), *Computerised Data Systems for Nonclinical Safety Assessment—Current Concepts and Quality Assurance,* (known as the Red Apple Document), Maple Glenn: Drug Information Association.

Part 1

Appendices

Appendix 1

Abbreviations

ABPI	Association of the British Pharmaceutical Industry
ADE	Application Development Environment
ANSI	American National Standards Institute
APV	Arbeitsgemeinschaft fur Pharmazeutische Verfahrenstechnik (Germany)
ASCII	American Standard Code for Information Interchange
BASEEFA	British Approvals Service for Electrical Equipment in Flammable Atmospheres
BASIC	Beginners All-purpose Symbolic Instruction Code
BCS	British Computer Society
BGA	Bundesgesundheitsamt (German Federal Health Office)
BOM	Bill of Materials
BMS	Building Management System
BPC	Bulk Pharmaceutical Chemical
BS	British Standard
CAD	Computer Aided Design
CAM	Computer Aided Manufacturing
CANDA	Computer Assisted NDA (United States)
CASE	Computer Aided Software Engineering

CDER	Center for Drug Evaluation and Research (FDA)
CD	Compact Disc
CDS	Chromatography Data System
CE	Cummunaute Europeenne (European Union)
CEFIC	Chemical European Federation Industry Council
CENELEC	Comité Européen de Normalisation Electrotechnique
CFR	Code of Federal Regulations (United States)
cGAMP	Current GAMP
cGMP	Current GMP
CGP	Code of Good Practice
CHAZOP	Computer HAZOP
CIM	Computer Integrated Manufacturing
CMM	Capability Maturity Model
COTS	Commercial OTS
CRC	Cyclic Redundancy Check
CRM	Certified Reference Material
CSA	Canadian Standards Association
CSV	Computer System Validation
CSVC	Computer Systems Validation Committee (of PhRMA)
DCS	Distributed Control System
DIA	Drug Information Association
DOS	Disk Operating System
DQ	Design Qualification
DSP	Digital Signal Processing
EBRS	Electronic Batch Record System
EC	European Commission
EDMS	Electronic Document Management System
EEC	European Economic Community
EEPROM	Electronically Erasable Programmable ROM
EFPIA	European Federation of Pharmaceutical Industry Association

EFTA	European Free Trade Association
ELD	Engineering Line Diagram
EMC	Electro-Magnetic Compatibility
EMEA	European Medicines Evaluation Agency
EMI	Electro-Magnetic Interference
EMS	Engineering Management System
ENCRESS	European Network of Clubs for Reliability and Safety of Software
EPA	Environmental Protection Agency (United States)
EPROM	Erasable Programmable ROM
ERP	Enterprise Resource Planning
ESD	Electro-Static Discharge
EU	European Union
FAT	Factory Acceptance Testing
FATS	Factory Acceptance Test Specification
FDA	Food and Drug Administration (United States)
FDS	Functional Design Specification
FFT	Fast Fourier Transform
FM	Factory Mutual Research Corporation
FMEA	Failure Modes and Effects Analysis
4GL	Fourth Generation Language
FRESCO	Framework for Evaluation of Safety-Critical Objects
FS	Functional Specification
GALP	Good Automated Laboratory Practice
GAMP	Good Automated Manufacturing Practice
GAP	Good Automation Practice
GATT	General Agreement on Tariffs and Trade
GC	Gas Chromatography
GCP	Good Clinical Practice
GEP	Good Engineering Practice

GIGO	Garbage In, Garbage Out
GITP	Good Information Technology Practice
GLP	Good Laboratory Practice
GMA	Gesellschaft Meβ- und Automatisierungstechnik (Germany)
GMP	Good Manufacturing Practice
GPP	Good Programming Practice
GXP	Acronym for general Good Practice
GUI	Graphical User Interface
HAZOP	HAZard and OPerability Study
HATS	Hardware Acceptance Test Specification
HDS	Hardware Design Specification
HIV	Human Immunodeficiency Virus
HMI	Human-Machine Interface
HP	Hewlett-Packard
HPLC	High Performance Liquid Chromatography
HSE	Health and Safety Executive (United Kingdom)
HVAC	Heating, Ventilation, and Air-Conditioning
I/O	Input/Output
IBM	International Business Machines
ICH	International Conference on Harmonization of Technical Requirements of Pharmaceuticals for Human Use
IChemE	Institution for of Chemical Engineers (United Kingdom)
ICI	Imperial Chemical Industries (United Kingdom)
ICS	Integrated Control System
ICSE	Interdepartmental Committee on Software Engineering (United Kingdom)
IEC	International Electrotechnical Commission
IEE	Institution for Electrical Engineers (United Kingdom)
IEEE	Institute of Electrical and Electronic Engineers (United States)
IMechE	Institution for Mechanical Engineers (United Kingdom)
InstMC	Institution for Measurement and Control (United Kingdom)

IP	Index of Protection
IP	Ingress Protection
IPC	Industrial Personal Computer
IPR	Intellectual Property Rights
IPSE	Integrated Project Support Environment
IQ	Installation Qualification
IQA	Institute of Quality Assurance (United Kingdom)
IRCA	International Register of Certificated Auditors
IS	Intrinsically Safe
ISA	Instrument Society of America
ISM	Industrial, Scientific, and Medical
ISO	International Standards Organisation
ISPE	International Society of Pharmaceutical Engineering
IT	Information Technology
JIT	Just-in-Time
JSD	Jackson Development Method
LAN	Local Area Network
LIMS	Laboratory Management Information System
L/R Ratio	Inductance-Resistance Ratio
MASCOT	Modular Approach to Software Construction, Operation, and Test
MCA	Medicines Control Agency (United Kingdom)
MES	Manufacturing Execution System
MHW	Ministry of Health and Welfare (Japan)
MIS	Management Information System
MMI	Man-Machine Interface
MODEM	Modulator-Demodulator Units
MORI	Market & Opinion Research International
MPI	Manufacturing Performance Improvement
MPS	Master Production Scheduling
MQ	Manufacturing Qualification

MRP	Materials Requirements Planning
MRP II	Manufacturing Resource Planning
MTTF	Mean Time to Failure
NAFTA	North American Free Trade Agreement
NAMAS	National Measurement Accreditation Service (United Kingdom)
NAMUR	Normenarbeitsgemeinschaft für Meß- und Regelungstechnik (Germany)
NDA	New Drug Application (United States)
NIR	Near Infrared
O&M	Operation and Maintenance
OCR	Optical Character Recognition
OECD	Organisation for Economic Co-operation and Development
OEM	Original Equipment Manufacturer
OICM	Office Intercantonal de Controle des Medicaments (Switzerland)
OQ	Operational Qualification
OS	Outline Specification
OTC	Over-the-Counter
OTS	Off-the-Shelf
PC	Personal Computer
PDA	Parenteral Drug Association (United States)
PhRMA	Pharmaceutical Research & Manufacturers Association (United States)
PIC	Pharmaceutical Inspection Convention
PIC/S	Pharmaceutical Inspection Cooperation Scheme
PICSVF	Pharmaceutical Industry Computer System Validation Forum (United Kingdom) (now known as the GAMP Forum)
P&ID	Piping and Instrument Diagram
PID	Proportional, Integral, Derivative (Loop)
PLC	Programmable Logic Controller
PMA	Pharmaceutical Manufacturers Association (United States)

PMS	Paperless Manufacturing Systems
PSU	Power Supply Unit
PTB	Physikalische-Technische Bundesanstalt
PQ	Performance Qualification
PQG	Pharmaceutical Quality Group (part of IQA)
PV	Performance Verification
QA	Quality Assurance
QC	Quality Control
QMS	Quality Management System
R&D	Research and Development
RAM	Random Access Memory
RDBMS	Relational Database Management System
RDS	Rapid Development Software
RFI	Radio Frequency Interference
RFP	Request for Proposal
ROM	Read Only Memory
RPharmS	Royal Pharmacy Society (United Kingdom)
RSC	Royal Society of Chemists (United Kingdom)
RTL/2	Real-Time Language, Version 2
RTSASD	Real-Time System-Analysis System-Design
S&OP	Sales and Operations Planning
SAA	Standards Association of Australia
SaRS	Safety and Reliability Society (United Kingdom)
SCADA	Supervisory Control And Data Acquisition
SAM	Software Assessment Method
SAT	System Acceptance Testing
SATS	System Acceptance Test Specification
SCR	Source Code Review
SDS	Software Design Specification
SEI	Software Engineering Institute (Carnegie-Mellon University)

SLA	Service Level Agreement
SOP	Standard Operating Procedure
SPC	Statistical Process Control
SPICE	Software Process Improvement and Capability Determination
SQAP	Software Quality and Productivity Analysis
STARTS	Software Tools for Large Real-Time Systems
STD	Software Technology Diagnosis
T&C	Threats and Controls
TBT	Technical Barriers to Trade
TGA	Therapeutic Goods Administration (Australia)
TIR	Test Incident Report
TÜV	Technischer Uberwachungs-Verein (Germany)
UK	United Kingdom
UL	Underwriters Laboratories Inc.
ULD	Utility Line Diagram
UPS	Uninterruptible Power Supply
URS	User Requirement Specification
U.S.	United States (of America)
VDU	Visual Display Unit
V-MAN	Validation Management Manual (United Kingdom)
VMP	Validation Master Plan
WAN	Wide Area Network
WFI	Water for Injection
WHA	World Health Assembly
WHO	World Health Organisation
WORM	Write Once, Read Many
WWW	World Wide Web
Y2K	Year 2000

Appendix 2

Glossary of Terms

The following pages contain a list of validation definitions for computer-related systems within manufacturing. The definitions presented are, wherever possible, established definitions taken from the pharmaceutical industry or Good Manufacturing Practice (GMP) regulatory authorities:

Acceptance Criteria
ANSI/IEEE (1983): The criteria a software product must meet to successfully complete a test phase or to achieve delivery requirements.

Actuator
FDA (1995): A peripheral output device which translates electrical signals into mechanical actions, e.g., a stepper motor which acts on an electrical signal received from a computer system to turn its shaft a certain number of degrees or a certain number of rotations.

Alpha Testing
FDA (1995): Acceptance testing performed by the customer in a controlled environment at the developer's site. The software is used by the customer in a setting approximating the target environment with the developer observing and recording errors and usage problems.

As-Built
FDA (1995): Pertaining to an actual configuration of software code resulting from a software development project.

Assembly Language

FDA (1995): A low level programming language that corresponds closely to the instruction set of a given computer, allows symbolic naming of operations and addresses, and usually results in a one-to-one translation of program instructions (mnemonics) into machine instructions.

Audit

GMA-NAMUR (1996): An activity to determine through investigation the adequacy of, and adherence to, established procedures, instructions, specifications, codes, and standards or other applicable contractual and licencing requirements, and the effectiveness of implementation.

Automation System

A system based on a computer technology with input devices (e.g., sensors), output devices (e.g., actuators) and communication links (e.g., telemetry and cable networks) which are collectively designed to perform a specific function or group of functions (e.g., control, protection, or monitoring). Automation systems may be linked into larger integrated systems. [Defined for this document]

Baseline

FDA (1995): A specification or product that has been formally reviewed and agreed upon, that serves as the basis for further development, and that can be changed only through formal change control procedures.

Batch Record

IQA (1994): Documents (including those stored in photographic and electronic form) which record stages in the manufacture of a batch, details of ingredients and process equipment used, methods followed, in-process controls carried out, test results obtained, dates of manufacture and testing, and history of the storage of the pharmaceutical raw material.

Bespoke Software

GAMP Forum (1996): A system produced for a customer, specifically to order, to meet a defined set of user requirements.

Beta Testing

FDA (1995): Acceptance testing performed by the customer in a live application of the software, at one or more end user sites, in an environment not controlled by the developer.

Black Box Testing (see Functional Testing)

Bomb
FDA (1995): A trojan horse which attacks a computer system upon the occurrence of a specific logical event ("logic bomb"), the occurrence of a specific time-related logical event ("time bomb"), or is hidden in electronic mail or data and is triggered when read in a certain way ("letter bomb").

Bootstrap
FDA (1995): A short computer program that is permanently resident or easily loaded into a computer and whose execution brings a larger program, such as an operating system or its loader, into memory.

Calibration
FDA (1995): Ensuring continuous adequate performance of sensing, measurement, and actuating equipment with regard to specified accuracy and precision requirements.

Certification
FDA (1995): In computer systems, a technical evaluation, made as part of and in support of the accreditation process, that establishes the extent to which a particular computer system or network design and implementation meet a prescribed set of requirements.

Change Control
FDA (1995): The processes, authorities for, and procedures to be used for all changes that are made to the computerized system and/or the system's data. Change control is a vital subset of the Quality Assurance program within an establishment and should be clearly described in the establishment's Standard Operating Procedures.

GAMP Forum (1996): A formal system by which qualified representatives of appropriate disciplines review proposed or actual changes that might affect a validated status. The intent is to determine the need for action that would ensure and document that the system is maintained in a validated state.

OECD (1995): Ongoing evaluation and documentation of system operations and changes to determine whether a validation process is necessary following any changes to the computerised system.

CHAZOP (see Hazard Study)

Client-Server
FDA (1995): A term used in a broad sense to describe the relationship between the receiver and provider of a service . . . a networked system where

front-end applications, as the client, makes service requests upon another networked system.

Code (see Software)

Comment

FDA (1995): In programming languages, a language construct that allows explanatory text to be inserted into a program and that does not have any effect on the execution of the program.

Computer Aided Software Engineering (CASE)

Tools designed to support the analysis and design phases of the software development life cycle. The tools are usually oriented towards the support of graphical notations. [Defined for this document]

Computerised System (see Automation System)

Computer-Related System (see Automation System)

Computer System (see Automation System)

Configuration

FDA (1995): The arrangement of a computer system or component as defined by the number, nature, and interconnection of its constituent parts.

Crash

FDA (1995): The sudden and complete failure of a computer system or component.

Data Integrity

FDA (1995): The degree to which a collection of data is complete, consistent, and accurate.

Data Validation

FDA (1995): A process used to determine if data are inaccurate, incomplete, or unreasonable. The process may include format checks, completeness checks, check key tests, reasonableness checks, and limit checks.

Dead Code

FDA (1995): Program code statements which can never execute during program execution. Such code can result from poor coding style, or can be an artifact of previous versions or debugging efforts. Dead code can be confusing, and is a potential source of erroneous software changes. [Note: Dead code does not include unused features (including diagnostic programs) of a standard product, which should be clearly identified and defined as such.]

Debugging

FDA (1995): Determining the exact nature and location of a program error, and fixing the error.

Design

FDA (1995): The process of defining the architecture, components, interfaces, and other characteristics of an [automation] system or component.

Design Qualification (DQ)

GAMP Forum (1996): Formal and systematic verification that the requirements defined during specification are completely covered by the succeeding [design] specification or implementation.

GMA-NAMUR (1996): Formal and systematic verification that the requirements determined at the functional specification phase were completely met in the subsequent specification or implementation phase and that the higher authority of guidelines or laws have been taken into account.

Design Review

Meeting held to conduct a Design Qualification. [Defined for this document]

Drug (Medicinal) Product

IQA (1994): Any substance or article (not being an instrument, apparatus, or appliance) which is manufactured, sold, supplied, imported, or exported for use by being administered to one or more human beings or animals for a medicinal purpose, or for use as an ingredient in the preparation of a substance or article which is to be administered to one or more human beings or animals for a medicinal purpose.

Electronic Record

FDA (1997): Any combination of text, graphics, data, audio, pictorial, or other information representation in digital form that is created, modified, maintained, archived, retrieved, or distributed by a computer system.

Electronic Signature

OECD (1995): The entry in the form of magnetic impulses or computer data compilation of any symbol or series of symbols, executed, adapted, or authorised by a person to be equivalent to the person's handwritten signature.

FDA (1997): A computer data compilation of any symbol or series of symbols executed, adopted, or authorised by an individual to be the legally binding equivalent of the individual's handwritten signature.

Embedded System

GAMP Forum (1996): A system, usually microprocessor or PLC based, whose sole purpose is to control a particular piece of automated equipment. This is contrasted with a stand-alone computer system.

Emulation

FDA (1995): A model that accepts the same inputs and produces the same outputs as a given system. To imitate one system with another.

Escrow

Held in trust by a third party, to be turned over to the grantee only upon fulfillment of a condition.

Firmware

FDA (1995): The combination of a hardware device, e.g., an Integrated Circuit, and computer instructions and data that reside as read only software on that device. Such software cannot be modified by the computer during processing.

Functional Specification

A written definition of the function that a system or system component can perform. [Defined for this document]

Functional Testing

GAMP Forum (1996): Also known as "Black Box" testing, since source code is not needed. Involves inputting normal information and abnormal test cases; then, evaluating outputs against those expected. Can apply to computer system or to a total system. [Adapted]

Good Manufacturing Practice (GMP)

EU (1991): That part of quality assurance which ensures that products are consistently produced and controlled to the quality standards appropriate to their intended use.

IQA (1994): [supplement EU definition with . . .] It concerns production, quality control, and warehousing and distribution procedures.

GMP Critical
An aspect of the manufacturing process that if not properly managed can impact product quality. [Defined for this document]

Handshake
FDA (1995): An interlocked sequence of signals between connected components in which each component waits for the acknowledgement of its previous signal before proceeding with its action, such as data transfer.

Hardware
FDA (1995): The physical equipment [making up an automation system], as opposed to programs, procedures, rules, and associated documentation. [Adapted]

Hardware Design (see Design)

Hazard Study
Computer hazard and operability study to assess the threats and their control between Automation Systems, their users and operational environments, and the manufacturing process. Hazard Studies for IT systems concentrate on the threats and their controls affecting data integrity. [Defined for this document]

Industry Standard
FDA (1995): Procedures or criteria recognised as acceptable practices by peer, professional, credentialing, or accrediting organisations.

In-Process Control
EU (1991): Checks performed during production in order to monitor and, if necessary, to adjust the process to ensure that the product conforms to its specification. The control of the environment or equipment may also be regarded as part of in-process control.

Installation Qualification (IQ)
FDA (1995): Establishing confidence that process equipment and ancillary systems [including automation systems] are compliant with appropriate codes and approved design intentions, and that manufacturer's recommendations are suitably considered.

PMA (1990): Documented verification that all key aspects of hardware installation adhere to appropriate codes and approved design intentions and that the recommendations of the manufacturer have been suitably considered.

Integrated Project Support Environment (IPSE)
Tools supporting the configuration management of documentation and programming during the software development life cycle. [Defined for this document]

Intermediate Product
EU (1991): Partly processed material which must undergo further manufacturing steps before it becomes a finished product.

Manufacture
EU (1991): All operations of purchase of materials and products—production, Quality Control, release, storage, distribution of medicinal products, and related controls.

Millenium Friendly
The operability of an automation system must not be adversely affected by dates associated with the year 2000; either prior to, during and after the year 2000. Interfaces and data storage must specify the year 2000 either explicitly or by unambiguous derivations. The year 2000 must also be recognised as a leap year. [Defined for this document]

Object Code
A computer program that is the output of translated [assembler or compiler] source code. [Defined for this document]

Operational Qualification (OQ)
FDA (1995): Establishing confidence that process equipment and subsystems [including automation systems] are capable of consistently operating within established limits and tolerances.

PMA (1990): Documented verification that the equipment-related system or subsystem performs as intended throughout all anticipated operating ranges.

Patch
A change made directly to object code without retranslating [assembler or compiler] the source code. [Defined for this document]

Performance Qualification (PQ)
EPA (1995): Documented verification that the process-related system performs as intended throughout representative or anticipated operating ranges.

FDA (1995): Establishing confidence that the [manufacturing] process is effective and reproducible.

Pharmaceutical Manufacturer

IQA (1994): An organisation named as the manufacturer of a medicinal product in a manufacturing authorisation granted by a competent national drugs or medicines control authority.

Platform

FDA (1995): The hardware and software which must be present and functioning for an application program to perform as intended. A platform includes, but is not limited to, the operating system or executive software, communication software, microprocessor, network, input/output hardware, any generic software libraries, database management, user interface software, and the like.

Procedures

EU (1991): Description of the operations to be carried out, the precautions to be taken and measures to be applied directly or indirectly related to the manufacture of a medicinal product.

Process Qualification

FDA (1995): Establishing confidence that a process is effective and reproducible.

Production

EU (1991): All operations involved in the preparation of a medicinal product, from receipt of material, through processing and packaging, to its completion as a finished product.

Product Qualification

FDA (1995): Establishing confidence through appropriate testing that the finished product produced by a specified process meets all release requirements for functionality and safety.

Program (see Software)

Project Plan

Similar to Quality Plan but including a detailed schedule of project activities and deliverables. [Defined for this document]

Prospective Validation

FDA (1995): Validation conducted prior to the distribution of either a new [drug] product, or [drug] product made under a revised manufacturing process, where the revisions may affect the [drug] product's characteristics.

GMA-NAMUR (1996): Documented evidence that a system does what it was planned to do before it is used in production. Also referred to as validating new systems.

Prototyping
FDA (1995): An approach to accelerate the software development process by facilitating the identification of required functionality during analysis and design phases. A limitation of this technique is the identification of system and software problems and hazards. [Adapted]

Quality Assurance (QA)
ANSI/IEEE (1983): A planned and systematic pattern of all actions necessary to provide adequate confidence that the item conforms to established technical requirements.

Quality Control (QC)
GAMP Forum (1996): The regulatory process through which industry measures actual quality performance, compares it with standards, and acts on the differences.

Quality Plan
GAMP Forum (1996): A plan created by the supplier to define actions, deliverables, responsibilities, and procedures to satisfy the customer's quality and validation requirements.

Raw Data
GAMP Forum (1996): Any worksheets, records, memoranda, notes, or exact copies thereof that are the result of original observations and activities of a study and are necessary for the reconstruction and evaluation of a work project, process or study report, etc. Raw data may be hard/paper copy or electronic but must be known and defined in the system procedures.

Real-Time
FDA (1995): Pertaining to a system or mode of operation in which computation is performed during the actual time that an external process occurs, in order that the computation results can be used to control, monitor, or respond in a timely manner to the external process.

Redundant Code (see Dead Code)

Retrospective Validation
FDA (1995): Validation of a process for a [drug] product already in distribution based upon accumulated production, testing, and control data.

GMA-NAMUR (1996): Documented evidence that a system does what it purports to do based on an analysis of historical information. Also referred to as validating existing systems.

Revalidation
GMA-NAMUR (1996): Repetition of the validation process or a specific portion of it [in response to a change].

Security
OECD (1995): The protection of computer hardware and software from accidental or malicious access, use, modification, destruction, or disclosure. Security also pertains to personnel data, communications, and physical protection of computer installations.

Sensor
FDA (1995): A peripheral input device which senses some variable in the system environment, such as temperatures, and converts it to an electrical signal which can be further converted to a digital signal for processing by the computer.

Simulation
FDA (1995): A model that behaves or operates like a given system when provided a set of controlled inputs.

Software
GAMP Forum (1996): A collection of programs, routines, and subroutines that controls the operation of an automation system. [Adapted]

Software Design (see Design)

Software Inspection
FDA (1995): A manual testing technique in which program documents (including source code) are examined in a very formal and disciplined manner to discover errors, violations of standards, and other problems.

Source Code
GAMP Forum (1996): An original computer program expressed in human readable form (programming language) which must be translated into machine readable form before it can be executed by the computer.

Source Code Review (see Software Inspection)

Standard (see Industry Standard)

Standard Operating Procedures (see also Procedures)
FDA (1995): Written procedures prescribing and describing the steps to be taken in normal and defined conditions which are necessary to assure control of production and processes.

GMA-NAMUR (1996): Instruction which describes how something is to be accomplished. SOPs regulate the operation and maintenance of a computerised [automated] system in order to use it in a correct way and also to fulfill its real purpose permanently.

Stepwise Refinement
FDA (1995): A structured software design technique; data and processing steps are defined broadly at first, and then further defined with increasing detail.

Structural Testing
GAMP Forum (1996): Also known as "White Box" testing and involves examining the internal structure of the source code. Includes low-level and high-level code review, path analysis, auditing of programming procedures, and standards actually used, inspection for extraneous "dead code", boundary analysis and other techniques. Requires specific computer science and programming expertise. [Adapted]

Superfluous Code
Software code which unnecessarily recalculates, rechecks, or reperforms calculations or actions which are unnecessary or which have already been done. [Defined for this document]

Supplier
GMA-NAMUR (1996): The company or group responsible for developing, constructing, and delivering a system or part of a system. A supplier can be an [equipment] vendor, a contractor [including system's application integrator], or a consultant.

Testing
FDA (1995): The process of operating a system or component under specified conditions, observing or recording the results, and making an evaluation of some aspect of the system or component.

Trojan Horse
FDA (1995): A method of attacking a computer system, typically by providing a useful program which contains code intended to compromise a computer system by secretly providing for unauthorised access, the unauthorised collection of privileged system and user data, the unauthorised reading or altering of files, the performance of unintended and unexpected functions, or the malicious destruction of software and hardware.

User
GMA-NAMUR (1996): The company or group responsible for the operation of a system.

User Requirements Specification
The customer's written functional needs in regard to an automation system. [Defined for this document]

Validation
EU (1991): Action of proving, in accordance with the principles of Good Manufacturing Practice, that any procedure, process, equipment, material, activity, or system actually leads to the expected results.

FDA (1995): Establishing documented evidence which provides a high degree of assurance that a specific process will consistently produce a product meeting its pre-determined specifications and quality attributes.

GMA-NAMUR (1996): Documented evidence that a specific process will consistently produce a product meeting its pre-determined specification and quality attributes.

IQA (1994): The process of establishing documentary evidence which provides a high degree of assurance that any product, process, activity, procedure, system, equipment, or software used in the control or manufacture consistently meets its predetermined specification.

OECD (1995): The demonstration that a computerised system is suitable for its intended purpose.

Validation Master Plan
A high-level plan coordinating a number of validation plans. [Defined for this document]

Validation Plan
GMA-NAMUR (1996): A prospective plan of action whose implementation should produce formal and documented proof that the system is validated.

Vendor (see Supplier)

Virus

FDA (1995): A program which secretly alters other programs to include a copy of itself, and executes when the host program is executed. The execution of a virus program comprises a computer system by performing unwanted or unintended functions which may be destructive.

White Box Testing (see Structural Testing)

White Space

Blank lines of code which have been purposely inserted into the software listing to make it easier to read. [Defined for this document]

WORM

FDA (1995): An independent program which can travel from computer to computer across network connections replicating itself in each computer. They do not change other programs, but compromise a computer system through their impact on system performance.

REFERENCES

ANSI/IEEE (1983)

Glossary of Software Engineering Terminology, Standard 729.

EPA (1995)

United States Environmental Protection Agency (1995), *Good Automated Laboratory Practices: Principles and Guidance to Regulations for Ensuring Data Integrity in Automated Laboratory Operations with Implementation Guidance,* Document Reference 2185, 1995 Edition.

EU (1991)

European Union Directive 91/356/EEC (Good Manufacturing Practice).

FDA (1995)

United States Food and Drug Administration, *Glossary of Computerized System and Software Development Terminology,* Issued August.

GAMP Forum (1996)

UK GAMP Forum (1996), *Supplier Guide for Validation of Automation Systems in Pharmaceutical Manufacture,* Second Version, The Hague: International Society for Pharmaceutical Engineers.

GMA-NAMUR (1996)
NE 58: Abwicklung von qualifizierungspflichtigen PLT-Projekten (version 04.06.96); [including . . .] Dannapel, B., Hensel, H., Mockel, B., Muhlenkamp, J., Muller-Heinzerling, T., Otto, A., and Teuchert, V., Qualifizierung von Leitsystemen: Ein Gemeinschaftsprojekt von GMA und NAMUR zur Validierung, *ATP—Automatisierungstechnische Praxis,* Vol. 37 (1995), No. 10, pp. 64–76.

IQA (1994)
United Kingdom Institute of Quality Assurance (Pharmaceutical Quality Group), *Pharmaceutical Supplier Code of Practice Covering the Manufacture of Pharmaceutical Raw Materials, Active Ingredients and Excipients,* Document Reference No. P00020, Issue 2.

OECD (1995)
Organisation for Economic Co-operation and Development, *The Application of the Principles of GLP to Computer Systems,* GLP Consensus Document, Environmental Monograph No. 116, (No. 10 in OECD Series on Principles of GLP and Compliance Monitoring).

PMA (1990)
Computer System Validation—Staying Current: Installation Qualification, *Pharmaceutical Technology,* September, pp. 88–104.

Appendix 3

Selected GLP/GMP Regulation Quotes

The following selection of GLP and GMP regulations quotes have been chosen as a representative sample of validation requirements. The reader is encouraged to refer to the original sources for more information and to see the quotes given here in the context of their corresponding regulations.

THE VALIDATION OF AUTOMATED SYSTEMS

Australian Code of GMP for Therapeutic Goods—Medicinal Products—Part 1, Use of Computers

900. Where a computer is used in connection with any procedure or process associated with the production of therapeutic goods, the computer system employed should meet the requirements of this Code for those manual functions which it replaces.

Australian Code of GMP for Therapeutic Goods—Medicinal Products—Part 1, Use of Computers

903. The development, implementation, and operation of a computer system should be carefully documented at all stages and each step proven to achieve its written objective under challenging test conditions.

Australian Code of GMP for Therapeutic Goods—Medicinal Products—Part 1, Use of Computers

907. A change to an existing computer system should be made in accordance with a defined change control procedure which should document the details of each change made, its purpose, and its date of effect, and it should provide for a check to confirm that the change has been applied correctly.

EU Directive 91/356/EEC—Chapter 3, Premises and Equipment, Principle

Premises and equipment must be located, designed, constructed, adapted, and maintained to suit the operation to be carried out. Their layout and design must aim to minimize the risk of errors and permit effective cleaning and maintenance in order to avoid cross-contamination, build up of dust or dirt, and, in general, any adverse effect on the quality of products.

EU Directive 91/356/EEC—Annex 11, Computerised Systems, Principle

The introduction of computerised systems into systems of manufacturing, including storage, distribution, and quality control, does not alter the need to observe the relevant principles given elsewhere in the Guide. Where a computerised system replaces a manual operation, there should be no resultant decrease in product quality or quality assurance. Consideration should be given to the risk of losing aspects of the previous system which could result from reducing the involvement of operators.

EU Directive 91/356/EEC—Annex 11, Computerised Systems, Validation

2. The extent of validation necessary will depend on a number of factors including the use to which the system is to be put, whether the validation is to be prospective or retrospective and whether or not novel elements are incorporated. Validation should be considered as part of the complete life cycle of a computer system. This cycle includes the stages of planning, specification, programming, testing, commissioning, documentation, operation, monitoring, and modifying.

EU Directive 91/356/EEC—Annex 11, Computerised Systems, System

3. Attention should be paid to the siting of equipment in suitable conditions where extraneous factors cannot interfere with the system.

EU Directive 91/356/EEC—Annex 11, Computerised Systems, System

4. A written detailed description of the system should be produced (including diagrams as appropriate) and kept up to date. It should describe the principles, objectives, security measures, and scope of the system and the main features of the way in which the computer is used and how it interacts with other systems and procedures.

EU Directive 91/356/EEC—Annex 11, Computerised Systems, System

5. The software is a critical component of a computerised system. The user of such software should take all reasonable steps to ensure that it has been produced in accordance with a system of quality assurance.

EU Directive 91/356/EEC—Annex 11, Computerised Systems, System

11. Alterations to a system or to a computer program should only be made in accordance with a defined procedure which should include provision for validating, checking, approving, and implementing the change. Such an alteration should only be implemented with the agreement of the person responsible for the part of the system concerned, and the alteration should be recorded. Every significant modification should be validated.

Japanese Guideline on Computer Systems in Drug Manufacturing—Scope of Application

This guideline shall apply to the drug manufacturing plants governed by Drug GMP and other regulations where any of the following systems are introduced. However, the system with limited function and are operated simply by inputting the parameters to the programme fixed by the supplier of the hardware (including every device and equipment controlled by a computer) as general functions of the devices shall be exempted from this guideline.

(1) The system for manufacturing process control and management including that for recording these data.

(2) The system for production control such as storage and inventory of starting materials and final products including intermediates.

(3) The system for documentation of manufacturing directions, testing protocols, or records.

(4) The system for quality control and recording these data.

Japanese Guideline on Computer Systems in Drug Manufacturing—System Designing

3.1.2 The manufacturer shall document a system development manual which shall normally include:

(A) Procedures of system development

(B) Documents to be prepared during each step of the system development and the methods of maintaining these documents

(C) Procedures for evaluation and approval of each step of system development

(D) Procedures for amending or repeal of the system development manual

Japanese Guideline on Computer Systems in Drug Manufacturing—Operation Control

4.1.3 (A) The manufacturer shall prepare a system alteration standard code which includes, in principles, the following:

a) Procedures for alteration application and approval of alteration

b) Examination after system alteration

c) Amendment of operation procedures

d) Notification of the amended parts to the persons concerned

e) Title or name of the manager and person/s in charge

(B) The provisions [. . . during . . .] "development of the system" shall generally apply to the system alteration when associated with programme change after its introduction.

Japanese Guideline on Computer Systems in Drug Manufacturing—Accidents

4.4.1 The manager shall ensure that the peron/s in charge take immediate actions when accidents occur in the system in accordance with the provisions of the operation procedures and let him/her conduct a cause finding study as well as take necessary actions for the prevention of these accidents.

Japanese Guideline on Computer Systems in Drug Manufacturing—Self-Inspection

4.6.1 The manufacturer shall ensure that the operation of the system is consonant with this guideline through periodical inspection by its manager.

U.S. CFR Title 21, 11.10—Controls for Closed Systems

Persons who use closed systems to create, modify, maintain, or transmit electronic records shall employ procedures and controls designed to ensure authenticity, integrity, and, when appropriate, the confidentiality of electronic records, and to ensure the signer cannot readily repudiate the signed record as not genuine.

U.S. CFR Title 21, 11.30—Controls for Open Systems

Persons who use open systems to create, modify, maintain, or transmit electronic records shall employ procedures and controls designed to ensure authenticity, integrity, and, as appropriate, the confidentiality of electronic records from the point of their creation to the point of their receipt.

U.S. CFR Title 21, 58.61—Equipment Design

Automatic, mechanical, or electrical equipment used in the generation, measurement, or assessment of data shall be of appropriate design and adequate capacity to function according to the protocol and shall be suitably located for operation, inspection, cleaning, and maintenance.

U.S. CFR Title 21, 58.63—Maintenance and Calibration of Equipment

(a) Equipment used for the generation, measurement, or assessment of data shall be adequately tested, calibrated, and/or standardized.

(b) The written standard operating procedures required under section 58.81(b)(11) shall set forth in sufficient detail the methods, materials, and schedules to be used in the routine inspection, cleaning, maintenance, testing, calibration, and/or standardization of equipment, and shall specify remedial action to be taken in event of failure or malfunction of equipment.

(c) Written records shall be maintained of all inspection operations.

U.S. CFR Title 21, 58.130—Conduct of a Nonclinical Laboratory Study

(e) In computer driven data collection systems, the individual responsible for the direct data input shall be identified at the time of data input. Any change in the computer entries shall be made so as not to obscure the original entry, shall indicate the reason for the change, and shall be dated, and the responsible individual shall be identified.

U.S. CFR Title 21, 211.68—Automated Equipment and Electronic Equipment

(a) Automatic, mechanical, or electronic equipment or other types of equipment, including computers, or related systems that will perform a function satisfactorily, may be used in the manufacture, processing, packaging, and holding of a drug product. If such equipment is so used, it shall be routinely calibrated, inspected, or checked according to a written program designated to assure proper performance. Written records of those calibration checks and inspections shall be maintained.

(b) Appropriate controls shall be exercised over computer or related systems to assure that changes in master production and control records or other records are instituted only by authorised personnel. Input to and output from the computer or related system of formulas or other records or data shall be checked for accuracy. The degree and frequency of input/output verification shall be based on the complexity and reliability of the computer or related system. A backup file of data entered into the computer or related system shall be maintained except where certain data, such as calculations performed in conjunction with laboratory analysis, are eliminated by computerisation or other automated processes. In such instances a written record of the program shall be maintained along with appropriate validation data. Hard copy or alternative systems, such as duplicates, tapes, or microfilm, designed to assure that backup data are exact and complete and that it is secure from alteration, inadvertent erasures, or loss shall be maintained.

U.S. CFR Title 21, 820.195—Critical Devices, Automated Data Processing

When automated data processing is used for manufacturing or quality assurance purposes, adequate checks shall be implemented to prevent inaccurate data output, input, and programming errors.

U.S. CFR Title 21, 820.61—Measurement Equipment

All production and quality assurance measurement equipment, such as mechanical, automated, or electronic equipment, shall be suitable for its intended purposes and shall be capable of producing valid results. Such equipment shall be routinely calibrated, inspected, and checked according to written procedures. Records documenting the activities must be maintained. When computers are used as part of an automated production or quality assurance system, the computer software programs shall be validated by adequate and documented testing. All program changes shall be made by a designated individual(s) through a formal approval procedure.

PERSONNEL CONDUCTING VALIDATION

Australian Code of GMP for Therapeutic Goods—Medicinal Products—Part 1, Use of Computers

902. Persons with appropriate expertise should be responsible for the design, introduction, and regular review of a computer system.

EU Directive 91/356/EEC—Annex 11, Computerised Systems, Personnel

It is essential that there is the closest cooperation between key personnel and those involved with computer systems. Persons in responsible positions should have the appropriate training for the management and use of systems within their field of responsibility which utilizes computers. This should include ensuring that appropriate expertise is available and used to provide advice on aspects of design, validation, installation, and operation of computerized system.

Japanese Guideline on Computer Systems in Drug Manufacturing—System Designing

3.1.1 (A) The manufacturer shall designate a manager and person/s in charge of each step of the system development ranging from "system engineering" to "installation and operation test". The same person may also assume the responsibility for several steps of the system development.

(B) The manager shall specify individual duties of person/s in charge.

Japanese Guideline on Computer Systems in Drug Manufacturing—Operation Control

3.1.1 (A) The manufacturer shall designate a manager and person/s in charge of each step of the system development ranging from "operation of hardware" to "self-inspection". The same person may also assume the responsibility for several steps of the system development.

(B) The manager shall specify individual duties of person/s in charge.

Japanese Guideline on Computer Systems in Drug Manufacturing—Others

All or part of the activities described in "development of the system" can be entrusted to other firms on condition that the manufacturer concerned shall obtain and maintain the relevant documents of the activities from the contracting firm or otherwise ensure that these documents are properly retained by the contracting firm. However, the contracted activities which fall within "system performance test" or "installation and operation test" shall be directly supervised, evaluated, and accordingly approved by the responsible person designated by the manufacturer concerned.

U.S. CFR Title 21, 211.34—Consultants

Consultants advising on the manufacture, processing, packaging, or holding of drug products shall have sufficient education, training, and experience, or any combination thereof, to advise on the subject for which they are retained. Records shall be maintained stating the name, address, and qualifications of any consultants and the type of service they provide.

Appendix 4

Contributors' Biographies

ROB ALMOND
Computer Validation Manager, Glaxo Wellcome, UK

Mr. Almond is the external liaison manager for Glaxo Wellcome's manufacturing IT systems with special responsibility for validation compliance. Between 1991 and 1996, he was responsible for retrospective validation of manufacturing and laboratory computer and control systems. Mr. Almond has 20 years' experience of Quality Assurance within the Pharmaceutical Industry, during the last six he has become involved with computer validation applied to process automation and business IT systems. He is a member of the UK Good Automated Manufacturing Practice (GAMP) Forum and has contributed to the various versions of the GAMP Supplier Guide *Good Automated Manufacturing Practice* (GAMP) published between 1994 and 1996.

Address:
Glaxo Wellcome Operations
Harmire Road
Barnard Castle
County Durham, DL2 8DT, England
Tel: +44-1833-690600
Fax: +44-1833-692300

JOHN BIANCULLI
Total Quality Manager, Beckman Instruments, USA

Mr. Bianculli has a bachelor's degree in Chemical Engineering from the University of Delaware. As a LIMS customer, he has implemented commercial LIMS systems. Upon joining Beckman Instruments, Mr. Bianculli delivered LIMS implementation consulting, ultimately leading the consulting team responsible for North American implementation work. In his current role as Total Quality Manager, Mr. Bianculli has responsibility for maintaining Beckman Instruments Laboratory Automation Operations ISO 9001 Quality System registration and conducting product verification and validation testing.

Address:
Beckman Instruments Inc.
90 Bordine Road
Allendale, NJ 07401-1613, U.S.A.
Tel: +1-201-818-8900
Fax: +1-201-818-8698

PETER BOSSHARD
Manager Quality Assurance, Hoffmann-La Roche, Switzerland

Dr. Bosshard joined the Quality Assurance Department at Hoffmann-La Roche in 1994. He is responsible for ensuring computer system validation documentation is compliant with GMP regulatory requirements and internal company guidelines. Dr. Bosshard's background includes six years of industrial experience as an electronic-mechanical technician before studying for his doctorate in pharmacy at Fribourg and Bern in Switzerland. Prior to joining Hoffmann-La Roche, Dr. Bosshard worked for two years with Sandoz as a scientific coordinator.

Address:
Hoffmann-La Roche
PS1B, Business Relations, Building 224/35
4070 Basel, Switzerland
Tel: +41-61-687-3525
Fax: +41-61-687-2849

PETER COADY
Consultant Engineer, P.J. Coady & Associates, UK

Mr. Coady is a Consultant Engineer specialising in process control and instrumentation working in the pharmaceutical industry. He has over 20 years of industrial experience, with a career centred on project management, and he was employed as Manager of the Electrical, Instrumentation, and Systems Group at AMEC (formerly Matthew Hall Engineering), prior to moving into consultancy. He is currently working with SmithKline Beecham Pharmaceuticals on a major capital R&D project, which includes the provision of specialist validation assistance for process control systems. Mr. Coady has a B.Sc. Honours degree and is a Chartered Engineer and a European Engineer. He is a Fellow of the InstMC, a Fellow of the IMechE, a Member of the ISPE, a Member of the PDA, a Senior Member of the ISA, and a registered TickIT Auditor.

Address:
P.J. Coady & Associates
15 Cutter Avenue
Warsash
Southampton, Hampshire, SO31 9BA, England
Tel/Fax: +44-1489-572047

TONY DE CLAIRE
Control & Automation Manager, SmithKline Beecham, UK

Mr. de Claire is Manager, Process Control and Automation Group, Worldwide Supply Operations for SmithKline Beecham Pharmaceuticals. The group provides worldwide project support and technology transfer on the company's strategic capital investments and product development. Mr. de Claire has been responsible for numerous process computer system validation projects. He is a Member of InstMC, a Senior Member of the ISA, a Member of the ISPE and a trained TickIT Auditor. During the last 30 years, he has progressed through a career in control and instrument engineering in the chemical, steel, and pharmaceutical industries.

Address:
SmithKline Beecham Pharmaceuticals
Clarendon Road
Worthing, West Sussex, BN14 8QN, England
Tel: +44-1903-822551
Fax: +44-1903-822670

CHRIS EVANS
Senior Validation Engineer, Eutech Engineering, UK

Mr. Evans is a Senior Validation Engineer working for Eutech Engineering Solutions Limited. He has over 24 years experience in engineering instrumentation and process control systems within the chemicals and pharmaceuticals industry. During the last decade, Mr. Evans has developed specialist skills integrating Distributed Control Systems (DCSs) and more recently has been responsible for ensuring GMP compliance of these and other automation systems to FDA and MCA requirements.

Address:
Eutech Engineering Solutions Ltd
Belasis Hall Technology Park
Billingham, Cleveland, TS23 4YS, England
Tel: +44-1642-372126
Fax: +44-1642-372166

JOHN GOUGH
Production Engineering Manager, Pfizer, UK

Mr. Gough is Production Engineering Manager for the Manufacturing Division of Pfizer Limited, Sandwich, UK. He is responsible for the project engineering required for capital projects in the Bulk Pharmaceutical Manufacturing plant at Sandwich. He also manages an automation group responsible for process control systems across the manufacturing site. After four years as a Research Chemical Engineer with Courtaulds, Mr. Gough moved to Pfizer in 1977 as a production manager. He became involved with process automation in 1980, project managing the first major DCS on site. Since that time he has become involved in, and finally responsible for, all automation and its ramifications within the Manufacturing Division.

Address:
Pfizer Ltd
Ramsgate Road
Sandwich, Kent, CT13 9NJ, England
Tel: +44-1304-616161
Fax: +44-1304-616525

PETER GOUGH
Quality Assurance Advisor, Eli Lilly, UK

Mr. Gough is currently Quality Assurance Advisor and a Qualified Person at Eli Lilly where he has worked for the past 22 years. He became involved with computer validation early in 1993 when Eli Lily implemented a new worldwide computer systems validation policy. He has been providing QA oversight of computer validation at the company's Basingstoke site, and he has been a member of the site's Computer Validation Committee since its inception. Mr. Gough holds an M.Sc. in analytical chemistry, and he is a Chartered Chemist, a member of the RSC, and a committee member of the UK IQA-PQG.

Address:
Eli Lilly and Company Ltd
Kingsclere Road
Basingstoke, Hampshire, RG21 6XA, England
Tel. +44-1256-315378
Fax: +44-1256-315738

THOMAS HEFTI
Quality Manager, Hoffmann-La Roche, Switzerland

Mr. Hefti joined Hoffmann-La Roche in 1992, where he is currently responsible for the implementation and operation of the ISO 9000 certified quality system of the central information technology service unit in Basel, Switzerland. He studied business administration at the University of St. Gallen, Switzerland. Mr. Hefti is currently working on a doctorate thesis in the area of computerised system validation.

Address:
Hoffmann-La Roche
PS1B, Business Relations, Building 224/35
4070 Basel, Switzerland
Tel: +41-61-687-3525
Fax: +41-61-687-2849

LUDWIG HUBER
Product Manager, Hewlett-Packard, Germany

Dr. Huber began work at Hewlett-Packard as an Applications Chemist for GC and HPLC in 1978. His current position is product manager for HPLC products and environmental, food and pharmaceutical industry markets. In this position he has developed HP's compliance program. He is the author of more than 50 publications dealing with chromatography and regulatory and quality standard compliance in the analytical laboratory. His most extensive publication is the book *Validation of Computerized Analytical Systems,* published by Interpharm in May 1995. Dr. Huber also provides consultancy to a regulatory agency in Europe on the use computers in regulated environments. Dr. Huber received an M.Sc. in Chemistry in 1975 and a Ph.D. in Chemical Engineering in 1978 from the University of Karlsruhe, Germany.

Address:
Hewlett-Packard GmbH
Hewlett-Packard Strasse
D-76337 Waldbronn, Germany
Tel: +49-7243-602209
Fax: +49-7243-602501
E-mail: ludwig_huber@hp.com

TERRY LUCY
Senior Controls Engineer, Glaxo Wellcome, UK

Mr. Lucy is the Senior Controls Engineer with Glaxo Wellcome Operations where he is responsible for the management of the computer systems validation for control systems. He joined Wellcome in 1977 from AKZO Chemicals as a process engineer in the project group. This section was responsible for the design, installation, and commissioning of all control systems used on process plant projects on a worldwide basis. In 1993 as the control systems expert, he was a member of the team that wrote the computer systems validation SOPs currently in use at Glaxo Wellcome Operations. Recently, he has been the "systems expert" for a number of prospective computer validation exercises for process plants being installed in the company's sterile facility. Mr. Lucy is a Chartered Engineer and a member of the IChemE and InstMC.

Address:
Glaxo Wellcome Operations
Temple Hill
Dartford, Kent, DA1 5AH, England
Tel: +44-1322-223488
Fax: +44-1322-291840
E-mail: terry_r_lucy@gb.wfl.com

RICHARD MITCHELL
Validation Coordinator, Pfizer, UK

Mr. Mitchell is Validation Coordinator for the Bulk Pharmaceutical Manufacturing plants in the Manufacturing Division of Pfizer Limited, Sandwich, UK. He is involved in all aspects of the validation of bulk pharmaceutical chemical manufacture with particular responsibility for the validation of process computer systems and equipment qualification. A microbiologist by training, he joined Pfizer Limited in 1987 as a Fermentation Technologist in the fermentation development laboratory. He managed the laboratory for four years before moving into his current role in 1993. Mr. Mitchell has gained practical experience of automated systems in bulk pharmaceutical chemical manufacture and the development of strategies to validate them.

Address:
Pfizer Ltd
Ramsgate Road
Sandwich, Kent, CT13 9NJ, England
Tel: +44-1304-616161
Fax: +44-1304-616926

PETER OWEN
Computer Validation Coordinator, Eli Lilly, UK

Mr. Owen is an experienced engineer having spent 20 years working in the field of control and instrumentation engineering, with 7 years specialising in the validation of computer systems in the pharmaceutical industry. He has worked on a number of different environments, including industrial and medical gases, fine chemicals, multidose inhalation, and solid dose facilities. Mr. Owen's experience with Eli Lilly includes the successful completion of approximately 70 validation projects, both prospective and retrospective. These have included PLCs, SCADA, DCS, LIMS, EMS, and warehouse management systems.

Address:
Eli Lilly and Company Ltd
Kingsclere Road
Basingstoke
Hampshire, RG21 6XA, England
Tel: +44-1256-315378
Fax: +44-1256-315738

BOB PAIGE
Validation Consultant, Eutech Engineering, UK

Mr. Paige is a senior validation consultant with Eutech Engineering. He has extensive practical validation experience developed initially with ICI Pharmaceuticals and more recently with Zeneca. Mr. Paige is currently involved with the overall coordination and management of the validation of a medical device undergoing GMP regulatory approval. Mr. Paige has been involved with the UK GAMP Forum's Validation Guide for Suppliers since its inception through to its current issue. He is a Member of the BCS and a Chartered Engineer. Mr. Paige has made presentations on the topic of computer systems validation at numerous UK conferences.

Address:
Eutech Engineering Solutions Ltd
Belasis Hall Technology Park
Billingham
Cleveland, TS23 4YS, England
Tel: +44-1642-372000
Fax: +44-1642-372166

CHRIS REID
Pharmaceutical Controls Manager, ICI, UK

Mr. Reid joined ICI in 1987 and is now Manager of Pharmaceutical Manufacturing Controls, which encompasses manufacturing automation. Mr. Reid was originally involved with the development of process control systems for control of bulk chemical plants. He later transferred to ICI's Informational Technology Group where he was engaged in the development for bespoke

SCADA systems utilised in bulk chemical and pharmaceuticals industries and was appointed Product Manager. In this role, he was responsible for control of product development and support, which necessitated establishing a quality management framework that satisfied stringent pharmaceutical regulatory requirements and customer expectations. Mr. Reid graduated with a B.Sc. (Honours) in Computer Science from North Staffordshire University.

Address:
c/o Eutech Engineering
Belasis Hall Technology Park
Billingham
Cleveland, TS23 4YS, England
Tel: +44-1642-372133
Fax: +44-1642-372100

OWEN SALVAGE
Senior Validation Engineer, Eutech Engineering, UK

Mr. Salvage is a senior validation engineer with Eutech Engineering Solutions Limited. Having spent 10 years with ICI and Zeneca installing pharmaceutical process control and information systems, Mr. Salvage now supplies project management and advice to the industry on matters relating to computer systems validation. In particular, he has expertise with batch control systems. Mr. Salvage holds a B.Sc. in Electronic Engineering from Salford University, and he is an Associate Member of the IEE.

Address:
Eutech Engineering Solutions Ltd
Belasis Hall Technology Park
Billingham
Cleveland, TS23 4YS, England
Tel: +44-1642-372007
Fax: +44-1642-372166

KATE SAMWAYS
Computer & Control Systems Validation Manager, Rhône-Poulenc Rorer, UK

Ms. Samways is responsible for setting standards within the company for the validation of computer and control systems of all types used in the support of manufacture, control, quality, and distribution of pharmaceutical products. She provides direction and support to the worldwide affiliates to ensure their compliance with the company and regulatory requirements. Previously, Ms. Samways worked for Rhône-Poulenc Rorer Nenagh, Republic of Ireland, as Business Systems Development Manager. Ms Samways holds a BPharm from the School of Pharmacy at the University of London, and she is a Member of the RPharmS.

Address:
Rhône-Poulenc Rorer
Rainham Road
South Dagenham
Essex, RM10 7XS, England
Tel: +44-181-9192320
E-mail: kate.samways@rp.fr

MARTIN SMITH
Computer Validation Manager, Zeneca Pharma, France

Mr. Smith is the Computer Systems Validation Manager at Zeneca Pharma's Reims site. He originally joined ICI in 1986 and was soon transferred to ICI Pharmaceuticals which was later demerged to become Zeneca Pharmaceuticals. Mr. Smith began his career as a Systems Analyst gaining experience of IT production systems before moving on to work in computer validation. Mr. Smith is particularly knowledgeable about validating PLC, EBRS, and MES computer systems supporting pharmaceutical manufacturing. He has a B.Eng. (Honours) in Mechanical Engineering from Leeds University.

Address:
Zeneca Pharma France
Zl La Pompelle
Chemin de Vrilly
BP 401
51804 Reims Cedex, France
Tel: +33-26-61-68-98

HANS SUCKER
Project Manager, Hoffmann-La Roche, Switzerland

Mr. Sucker joined Hoffmann-La Roche in 1990 where he is involved in computer applications and projects in the galenical production department. Mr. Sucker has previously worked at for the Federal Institute of Technology's Department of Pharmacy in Zurich and for Cilag Limited, leading the production of semisolid and nonsterile liquid dosage forms at Schaffhausen in Switzerland.

Address:
Hoffmann-La Roche
PS1B, Business Relations, Building 224/35
4070 Basel, Switzerland
Tel: +41-61-687-3525
Fax: +41-61-687-2849

NICK TOWNSEND
Business Manager, Beckman Instruments, UK

Mr. Townsend is Business Manager of Beckman Instruments' European Laboratory Automation Operations. He has over 16 years' experience of Laboratory Information Management Systems (LIMS) in regulated environments. Originally a Biochemist in a leading pharmaceutical company, he developed a strong interest in LIMS whilst helping introduce a data system into the laboratory in which he was working. He left the laboratory to become a LIMS programmer and implementation specialist. Later he moved into LIMS sales and marketing and he is now responsible for the sales and implementation of Beckman Instruments LIMS and data acquisition systems across Europe. Mr. Townsend holds a B.Sc. in Biochemistry from the University of Manchester.

Address:
Beckman Instruments Ltd
Oakley Court
Kingsmead Business Park
London Road
High Wycombe
Buckinghamshire, HP11 1JL, England
Tel: +44-1494-441181
Fax: +44-1494-461935

ANTHONY TRILL
Specialist Principal Inspector, Medicines Control Agency, UK

Mr. Trill joined the Medicines Inspectorate in 1984 and since 1988 has had national responsibility for MCA standards and inspection guidance relating to computerised systems, in addition to routine regional GMP inspection work, both at home and abroad. Before joining the MCA, he worked in the pharmaceutical industry for 18 years in R&D, new product and process development, production, QA, and technical services in management and technical roles. Mr. Trill has lectured widely and published on the topic of validating automated systems and GMP guidance, and he is a member of several review panels for quality critical guidance, including ICSE, TickIT, FRESCO, and GAMP Forum. Mr. Trill is also a member of the Editorial Advisory Board to *Pharmaceutical Technology—Europe* (Advantstar Publications). Mr. Trill holds a B.Sc. (Honours) in Pharmacy from the University of Aston and an M.Sc. in Pharmaceutical Technology from the University of London. He is an IRCA Lead Auditor and an EC Qualified Person.

Address:
MCA (Inspection and Enforcement)
North-West Regional Office, Room 209
Chantry House
City Road
Chester, CH1 3AQ, England
Tel: +44-1244-351515
Fax: +44-1244-319762

MARK WHITEHOUSE
Senior Project Manager, Yokogawa, UK

Mr. Whitehouse is responsible for managing DCS integration projects for a variety of pharmaceutical and process plants. He graduated in 1985 with an M.Sc. in Chemical Engineering from Nottingham University. Mr. Whitehouse is a Member of the BCS and is a Chartered Engineer.

Address:
Yokogawa UK Ltd
Stuart Road
Manor Park
Runcorn
Cheshire, WA7 1TR, England
Tel: +44-1928-579879
Fax: +44-1928-579899

GUY WINGATE
Validation Manager, Eutech Engineering, UK

Dr. Wingate heads the Validation Services Group at Eutech Engineering. Eutech provides engineering services and consultancy to the chemicals and pharmaceuticals industry and has assisted many leading pharmaceutical manufacturers with the validation of their automation systems. Dr. Wingate's personal validation experience covers more than 60 validation projects dealing with process control systems, laboratory systems, MRP II, and document management systems. He is a Chartered Engineer, a Member of the ISPE, a Member of the PDA, a Member of the SaRS, and a Member of the IEE. He holds a B.Sc., an M.Sc., and a Ph.D. from the University of Durham in Computing, Advanced Electronics, and Engineering, respectively. Dr. Wingate has published papers widely on the subjects of dependability and validation of automation systems, and regularly chairs and speaks at validation conferences in the UK and Europe. Dr. Wingate is also a Visiting Lecturer for the University of York's M.Sc. course on Safety Critical Systems and a Tutor for the University of Manchester's M.Sc. course on Pharmaceutical Engineering Advanced Technology.

Address:
Eutech Engineering Solutions Ltd
Belasis Hall Technology Park
Billingham
Cleveland, TS23 4YS, England
Tel: +44-1642-372124
Fax: +44-1642-372166
E-mail: guy.wingate@gbeut02.eutech.com

SION WYN
Director, Activa Systems, UK

Mr. Wyn has specialised in software for the pharmaceutical industry for over 10 years, focusing on electronic record and document management, computer validation, and regulatory compliance. He is also a trained ISO 9001 and TickIT auditor. Mr. Wyn has been closely involved in the development of the GAMP Guide for Validation of Automated Systems in the Pharmaceutical Manufacture, and he is a member of the GAMP Forum Specialist Group on Electronic Documents, Records, and Signatures. Mr. Wyn has chaired seminars on Good Automated Manufacturing Practice and is an Honorary Lecturer in Software Engineering at the University of Wales, Aberystwyth.

Address:
Activa Systems Ltd
Hanover House
The Roe. St. Asaph
Clywd, LL17 OLT, Wales
Tel: +44-1745-582600
Fax: +44-1745-584348

Part 2

Case Studies

Case Study A

Instrument Application Design and Validation

Tony de Claire
SmithKline Beecham
Worthing, UK

Peter Coady
P.J. Coady & Associates
Southampton, UK

SUMMARY

Measurement and control instrumentation must be applied and maintained in support of computerised system validation. Unsatisfactory instrumentation can cause significant operational problems. This case study embraces the design and validation of both standard and intelligent instrument applications, and briefly discusses special instrument systems (shutdown systems and analyser packages). Particular attention is focussed on producing auditable documentation in compliance with GMP requirements [1].

INTRODUCTION

Instrumentation is the critical link between the manufacturing process and the control system. Instruments are the eyes (i.e., transmitters, sensors) and limbs (i.e., actuators, positioners) of a process control system and enable it to perform the actions that were once performed by operators and/or laboratory technicians. The number of instruments that can be involved with the dynamic operation of a pharmaceutical manufacturing process can be large (2000–3000 items). In most cases, they are remotely installed from the control room environment and operate unsupervised except during routine maintenance work.

The correct operation of any computer control and data acquisition system is totally reliant on the information it receives from the instrumentation. If an instrument should malfunction, data integrity and the predefined control actions will be affected. Therefore, it is essential that an instrument is carefully chosen to be fit for purpose (i.e., correct type, size, materials, accuracy, repeatability, reliability, documentation, etc.) to enable confidence to be gained in its ability to perform its intended function [2,3].

SUPPLIER SELECTION

Instrument suppliers are generally selected based on company or site "standards". Where there is no stated preference or knowledge of a particular instrument, selection can be made using a technical evaluation and a tender process. Companies that supply special instrument systems (e.g., shutdown systems, analysers), companies that provide design/validation consultancy, and subcontractors (engineering design contractors, site installation contractors, panel manufacturers) should be prequalified to determine their suitability, from both an engineering and a commercial perspective, to receive the tender enquiry documents. Specialist instrument suppliers and consultants would generally be subject to a Supplier Audit prior to any order being placed. Similarly, suppliers wishing to be included on the preferred vendor list for the site will also be subject to a Supplier Audit.

Audits should be conducted by suitably trained/qualified personnel against the applicable ISO 9000 [4] series standard, with special reference being made to software quality guidelines (e.g., ISO 9000-3 [5], TickIT [6]) for instrument systems involving software. The software audit may cover the development of both application software and core (operating system level) software, depending on the type of system to be supplied. Follow-up audits should be considered.

INSTRUMENT APPLICATION DESIGN

The design of instrument applications is an interactive process centred around an instrument schedule and process data. The instrument application design process is shown diagrammatically in Appendix 2 and its chronological position, in relation to an overall project development life cycle, is presented in Appendix 1.

The instrument schedule is generated from an approved set of Process and Instrument Diagrams (P&IDs) and is used to identify all instruments associated with a manufacturing process. The instruments in the schedule are grouped in tag number (loop) order along with an identification of all associated documentation on which they appear.

Process data are provided by the end user and include critical process data that are generated from, or with reference to, the end user's pharmaceutical product manufacturing specifications.

A HAZOP study (sometimes known as a Hazard Study or Hazard Analysis) normally carried out on the P&IDs during the design phase to determine where potentially hazardous conditions could occur during the operation of the process and the circumstances that lead to them. The results of the HAZOP study are used to generate safe working practices and the selection of suitable safety devices including rupture disks, safety relief valves, dedicated safety shutdown systems (solid state or PLC– [Programmable Logic Controller] based systems), and hard-wired (relay-based) trip systems.

The types of documentation produced during the instrument application design process are listed below, and the content of each document is described in more detail in Appendix 5.

- Instrument schedule
- Instrument specification/data sheets
- Cable block diagrams
- Cable schedule
- Pneumatic tubing schedules
- Termination drawings
- Miscellaneous label schedules
- Field panel specification and drawings
- Field junction box drawings
- Electrical hook-up (loop or wiring diagrams) drawings
- Pneumatic hook-up drawings
- Process hook-up drawings
- Instrument layout (location) and cable/tubing routing drawings

- Earthing schedules and drawings
- Miscellaneous drawings (control room/instrument room layouts)
- Instrument installation specification
- Package plant instrument specification
- Electrical and instrumentation interface panel
- Any special instrument specifications and wiring diagrams

Due to the interactions between the various types of instrument design documentation, and the sharing of input information, many of the documents can be produced in parallel. Each document should contain the required content (see Appendix 5), presented precisely and completely, to enable that part of the plant to be constructed and/or maintained in a proper and auditable manner.

MANUFACTURING INSPECTIONS

Equipment that is either high cost or complex is often inspected during manufacture by either the customer, an engineering design contractor, or a third-party inspection agency. During the inspection visit, the equipment is checked against its design specification, and the manufacturing/fabrication progress is assessed against the delivery programme. Any problems found are recorded on an inspection report form, along with agreed-on corrective actions; copies are given to the manufacturer and the inspector's employer/customer, as applicable.

PREDELIVERY TESTING AND CALIBRATION

Calibration and Test Equipment Requirements

The manufacturer should possess test equipment to enable all manufacturing tests and inspections to be performed. All test equipment used by the manufacturer must have a standard of accuracy better than the stated accuracy for the instrument(s) to be tested. All applicable test equipment must have a valid calibration certificate issued by a calibration laboratory that is certified to either a national or international standard (e.g., NAMAS [National Measurement Accreditation Service]) for calibrating the specific types of instruments concerned.

Factory Testing

The manufacturer should have written test procedures and should test all equipment supplied against these procedures prior to delivery. The manufacturer's testing should comprise the physical checking and operational and functional testing of instrumentation (e.g., valves, transmitters) and equipment (e.g., panels, analysers) to be supplied. All tests must be fully documented, the results recorded, and the appropriate test sheets signed off by an authorised person.

Factory Calibration

Factory calibration should be carried out against the instrument specification/data sheets supplied. The calibration activities should address the following areas, as applicable:

- Process operating ranges
- Required accuracy
- Repeatability
- Hysteresis effects
- Switch set points
- Condition of switching (e.g., on a rising or falling measured variable)
- Switch action (e.g., open or close on fault condition)

In most cases, the manufacturer's own calibration procedures should be acceptable, as they form part of the manufacturer's own performance guarantees and/or quality certification. If special calibration is required, then companies with custom-built test facilities must be used (e.g., a magnetic flowmeter that requires a specific certification will require calibration in a flow rig that has been certified by an approved certifying authority).

DESIGN QUALIFICATION

Design Qualification (DQ) is the name given to the technical and quality audit of the instrument application design engineering, construction documentation package, vendor documentation, factory inspection report forms, and calibration data. The purpose of the DQ audit is to verify through defined procedures and support documentation that the individual items of instrument application design have been designed and approved so that they meet the needs of the customer and the contractor's project and quality plan. The findings of the DQ audit and the documentation inspected should be formally recorded, and a DQ report should be produced.

Manufacturing Documentation Requirements

The manufacturer should provide copies of the following documents prior to the delivery of the equipment. It should be specified that documents are written in the local national language wherever possible.

Factory Calibration Certificates

The calibration certificate should include the following information:

- Serial number
- Instrument specification/data sheet number
- Tag number
- Model number
- Certificate numbers of the test equipment used for the calibration
- Validity period of the calibration certificate
- Calibration data
- Limits of uncertainty (for critical instrumentation)

Equipment Test Records

Copies of the test records for panels and associated equipment should be provided. Equipment test records can include the following:

- Copies of the signed and approved test record sheets
- The manufacturer's own quality system compliance
- Electro-magnetic compatibility Declaration of Conformity certificates (self-certification) for equipment containing European Economic Community (EEC) CE-marked equipment (e.g., panels)

Hazardous Area Approval Certificates

Copies of hazardous area approval certificates for all applicable equipment should be provided. The approval certificates are issued by national or international approvals bodies, including

- British Approvals Service for Electrical Equipment in Flammable Atmospheres (BASEEFA) and Physikalische-Technische Bundesanstalt (PTB), West Germany, which, along with other European approvals bodies, provides certification to Comité Européen de Normalisation Electrotechnique (CENELEC) standards.
- Factory Mutual Research Corporation (FM) and Underwriters Laboratories Inc. (UL), United States

- Canadian Standards Association (CSA)
- Standards Association of Australia (SAA)

Material Certificates

Material certificates are normally only required where the materials of construction were specified on the instrument specification/data sheets to comply with process or environmental requirements (e.g., valve bodies and trims).

Construction Documentation Package

The construction documentation package comprises the instrument installation specification, drawings, and documentation listed in Appendix 5, "Instrument Installation Specification". During this phase, and thereafter, it is important that the drawing register for the manufacturing process is maintained on-site and that only the latest revisions of drawings are used.

The instrumentation construction documentation package may also reference supplementary information contained in the following documentation:

- Process design documentation (e.g., P&IDs, ELDs [Engineering Line Diagrams], ULDs [Utility Line Diagrams])
- Piping design documentation (e.g., piping isometric drawings)
- Process unit design documentation (e.g., vessel connections)
- Mechanical design documentation (e.g., package plant vendor installation drawings)
- Computerised control system documentation (e.g., termination and interconnecting cabling drawings)

EQUIPMENT DELIVERY, INSPECTION, PROTECTION, AND STORAGE

On arrival at site, instrumentation and equipment should be checked against the delivery note, checked for damage, and then either preinstallation tested and installed or put into a suitable store until required. Any discrepancy or damage should be recorded and reported to the supplier through the contractual channels established for the project. Rejected items should be stored and controlled separately from accepted items.

Instrumentation and equipment (e.g., panels, junction boxes) that cannot be installed on delivery must be housed in a properly constructed and conditioned store and protected from dust and moisture. Completion of control rooms should be programmed to permit the installation of panels immediately on receipt to minimise handling. If the control room heating system is not in operation, temporary heaters must be installed to ensure that the panels and instrumentation are kept within acceptable temperature and humidity limits.

Throughout the construction period, instruments that are not provided with housings must be adequately protected by covering with heavy duty plastic bags of an approved type or by applying more robust protection where necessary. The protection of instruments and the provision of covers is the responsibility of the installation contractor.

SITE PREQUALIFICATION

General

All instruments should, wherever possible, be subject to a preinstallation test; this test should commence as soon as practicable after the receipt of the instrument on-site. The object of preinstallation testing is to ensure that each instrument has been supplied in accordance with its specification, is functionally correct, and is in working order. Where the preinstallation test is not specified or where circumstances prohibit carrying out the prescribed test, the installation contractor must propose a suitable test method for approval by the customer.

The tests should be performed as described below and with due consideration given to the manufacturer's recommended test methods. Adjustments must be carried out in accordance with the manufacturer's instructions. Any deviation from this must be approved by the customer and supplier prior to testing. All tests must be fully documented, the results recorded, and the appropriate test sheets signed off by an authorised person.

Instrument testing should preferably be carried out in a calibration workshop. However, instruments that form part of an integrated system or control panel may be tested in the control room or instrument room after installation, using portable test gear and/or simulation equipment. All instruments that require calibration must be calibrated in both the upscale and downscale directions and, if necessary, adjusted until their accuracies are within the limits stated by the manufacturer. On completion of the tests, the instrument must be suitably cleaned and protected in accordance with the manufacturer's recommendations.

Preparation for Site Testing

The following checks should be carried out before preinstallation testing commences:

- All test equipment used by the installation contractor must be approved by the customer and/or engineering design contractor and must have a standard of accuracy better than the manufacturer's stated accuracy for the instrument(s) to be tested. Test equipment must have a valid calibration certificate issued by a calibration laboratory that is certified to either a national or international standard (e.g., NAMAS) for calibrating the specific types of instruments concerned.
- The instrument must be checked for damage (e.g., damage to doors, linkages). Any such damage must be rectified and approved before any tests are attempted.
- The data plate on the instrument must be checked for agreement with the information contained in the appropriate instrument specification/data sheet.
- A suitable means must be provided for simulating the required process conditions, and test gauges or meters must be made available with a sufficient degree of accuracy for the tests to be performed.
- The instrument to be tested should be mounted in the correct plane on a rigid and vibration-free stand or structure.
- The manufacturer's "Instruction Book" must be made available.
- All tests must simulate as closely as possible design process conditions.
- Tests must not be carried out on electronic instruments until an adequate warm-up period has elapsed. Wherever possible, instruments must be energised for at least 24 hours prior to testing.
- The instrument to be tested must be properly prepared prior to testing by the removal of any shipping stops and the installation of any miscellaneous components (e.g., charts, mercury, oil).

Test Status Indication

On completion of each site test, the stage reached in the testing procedure should be clearly indicated. A typical method would be affixing to each instrument or installation a coloured label conforming to the following code:

- Blue: Preinstallation tested
- Yellow: Pressure tested
- Green: Cables tested
- Red: Precommissioned

- White: Test failed (a written message may be added giving the reason for failure)

This identification must be shown on all components in the loop, thereby making all personnel aware of the current status of any instrument and its installation.

Connecting an Energy Supply

The following procedure is common to all instruments that require an energy supply source and that generate a signal output.

Pneumatic Instruments

Connect the air supply and adjust the air supply regulator to the correct setting (e.g., 1.4 bar for a standard transmitter with operating range of 0.2–1.0 bar, 20 psig for an operating range of 3–15 psig). Connect the output to a suitable test gauge via a capacity chamber (approximately 0.5 litre capacity).

Electronic Instruments

Connect a suitable power supply. Connect the output to a suitable test meter, preferably a digital voltmeter, installed across the circuit dropping resistor.

Connecting a Signal Generator for Process Simulation

Connect a signal-generating source with an accurate indicator to the sensing device, together with the means of isolating and regulating its output. The type of signal generator required will depend on the type of signal to be simulated and should conform to recognised instrument calibration standards and the supplier's instructions. When hazardous fluids or gases are involved (e.g., oxygen or ammonium nitrate), suitable safety precautions must be observed and the test method must be agreed on with the customer.

Site Calibration

The calibration procedures adopted on-site must be agreed on with the customer and conform to recognised industry instrument calibration standards and the supplier's instructions. These procedures must be applied to all in-line instrumentation, loop instrumentation, local controllers, analysers, and so on. Where the control and monitoring instrumentation is integrated with a computerised control system and where factory tests have been carried out, the installation calibration procedure should be agreed on with the customer.

Calibration checks are usually carried out on analysers by injecting known samples into the sample conditioning systems. This must be determined for each type of analyser, by reference to the manufacturer's handbook or by consultation with the instrument vendor, and it must be agreed on with the customer. Complex analyser systems usually require specialist personnel from the analyser manufacturer to assist in precalibration and commissioning and are generally outside the scope of the installation contractor's responsibility and experience.

The calibration results should be recorded (a sample instrument preinstallation calibration sheet has been provided for reference purposes in Appendix 3) and included with the site test records.

Instrument Mounting and Accessibility

Each instrument to be installed must be inspected to check that its data plate agrees with the specification and that it has been preinstallation tested, if applicable, as described in the preceding sections. The instrument should then be installed in its intended location on brackets, a subpanel, a mounting post, or a pedestal, ensuring that it is levelled, plumbed, and firmly secured. The installation must follow good instrument installation practice and the supplier's instructions, and the instrument should be protected from damage until it is put into service.

Indicating instruments and instruments requiring adjustments should be accessible for observation and servicing from the floor level, walkways, permanent ladders, or platforms. Where possible, actuated valves should be accessible from the floor or permanent platform level.

Instrument Piping and Tubing

The installation and pressure testing for air supply piping, transmission/ signal tubing, and process impulse piping must conform to, and be checked against, the instrument installation specification, the construction documentation package drawings, and recognised industry instrument standards.

Cable Installation and Testing

The installation and testing of signal transmission cabling and power cabling must conform to, and be checked against, the instrument installation specification, the construction documentation package drawings, and recognised industry standards. Immediately after cables have been laid and before connection, all electric and electronic instrument wiring must be checked for polarity, continuity, and insulation resistance between the conductors and between the conductors and earth. These tests should be carried out before final loop tests and should comply with industry standards and statutory regulations.

Coaxial cables used for data highways must be tested using sinewave reflective testing techniques. Circuits involving intrinsically safe (IS) instrumentation must be tested (e.g., loop impedance, inductance, I/R

[Inductance/Resistance] ratio) in accordance with the manufacturer's instructions and approved by the customer.

Wiring that connects field instrumentation to a computerised control system should be isolated from the computerised control system (e.g., at the control room/marshalling cabinets) during cable testing in order to safeguard against damage due to incorrect connections. Isolation from the computerised control system may be provided by the use of isolating (e.g., knife edge) field terminals and/or by disconnecting the computerised control system input/output (I/O) wiring termination blocks.

After the tests have been completed, the cables should be identified with a coloured label, which clearly indicates its test status (see above). Wiring should be reconnected on completion of cable testing and recorded as such.

Loop Testing

General Requirements

The object of loop testing is to ensure that all instrumentation components in a loop are in full operational order when connected together and are in a state ready for process commissioning and validation (Operational Qualification [OQ] and Performance Qualification [PQ]). Loop testing also encompasses the integration of instrumentation with any associated computerised control systems.

The procedure to be adopted in carrying out these tests is detailed below, but in general, the completed loop should be tested as one system and, where necessary, adjustments should be made to ensure that the loop is fully operational as a system and is correctly calibrated. Associated alarms and trips must be checked during loop testing.

The loop test results should be recorded (a sample instrument loop check sheet has been provided for reference purposes in Appendix 4) and included with the site test records. Checks for mechanical/electrical completeness are recorded using the upper section of the sheet and the dynamic loop test results are recorded on the lower section. The test results sheets will provide the documentary evidence essential for Installation Qualification (IQ). Representatives from the installation contractor and/or the customer will witness the final loop tests and countersign the test sheets. Any tests not witnessed must be accompanied by written confirmation from the customer that witnessing has been waived.

Loop testing of remote control loops is a two-person exercise, with one person located in the field and the other in the control room or instrument room. Each person must be provided with an adequate means of remote communication (e.g., field telephones or two-way radios) as approved by the customer.

Loop testing of instrumentation and any associated computerised control system should encompass the interfaces with electrical equipment (via the electrical and instrumentation interface panel) and its related operation. Loop testing must not be carried out on electronic equipment until an adequate warm-up period has elapsed. Where possible, equipment should be energised for at least 24 hours prior to testing.

On completion of loop testing, it is recommended that all control devices/functions are left set with the correct control action and with a 100 percent proportional band setting. Derivative and integral functions must be set at their minimum time values.

Loop Testing Procedure

The following test procedure should be carried out in order to test the correct operation of field instrumentation and equipment installed in a control loop, and to provide the necessary documentary evidence (test records) to satisfy the requirements of the IQ protocols:

- Inspect the loop and set air/electrical supplies where appropriate. Check in particular that control valve air supply pressures are set in accordance with the instrument specification/data sheet.
- For electronic loops, check polarities, measure the loop impedance, and make the necessary compensating adjustments. The compensating adjustments on smart instruments can be made using either a handheld terminal or directly at the instrument. Smart instruments, if supported, can also be adjusted using an instrument configuration page on a computerised control system.
- Transmitter output signals equivalent to 0, 50, and 100 percent of the instrument range should be generated, either manually (e.g., hot oil bath, dead weight tester) or by applying appropriate signals at the field terminals in order to check the response of all other instruments and control valves in the loop. Instrument zero settings and calibration checks/adjustments should be made as necessary.
- Switch the loop controller to manual operation and, by applying the appropriate output signals, ensure that the control valve(s) stroke correctly. Valve positioner gauges should also be checked during this stage.
- Apply an input signal to the loop controller equivalent to 50 percent of the instrument range and adjust the output of the manual pneumatic regulator to 50 percent. Adjust the loop controller setpoint to 50 percent and, by switching the auto/manual transfer switch, check for "bumpless" transfer. Using the manufacturer's instructions, adjust where necessary until a satisfactory "bumpless" transfer is achieved.
- Check all alarm and trip actions by varying the loop controller input signals and adjust as necessary.

After the tests have been completed, the loop controller must be switched to manual operation and then identified with a coloured label that clearly indicates its test status (see above).

Testing Computerised Control System Loops

Before this level of testing commences, the instrument loop must be prepared in accordance with the loop testing procedure outlined above. All test methods must be agreed on with the customer.

The operation of instrumentation must be checked from the field to the control room graphics display unit or local controller I/O registers, as applicable depending on the type of system installed, and vice versa. The operation of control instrumentation (e.g., control valves, actuated on/off valves) should be checked by energising each control system field output from either the control room display or local controller, as applicable, and observing and recording the results.

The operation of monitoring instrumentation (e.g., transmitters, switches) should be checked by either injecting a suitable signal at the field instrument terminals or by installing the instrument in a comparator (e.g., a hot oil bath, dead weight tester). The result received by the control system on the control room display or local controller I/O register, as applicable, should be recorded. Any problems should be reported to the company/companies responsible.

The results of all tests must be recorded on loop test sheets. A sample copy of a loop test sheet is provided in Appendix 4. As each test is completed, the tested item must be identified with a coloured label that clearly indicates its test status (see above).

Testing Safety Interlocks

Safety interlocking and shutdown systems require detailed test procedures based around the design documentation (e.g., cause and effect charts, binary logic diagrams) that must be formulated and agreed on in advance.

Site Modifications and As-Built Drawings

Any modifications, exceptions, or additions to the construction documentation must be confirmed in writing by the customer before such work is commenced by the installation contractor. This work must be properly organised, with clear definitions of responsibilities for checking and approval, and must be undertaken following a strict change control procedure that identifies all documentation affected by the change.

The installation contractor should assist in the provision of as-built drawings that may be completed by others (e.g., the engineering design contractor) at the end of the contract. To assist in this exercise, the installation contractor must keep a set of printouts of all documentation that must be marked up as and when changes are agreed.

QUALIFICATION

Installation Qualification

On completion of installation, all documentation associated with the installation, calibration, and testing of the field instrumentation, along with any associated computerised control system documentation, should be collated by the project manager/engineer ready for IQ. Most of this documentation will be in the pre-"as-built" condition at this stage of the project and will, therefore, contain site (red line) markups.

The documentation should typically include the following:

- Construction documentation package (see Appendix 5, "Instrument Installation Specification")
- Instrumentation and loop test records and reports
- Instrument calibration certificates
- Change control notices and supporting forms
- Manufacturer's operation and maintenance manuals

IQ should be carried out using a written protocol [7] that is completed during the inspection of the installation and its documentation. The protocol should typically describe how the documents inspected will be marked to show their IQ acceptance status, as well as the acceptance criteria for the items inspected, and it should have space to record the reference numbers of the documents seen and where they can be located.

Operational Qualification and Performance Qualification

General

OQ verifies that the control and monitoring instrumentation, as integrated with the process equipment and any associated computerised control system, meets the operational and functional requirements defined in the instrument application design documentation and/or computerised control system User Requirements Specification (URS) [7]. PQ verifies that the control and monitoring instrumentation, as integrated with the process equipment and any associated computerised control system, meets the operational and functional requirements defined in the instrument application design documentation and/or computerised control system URS, and produces pharmaceutical product consistently to specification [7].

OQ and PQ should be carried out using written protocols that are completed during the functional testing of the manufacturing process. The protocols should typically describe how the tests will be carried out, as well as the acceptance criteria for the items tested, and they should have space to record the reference numbers of the documents seen and where they can be located. The principal reference document for the OQ testing of the instruments will be the instrument site commissioning test procedures and results. Some points to consider during OQ and PQ are described below.

Recalibration

There may be a large time gap between the IQ, OQ, and PQ phases for instrumentation associated with particular manufacturing processes due to the site construction programme (e.g., unavailability of utilities, panels). As a result, some control and monitoring instrumentation may need to be recalibrated prior to commencing OQ, and possibly again prior to PQ, depending on their calibration frequencies. It would be advisable to recalibrate critical instrumentation anyway to ensure its status is known prior to OQ and PQ.

Recalibration must be carried out to agreed on standard procedures using calibration test equipment that is traceable back to national standards. All calibration tests must be fully documented, the results recorded, and the sheets signed off by an authorised person. Calibrated instruments must be provided with a full calibration certificate that details the test results and their limits of uncertainty.

Testing

The customer should be kept informed of all site tests and when they are to occur by the supplier/contractor so that arrangements can be made for the end user to attend for witnessing purposes. All testing must be fully documented using test record sheets and witnessed and signed off by the customer and the supplier. Copies of all test result sheets/test records and reports should be reviewed and approved by the supplier/contractor and suitably qualified customer representatives. Any document revisions necessary during OQ and PQ must be progressed through the site document management system and implemented under a formal change control procedure.

Handover

The completion of OQ marks the end of the site construction (installation and commissioning) phase for the project, and the manufacturing process is formally handed over to the customer by the signing of a handover certificate prepared by the engineering design contractor. The handover certificate should be accompanied by an "as-built" issue of the construction documentation package bound in a series of Operation and Maintenance (O&M) Manuals, along with all test results, calibration certificates, manufacturer's reference manuals, and so on, to enable the manufacturing process to be properly maintained for the rest of its operational life. Some of the information contained in the O&M Manuals (e.g., calibration certificates) may be removed and placed in a centralised maintenance system for ease of control.

Reporting

Testing occurs at many levels in a project, as described in the preceding sections of this case study, starting with design phase verification activities (design reviews) and ending with the testing associated with IQ, OQ, and PQ on-site. All reviews and tests must be fully documented using appropriate methods (e.g., minutes of design review meetings, test record sheets) and must have the required checking and approval signatures. These documents, along with change control documentation, calibration certificates, and so on, comprise the formal records generated to provide the necessary evidence to support validation.

MAINTENANCE QUALIFICATION—ONGOING EVALUATION

Maintenance Qualification (MQ) is the periodic review of the performance of the manufacturing process, including the control and monitoring instrumentation and any associated computerised control system, in the manufacture of quality product from the time it is handed over to a site until it is replaced and/or decommissioned [7]. The purpose of an MQ review, with regard to control and monitoring instrumentation, is to verify that it has been maintained in a validatable condition.

Typical activities associated with the MQ phase for instrumentation include establishing a recalibration programme [8] and conducting routine maintenance activities as part of a planned preventive maintenance scheme. All maintenance activities must be carried out under a formal change control procedure and any associated testing must be fully documented using test record sheets.

NOTES ON SPECIAL INSTRUMENTS AND TECHNOLOGIES

A number of special instrumentation systems may be required for a project. This section briefly describes some typical systems used in the industry.

Emergency Shutdown Systems

Emergency shutdown (ESD) safety systems are relatively new to the pharmaceutical industry but have been used for many years in the petrochemical and other industries. They provide an independent, reliable (high integrity) method for protecting plant and personnel from situations that could lead to a dangerous occurrence (e.g., runaway reactions, handling of dangerous substances). A typical application would be on a solvent recovery plant or tank farm for the isolation of solvent feeds to the process. ESD systems are often designed by the instrument discipline as part of trip system design and can be either solid-state or PLC based.

Solid-state systems comprise a number of cards, each of which contain a number of independent logic channels (i.e., AND, OR, NOT function blocks) and special functions (e.g., timer blocks) that are hard-wired to provide the shutdown logic required. The cards are monitored and controlled by dual redundant CPU cards and are interfaced to the field by high integrity/availability relays to prevent problems with contact welding and/or malfunctioning due to lack of use. The systems (cards, CPUs, etc.) are subject to inspection and testing by an independent certification body (e.g., the German TÜV [Technischer Überwachungs-Verein] in Europe) and issued with an approval certificate.

PLC–based systems are similar to solid-state systems—they use the same field interface cards and have the same level of certification—but the logic functions are performed by software. They are also easier to interface to other systems (via serial communications) in order to notify the system of a failure. The PLC used is subject to rigorous source code (machine level) inspection and testing by an independent certification body (e.g., TÜV in Europe) to examine the safety integrity of the code, including all possible failure paths. The PLC system (application software and hardware) should be developed and tested using a formal, life-cycle methodology [7,9].

The shutdown logic required is usually determined during a HAZOP and represented on either cause and effect charts or on binary logic diagrams. Cause and effect charts have a spreadsheet (matrix) type of presentation and show for each identified failure condition (e.g., high temperature alarm) the safety status required for all affected equipment. Binary logic diagrams perform a similar function but show the physical connections between each logic block in diagrammatic form. More detailed versions of the binary logic diagrams showing card numbers, addresses, and so on should be provided by the system supplier as part of the documentation package.

Analyser Packages

Analyser systems are now becoming more widely used in the pharmaceutical industry at all levels of product development (primary, secondary, and R&D). Some typical systems include mass spectrometers, gas chromatographs, and near infrared (NIR) systems.

Each analyser should have a URS and should be supplied with a detailed design specification, installation and maintenance documentation, and operator instruction manuals. Some special considerations include the following:

- *The sample loop:* The sample (fast) loop for off-line analysers must bring a representative sample to the analyser in the shortest acceptable time so that, accounting for the analysis time itself and the output response time of any corrective systems, the system response time is achieved.
- *Sample conditioning:* The need for sample conditioning (heating, cooling, drying) must be addressed and consideration given to the effect this could have on the system response time.
- *Analyser results:* The format of the data produced by the analyser must be specified.
- *Communications:* The ability of the analyser to send data or signals to other systems must be specified. Raw analysis data may need to be transmitted to another system for further analysis and/or presentation. Further, the analyser may also monitor for the occurrence of critical situations (e.g., the start of an exothermic reaction, high solvent content, high particulate count), in which case there may be a requirement to communicate (via communications link or hard-wiring) to a shutdown system or circuit.
- *Validation issues:* The analysis data usually form part of the manufacturing batch records. Consideration must be given to a Supplier Audit, and this will include a formal software audit if the analyser is controlled by a computer system. The design and testing of the analyser computer system (application software and hardware) will need to follow a formal, life-cycle methodology [7,9].

Intelligent Instruments

Intelligent instruments are widely used in the industry and include smart transmitters, loop controllers, chart recorders, machine monitoring systems, and fume cupboard controllers. These instruments contain embedded software in the form of nonuser programmable firmware that is configured either by "filling in the blanks" or by entering high level statements. These devices are considered to be "black boxes" in validation terms and are classified as "Category 2 Software" in the GAMP Supplier Guide [9].

Although these devices are not subject to the normal rigor of application software validation on a project, the manufacturers of these devices are still expected to have formal documented methods and records in place for developing and testing the software, for controlling and reporting changes due to bug fixes and upgrades, and for the configuration management of both the software and firmware products. Information on these and other areas may be obtained for the project validation records either by a manufacturer audit or by signed statements from the manufacturer in response to a questionnaire.

Intelligent devices are now becoming associated with the evolving Fieldbus standard [10] for data acquisition, device control, and configuration. Fieldbus™ is a multidrop network standard that allows both digital (serial) and analogue (4–20 mA) signals to share the same cable without interference. The main points to consider for validation are data integrity and security within the network (i.e., evidence to ensure data are not corrupted when being transmitted within the network between devices or to a computerised control system). This evidence should include formal documentation and records of the data transfer/communication standard used, and error and diagnostic checks.

In addition to the more commonplace monitoring instruments and measurement devices, technology continues to present the industry with a range of "super" instruments. Equipment such as robotics, spectrophotometers, bio-instruments, vision/imaging systems, colour recognition, particle monitoring, and other sophisticated analysers could be considered as in-line instruments with embedded software. With these devices, more complex calibration and qualification issues will have to be addressed in addition to the manufacturer's design and testing methods described above.

RETROSPECTIVE VALIDATION

This case study has concentrated on the design of new instrument applications subject to prospective validation. The validation of existing instrument applications will necessitate a retrospective validation approach. The main difference between the two approaches is in the use of historical design information to prove that the current installation is properly documented and maintained.

Retrospective validation invariably involves the verification of any existing documentation, and the generation of missing information/documentation. As the plant/process is existing, some of the documentation involved with the original site installation can be ignored, provided it does not contain information needed for operation or maintenance. Maintenance and effective records are the main considerations when deciding on whether a particular document is or is not required.

Considering the construction documentation package listed in Appendix 5, "Instrument Installation Specification", the minimum level of documentation that should be in place for retrospective validation is as follows:

- Instrument schedule
- Instrument specification/data sheets
- Cable schedules
- Pneumatic tubing schedules

- Field panel drawings (e.g., layout, wiring, termination, and piping drawings)
- Electrical hookup (loop or wiring diagrams) drawings
- Pneumatic hookup drawings
- Earthing drawings/details
- Electrical and instrumentation interface panel wiring diagrams
- Special instrument specifications and wiring diagrams
- Shutdown/safety system logic diagrams
- Junction box layouts

The following certification, operation, and maintenance documentation will be required:

- Instrument calibration certificates
- Instrument hazardous area classification certificates
- Materials certificates or other method of material verification
- EMC Declaration of Conformity certificates (self-certification) for equipment containing EEC CE-marked equipment (e.g., panels)
- Manufacturer's O&M instructions

The following supplementary documentation provided by other disciplines will also be required:

- Process design documentation (e.g., P&IDs, ELDs, ULDs)
- Mechanical design documentation (e.g., package plant vendor drawings)
- Computerised control system documentation (e.g., termination and wiring drawings)

CONCLUSION

Instrument application design is one of the most extensive activities, in terms of the number of types of instruments and the associated paperwork, and requires a logical, carefully controlled approach—a change to an instrument tag number or the addition/deletion of an instrument can affect up to 10 different documents. However, with good document control, it is possible to produce a system of documentation that will allow instrument applications, both simple and complex, to be validated and easily maintained. This case study has described the instrument application design process commonly used in the industry and how this can be used to support validation.

REFERENCES

1. U.S. Code of Federal Regulations Title 21, Part 210 (last amended 1994), *Current Good Manufacturing Practice in Manufacturing, Processing, Packaging, or Holding of Drugs;* Part 211 (last amended 1995), *Current Good Manufacturing Practice for Finished Pharmaceuticals.*

2. U.S. Code of Federal Regulations Title 21, 211.68(a).

3. U.S. Code of Federal Regulations Title 21, 820.61.

4. ISO 9001 (1994), *Quality Systems—Model for Quality Assurance in Design, Development, Production, Installation and Servicing.* Geneva: International Organisation for Standardisation.

   ISO 9002 (1994), *Quality Systems—Model for Quality Assurance in Production, Installation and Servicing.* Geneva: International Organisation for Standardisation.

5. ISO 9000-3 (1991), *Quality Management and Quality Assurance Standards*—Part 3: Guidelines for the Application of ISO 9001 to the Development, Supply and Maintenance of Software. Geneva: International Organisation for Standardisation.

6 *The TickIT Guide:* A Guide to Software Quality Management System Construction and Certification Using ISO 9001:1994, Issue 3.0 (1995). London: DISC TickIT Office.

7. Coady, P.J. and de Claire, A.P. (1995), Best Practice Engineering for Validation of Process Control Systems. *Pharmaceutical Engineering* (July/August): 18–30.

8. U.S. Code of Federal Regulations Title 21, 211.160(b)(4).

9. UK GAMP Forum (1996), *Supplier Guide for Validation of Automated Systems in Pharmaceutical Manufacture.* Version 2.0. The Hague: ISPE.

10. ISA SP50, IEC SC65C/WGr6. International Fieldbus Standard. Under development.

APPENDIX 1. THE INSTRUMENT APPLICATION DEVELOPMENT LIFE CYCLE

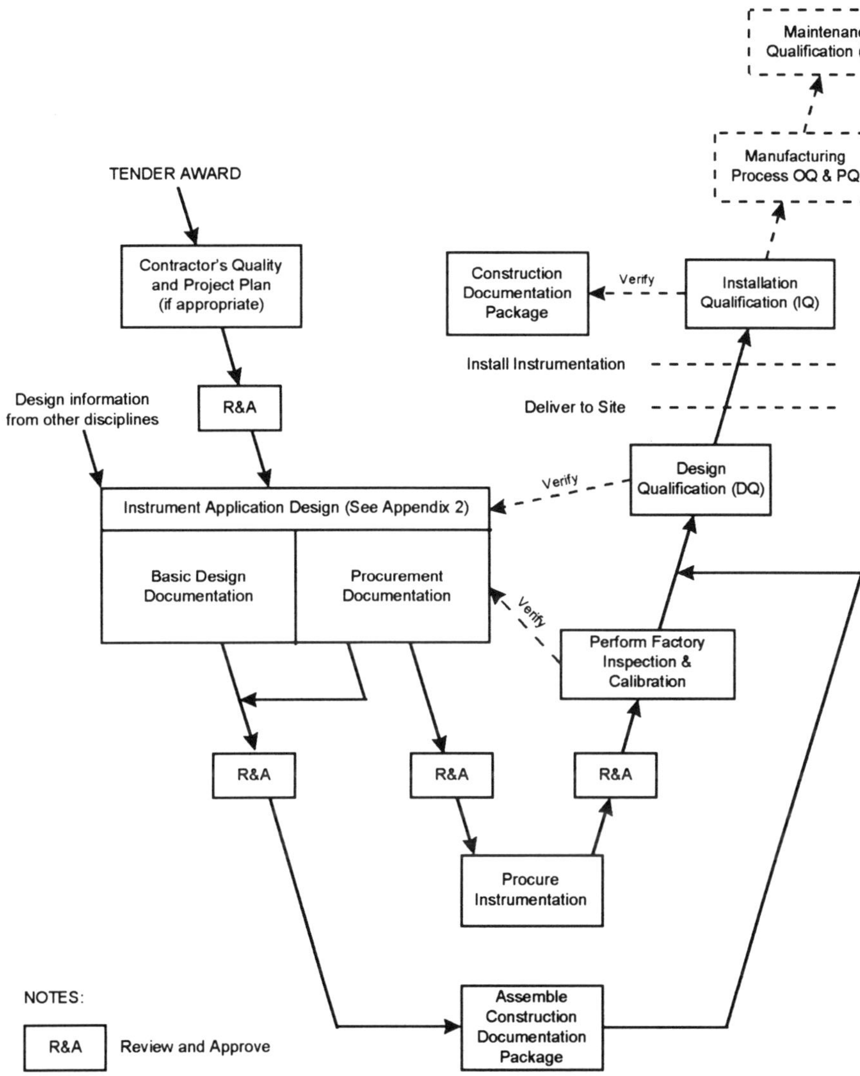

APPENDIX 2. OVERVIEW OF THE INSTRUMENT APPLICATION DESIGN PROCESS

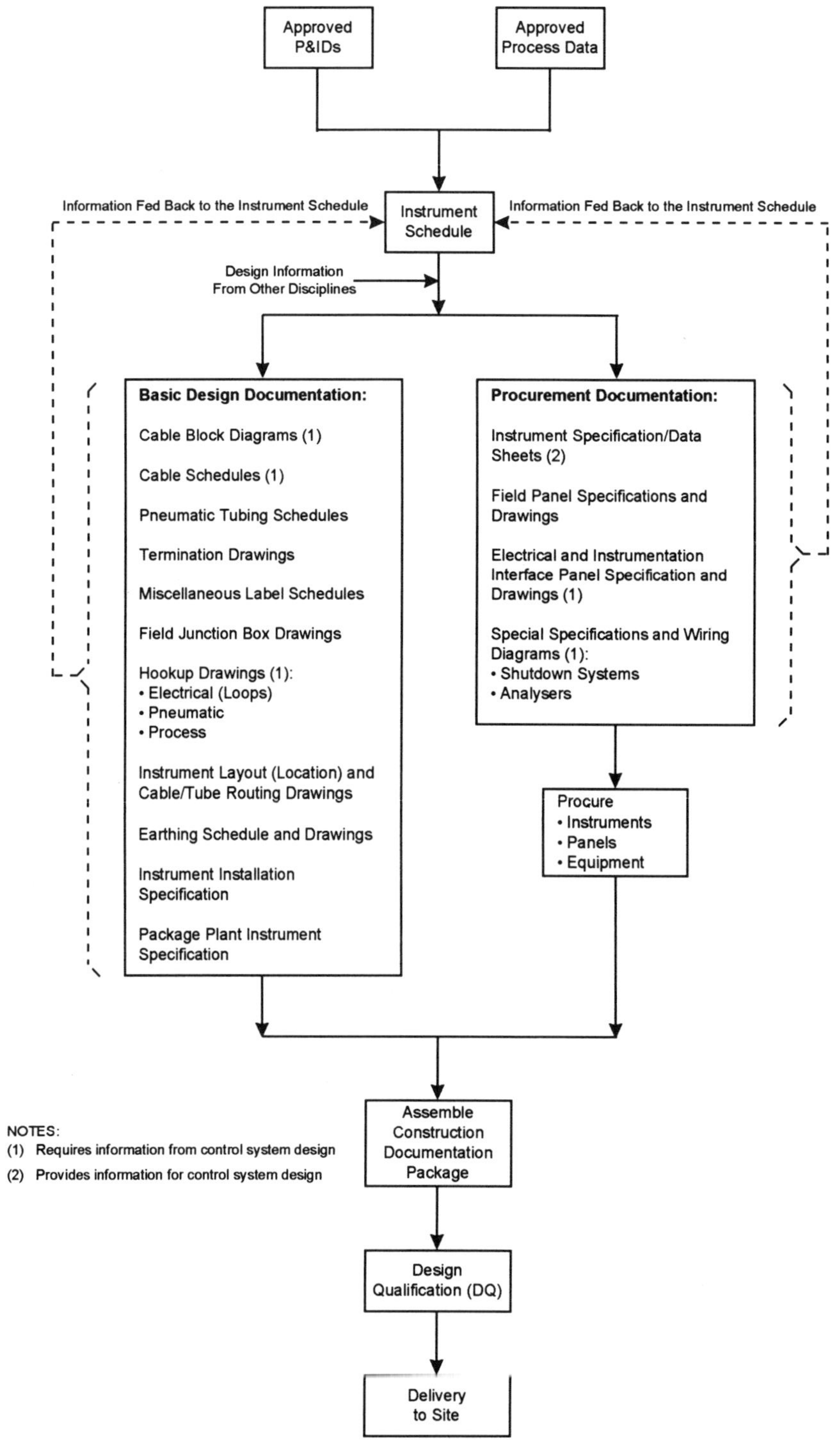

APPENDIX 3. SAMPLE INSTRUMENT PREINSTALLATION CALIBRATION SHEET

INSTRUMENT PREINSTALLATION CALIBRATION SHEET

CLIENT: PLANT:

CLIENT'S PROJECT No.: CONTRACTOR'S PROJECT No.:

INST. TAG No. ______ SERVICE: ______

TYPE: ______ MODEL No.: ______ SERIAL No.: ______

MANUFACTURER: ______ ORDER No.: ______ SPEC. No.: ______

SIGNAL RANGE: ______ DIAL/CHART RANGE: ______

PHYSICAL CHECK:

- PROCESS CONN. CORRECT ☐ — PNEU./ELECT. CONN. CORRECT ☐*
- BODY MATERIAL CORRECT ☐ — RANGE/SPAN CORRECT ☐
- ELECT. SUPPLY SETTING CORRECT ☐ — AIR SUPPLY SETTING CORRECT ☐
- GENERAL CONDITIONS SATISFACTORY ☐ — ANCILLARY EQUIPMENT SUPPLIED ☐

SHIPPING STOPS REMOVED ☐

CALIBRATION CHECK:

MAKER'S QUOTED ACCURACY ± ______%

INPUT		READING OR OUTPUT					
%SPAN	ACTUAL	RISING			FALLING		
		ACTUAL	%SPAN	ERROR%	ACTUAL	%SPAN	ERROR%
0							
25							
75							
100							

CONTROLLER CHECK: CONTROL MODE: PROPORTIONAL ☐ INTEGRAL ☐ DERIVATIVE ☐

ON-OFF ☐ DIFF. GAP ☐

CONTROLLER ALIGNMENT CORRECT ☐ AUTO/MANUAL CORRECT ☐

SETTINGS: CONTROL ACTION: DIRECT ☐ REVERSE ☐ DIFF. GAP ______%

ALARM SETTING ______ TIME DELAY SETTING ______

LIMIT SWITCH SETTING: HIGH ______ LOW ______

OUTPUT LIMIT SETTING: HIGH ______ LOW ______

CORRECTIONS: AUTOMATIC TEMPERATURE CORRECTION RANGE ______

S.G./DENSITY CORRECTION SETTING ______

ZERO ELEVATION/SUPPRESSION SETTING ______

THERMO-COUPLE BURNOUT DRIVES: UPSCALE ☐ DOWNSCALE ☐

SHIPPING STOPS REFITTED ☐

* ANCILLARY EQUIPMENT LIST:

REMARKS: ______

CHECKED BY:	DATE:	WITNESSED BY:	DATE:
ACCEPTED BY:		FOR:	DATE:
		INSTRUMENT TAG NO.	

APPENDIX 4. SAMPLE INSTRUMENT LOOP CHECK SHEET

INSTRUMENT LOOP CHECK SHEET

CLIENT:	PLANT:
CLIENT'S PROJECT No.:	CONTRACTOR'S PROJECT No.:
LOOP No.: ______	SERVICE: ______
LINE OR EQUIPMENT No.:	PIPE I.D.:

MECHANICAL/ELECTRICAL CHECKS

MEASURING ELEMENT:	INSTALLATION CORRECT	☐	LOCATION CORRECT	☐
	ISOLATING VALVES CORRECT	☐	MATERIALS CORRECT	☐
	TAPPING(S) POSITION CORRECT	☐	ORIFICE DIAMETER: ______	
IMPULSE CONNECTIONS:	CORRECT TO HOOK-UP	☐	MATERIALS CORRECT	☐
	PRESSURE TESTED	☐	TEST PRESSURE: ______	
	STEAM/ELECT. TRACED	☐	LAGGED	☐
FIELD INSTRUMENT(S):	INSTALLATION CORRECT	☐	AIR SUPPLY CORRECT	☐
	WEATHER PROTECTED	☐	POWER SUPPLY CORRECT	☐
PANEL INSTRUMENT(S):	INSTALLATION CORRECT	☐	AIR SUPPLY CORRECT	☐
	SCALE/CHART CORRECT	☐	POWER SUPPLY CORRECT	☐
CONTROL VALVE(S):	INSTALLATION & LOCATION CORRECT	☐	SIZE & TYPE CORRECT	☐
	STROKE TESTED	☐	POSITIONER CHECKED	☐
	LIMIT SWITCH(ES) SET	☐	I/P TRANSDUCER CHECKED	☐
AIR SUPPLIES:	CONNS. CORRECT TO DRAWINGS	☐	BLOWN CLEAR & LEAK TESTED	☐
TRANSMISSION PNEU:	LINES INSPECTED, BLOWN CLEAR & LEAK TESTED	☐		
ELECT:	INSULATION CHECKED - CORE TO CORE	☐	CORE TO EARTH	☐
	CONTINUITY CHECKED	☐	LOOP IMPEDANCE CHECKED	☐
	EARTH BONDING CHECKED	☐	ZENER BARRIERS CORRECT	☐
TEMPERATURE LOOPS:	T/C OR R/B CHECKED	☐	CABLE TO SPECIFICATION	☐
	CONTINUITY CHECKED	☐	LOOP IMPEDANCE CHECKED	☐
GENERAL:	SUPPORTS CORRECT	☐	TAGGING CORRECT	☐

CHECKED BY:	DATE:	WITNESSED BY:	DATE:

LOOP TEST:

MEASUREMENT	TRANSMITTER INPUT	TRANSMITTER OUTPUT	LOCAL INST. READING	PANEL INST. READING	
	0				
	50%				
	100%				

CONTROL	CONTROLLER INPUT	TRANSDUCER OUTPUT	VALVE POS'NR OUTPUT	CONTROL VALVE POSITION	
	0				
	50%				
	100%				

REMARKS: ______

CHECKED BY:	DATE:	WITNESSED BY:	DATE:
ACCEPTED BY:	FOR:		DATE:
		INSTRUMENT TAG NO.	

APPENDIX 5. INSTRUMENT–RELATED PLANT DOCUMENTATION

This appendix describes the typical contents of instrument application design documentation used by the industry. It is essential that the system of documentation used is suitable for its purpose, properly implemented, and auditable in order to support validation and future maintenance activities.

Document Control

Each document (drawing, schedule, specification, etc.) should contain a title block or front page (as appropriate) that contains the following information:

- Document title
- Document number
- Document revision number or code
- Project name and number
- Site name
- Plant area (if applicable)
- Type of document (e.g., instrument schedule, loop diagram, emergency shutdown system specification, temperature transmitter specification sheet)

Each document should contain the following change control and author information:

- Reason for issuing the document (e.g., "Issued for customer comment", "updated in accordance with change note 123")
- Name of the document originator or modifier, as applicable, and the date of completion
- Name of the document checker and the date checked
- Name of the document approver and the date approved

Each document should contain cross-references to other design and/or reference documents, as applicable. Examples include the following:

- Process design documentation (P&IDs, process data specifications, etc.)
- Instrument design documentation (schedules, drawings, and specifications)
- Customer site or company standards

Instrument Schedule

An instrument schedule lists all instrumentation on the project, grouped by its unique tag (loop) number. For each instrument, the instrument schedule will typically provide the following information:

- Unique tag number
- Service/duty description
- Equipment description/type
- Location (e.g., pipe, process unit, or panel number)
- Manufacturer
- Requisition number
- Process design drawing number (P&ID, ELD, ULD, etc.)
- Specification/data sheet number
- Electrical hookup (loop or wiring diagram) drawing number
- Pneumatic hookup drawing number
- Process hookup drawing number
- Control system I/O address or tag number
- Notes/comments

Instrument Specification/Data Sheets

Instrument specification/data sheets provide the technical specification and design data for each unique type of instrument on the instrument schedule. They are used for purchasing the equipment, for providing design information for other disciplines (e.g., the definition of instrument tag number, signal, and range that are essential for the design of any associated computerised control system), and as the basis for calibration data.

Similar items can be included on the same specification sheet in separate columns, and identical instruments can be listed by tag number under common specification details. There are three main classes of instruments: pipe mounted, process unit (e.g., vessel) mounted, and field/panel mounted.

Each specification sheet should contain the following instrument data:

- Unique tag number
- Instrument type
- Supply voltage/pneumatic supply details (as applicable)
- Electrical/pneumatic connection type (as applicable)

- Signal type (e.g., 4–20 mA, 0.2–1.0 bar, serial, Fieldbus™)
- Type of mounting
- Range of instrument (calibration range) or switch set point values
- Materials of construction of wetted parts
- Control characteristics
- Other requirements (e.g., smart or standard instrument, Fieldbus™)

Each specification sheet should contain the following environment information:

- Process connection details (e.g., chemical seals, capillary lengths, flange rating)
- Ingress protection (IP) rating of the housing (e.g., weatherproof, dust-tight)
- Type of hazardous area protection (e.g., intrinsically safe, explosion proof)
- Requirement to meet EMC regulations

Each specification sheet should contain the following process data:

- Process fluid/material
- Engineering units
- Working range (of all the process variables affecting the measurement)
- Maximum range (of all the process variables affecting the measurement)
- The fail-safe mode
- Duty requirements (applicable to modulating control or actuated on/off valves [e.g., trip service or normal operation])

Each specification sheet should contain the required documentation needs, for instance:

- Factory calibration certificates (full certificate or batch certificate of conformance)
- Testing/calibration equipment stipulations (e.g., traceable to national standards)
- Manufacturer's O&M Manuals
- Approval certificates for equipment in hazardous areas

- EMC Declaration of Conformity certificates (self-certification) for equipment containing EEC CE-marked equipment (e.g., panels)
- Layout drawings showing overall dimensions
- Electrical schematic wiring and/or pneumatic connection diagrams
- Valve sizing calculations
- Number of copies of each document required

Each specification sheet should contain the required calibration and testing needs. Consideration should be given to how any associated computerised control system will be tested to ensure conformance to the URS. Typical information to be considered includes the following:

- Reviews of algorithms and calculations (smart instruments, loop controllers)
- Representative testing across the full operating range, including range boundaries
- Testing of alarms and hard-wired interlocks
- The need for specific test data, conditions, or equipment
- Records of test results
- References to specific calibration and testing procedures

Cable Block Diagrams

Cable block diagrams show in schematic form the panels (e.g., field panels, computer system cabinets, marshalling racks) and large items of equipment (e.g., packaged plant), the cables connecting them, and any intermediate junction boxes through which cables are interconnected. Each diagram should contain the following:

- Blocks uniquely representing instruments, combined systems (e.g., panels, PLCs), and large equipment items (e.g., analysers)
- Interconnecting lines representing cables, referenced by unique cable numbers
- Clear representation of the location of each block in the plant

Cable Schedule

A cable schedule is a list of all field instrument cables in identification number order and is used for allocating cable numbers and providing installation information. Each schedule should contain the following for each cable:

- Unique cable reference number
- Cable source, location/routing, and gland type
- Cable destination, location/routing, and gland type
- Number of cores/pairs
- Estimated route length and route identification, if possible
- Cable specification/data sheet number
- Identification of special circuits (e.g., IS circuits)
- Any appropriate notes on segregation requirements for installation purposes (e.g., distance from electrical power cables)
- Other information if required (e.g., drumming details, termination details at each end)
- Notes/comments

Pneumatic Tubing Schedules

A pneumatic tubing schedule is a list of all field instrument pneumatic tubing (single and multitube) in identification number order and is used for allocating tubing numbers and providing installation information. Each schedule should contain the following for each tube/multitube:

- Unique tube reference number
- Tube source, location/routing, and bulkhead fitting type
- Tube destination, location/routing, and bulkhead fitting type
- Number of tubes
- Estimated route length and route identification, if possible
- Tube specification/data sheet number
- Notes/comments

Termination Drawings

Termination drawings are used to allocate cables to particular sets of terminals inside panels (e.g., field panels, system cabinets, marshalling racks), junction boxes, and plant equipment. Each drawing should contain the following for each core:

- Unique cable reference number
- Core reference number

- Terminal number at source and source location
- Terminal number at destination and destination location
- Core outer sheath colour/number
- Core size
- Any appropriate notes on segregation requirements (e.g., IS circuits, analogue signals, security)

Miscellaneous Label Schedules

A miscellaneous label schedule is a schedule of all labels used on the project (e.g., instrument labels, junction box labels) and their specifications. Each schedule should contain the following information for each label:

- Equipment reference
- Dimensions of label
- Dimensions of character height
- Engraving details (including line separators)
- The numbers of each type of label required
- Label material type (e.g., Traffolyte, stainless steel)
- Label colours (e.g., Traffolyte sandwich colours)

Field Panel Specification and Drawings

Each specification should contain the following panel data:

- Panel reference
- Details of mounting or fixing
- Materials of construction and surface finish
- IP rating (e.g., weatherproof, dust-tight)
- Type of hazardous area protection (e.g., increased safety, air purged)
- Requirement to meet EMC regulations

Each specification should refer to all associated drawings, for example,

- Front of panel layouts, including label information
- Interior layouts, including label information
- Internal wiring/pneumatic tubing drawings

Each specification should refer to appropriate standards, for instance,

- General panel/junction box specifications
- Cable/tubing standards

Each specification should refer to test requirements and certificates, covering

- Electrical power and/or pneumatic checks
- Functional checks

Field Junction Box Drawings

Field junction box drawings can range in complexity from a simple cable termination box or cabinet, to a local control station containing electrical/pneumatic equipment. Complex junction boxes may require information similar to that described above for instrument panels (e.g., specifications, drawings, test certificates), depending on the level of complexity involved.

Junction boxes used for cable termination/routing require the following drawing details:

- Junction box reference
- Details of mounting or fixing
- Materials of construction and surface finish
- IP rating (e.g., weatherproof, dust-tight)
- Type of hazardous area protection (e.g., increased safety, air purged)
- Interior layouts, including any label information
- Internal wiring details (cable and core identification, cable entry and glanding, etc.)

Electrical Hookup (Loop or Wiring Diagrams) Drawings

Instrument loop diagrams are the key design documents for instrumentation systems and are also the main troubleshooting tool for fault finding and maintenance activities on-site. Single loop diagrams, showing all items in the loop, tend to be the industry standard. Each loop diagram should contain the following functional information:

- All instrument items in the loop.
- All control items in the loop, including loop controllers and computerised control system I/O card address and termination details.

The I/O details would need to be provided by the computerised control system designers.

- The cables connecting each applicable item in the loop along with their identification numbers and, for multicore cables, pair number/identification.
- Termination details (terminal block identification and terminal numbers).
- Electro-pneumatic equipment/circuit information (e.g., control valves and other electro-pneumatic valve circuits) is usually shown on the electrical loop diagram.

As applicable, each loop diagram should contain the following additional information:

- Hazardous area classification zone, temperature classification, and gas group.
- Instrument type and tag number.
- The diagram should show the power flow from its source, often in a control room, through the various locations of any intermediary junction boxes, barriers, or switches, and out to the load and back. The different locations through which each cable passes (e.g., control room, interface room, field panel, junction box, etc.) should be represented clearly so that the full extent of the different environments is conveyed precisely.

Pneumatic Hookup Drawings

Pneumatic hookups are the pneumatic versions of instrument loop diagrams and serve a similar purpose. They are produced for control loops that are purely pneumatic. For loops with a small pneumatic element (e.g., control valves and other electro-pneumatic valve circuits) the pneumatic circuit is usually shown on the electrical loop diagram. Each drawing should contain the following:

- All filter/regulation sets, piping, valves, and so on relating to the pneumatic hookup
- Details of all components and their connections/fixings
- Air supply pressure before and after controlling devices and at strategic points in the circuit
- Installation notes

Process Hookup Drawings

Process hookups are drawings showing the physical method for connecting and mounting instruments connected directly to process piping and equipment. The drawings are used for costing purposes by installation contractors and for the subsequent installation of instrumentation. Each drawing should contain the following:

- The instrument and its method of connection to the process piping/equipment
- Instrument mounting arrangement
- All piping and fittings required to install the instrument (material takeoff)
- Installation notes

Instrument Layout (Location) and Cable/Tubing Routing Drawings

Layout and routing drawings are floor plans of the building/process area showing the locations of process equipment and instrument panels. Each drawing should contain the following:

- The "spot" location of each instrument and its tag number
- The location of all instrument panels and junction boxes and their identification numbers
- Main instrument tray/ladder rack routes for cables and tubing and all tray/trunking branches (the identification numbers of the cables/tubes on each route and branch should be shown for installation purposes)
- The size and specification of each instrument tray/ladder rack and its height above finished floor level
- Elevations, as necessary, to help prevent potential clashes with other items of tray work/ladder racking and with other services (e.g., pipework and HVAC [heating, ventilation, and air-conditioning] ducting)
- Separation distances from other cables and other services, on both plan and elevations, where compliance is necessary for safety reasons (e.g., intrinsic safety), for functional reasons (e.g., analogue signal integrity), or for electrical interference reasons
- Details of any transit frames or holes required through walls or floors to permit the installation of cables and tubing

Earthing Schedules and Drawings

Earthing schedules and drawings detail the preferred methods for earthing various types of equipment and its associated earth testing information. The documents should address the following (as applicable):

- Static earthing
- IS earthing
- Computer earthing

The earthing drawings should show how equipment should be connected for each of the above situations. Each item to be earthed should have an entry in the appropriate earthing schedule that details the following information:

- Plant item to be earthed and plant area location in which the item is to be found
- Earth bond size and location of earth bar to which the item is connected
- Earth test results (resistance in ohms) and date tested

Miscellaneous Drawings (Control Room/ Instrument Room Layouts)

There is usually a need to provide additional drawings to clarify certain aspects of the design. A typical example is the provision of layout drawings for instrument/interface rooms and for control rooms to show the location of key items of equipment and their relationship to other equipment that may already be installed.

Instrument Installation Specification

An installation specification should be prepared for issue to prospective installation contractors for tender. The specification forms the technical section of the construction documentation package that should be appended to the specification. Each specification should contain, or provide detailed reference to, the following information:

- Regulations and codes of practice
- Company/work rules
- Competence levels required of the installer
- Safety standards required of the installer
- Good practice guidelines for the installation of instrumentation
- Good practice guidelines for the installation of cabling

- Good practice guidelines for the installation of instrument piping/tubing

Each specification should incorporate a brief scope of work and refer to the construction documentation package that should be appended. The construction documentation package will typically comprise the following drawings and schedules:

- Instrument schedule
- Instrument specification/data sheets
- Cable schedules
- Pneumatic tubing schedules
- Termination drawings
- Miscellaneous label schedules
- Field panel specifications and drawings
- Field junction box drawings
- Electrical hookup (loop or wiring diagrams) drawings
- Pneumatic hookup drawings
- Process hookup drawings
- Instrument layout (location) and cable/tubing routing drawings
- Earthing schedules and drawings
- Miscellaneous drawings (control room/instrument room layouts)
- Electrical and instrumentation interface panel drawings
- Any special instrument wiring diagrams

Each specification should refer to the following test requirements and certificates:

- Loop test sheets
- Site calibration check sheets
- Earth loop tests
- Insulation tests
- Completion certificates

Package Plant Instrument Specification

The package plant instrument specification details the instrumentation requirements and standards to be applied to any equipment packages. Typical equipment packages include Water for Injection (WFI) systems, chiller packages, gas scrubber packages, tablet presses, packaging machines, freeze dryers, autoclaves, and so on. Each specification should contain, or provide detailed reference to, the following information:

- Regulations and codes of practice
- Company/work rules
- Safety standards required of the supplier
- Good engineering practice guidelines for the installation of instrument apparatus
- Good engineering practice guidelines for the installation of cabling
- Good engineering practice guidelines for the installation of pneumatic piping/tubing

Each specification should contain details of the local power supplies available and refer to the necessary drawings and schedules, for example,

- Supply voltage and air pressure
- Cable block diagrams describing the interface with the rest of the plant
- Cable schedules detailing interconnections with the rest of the plant

Each specification should refer to test requirements and certificates, for example,

- Instrument hazardous area certificates
- Calibration certificates
- Requirement to meet EMC regulations

Electrical and Instrumentation Interface Panel

The electrical and instrument interface (interposing relay) panel is the method used to interface low voltage control systems (e.g., PLCs, Distributed Control Systems [DCSs], shutdown systems, loop controllers) to electrical switch circuits for operating and monitoring items of electrical equipment, including equipment packages. The documentation requirements for the panel comprise a panel specification, panel layout drawings, and wiring schematics (see above).

Special Instrument Systems

A number of other instrumentation and control equipment may be required for a particular project. These could include

- ESD systems
- Analyser packages
- Laboratory instrumentation (mass spectrometers, gas chromatographs, etc.)

Each item would generally require a detailed specification and installation documentation. The standards and documentation detailed in the appropriate sections above should be applied to this equipment. In addition, if the equipment involves the use of a computerised system, the system (application software and hardware) should be developed and tested using a formal, life-cycle methodology [7,9].

Case Study B

Validating PLC–Based Computer Systems

Richard Mitchell and John Gough
Pfizer Limited
Sandwich, Kent, UK

This case study discusses the validation of Programmable Logic Controllers (PLCs) and the particular requirements within a bulk pharmaceutical chemical (BPC) environment. Emphasis is toward bespoke systems, but the requirements of prebuilt PLC package systems is discussed in the section on embedded PLCs.

PLCs are microcomputers that have input/output (I/O) connections that enable them to communicate with external devices, usually in an industrial environment. Communication includes detecting a change of state, monitoring a state, activation, or deactivation. Devices include actuators, switches, thermocouples, and other instruments. They can be programmed to process the incoming signal and, if required, respond with an appropriate output signal to enable control.

PLCs originated in the car industry in the 1970s where programmable logic devices were used to do repetitive tasks. Within the pharmaceutical industry, they have evolved over the past 15 years and their processing power has increased. Programming can now achieve complex nonrepetitive tasking as well as routine repetitive functionality. They are now used to control medium-sized manufacturing facilities. The worldwide market for PLCs is estimated to be $3 billion [1].

The use of PLCs provides an inherent flexibility for the automation of a production plant. They can be used as an independent control system either embedded into or remotely linked to one or more items of production equipment. Expanded automation can be achieved by networking PLCs together or using them as slave stations to a central Supervisory Control and Data Acquisition (SCADA) system or Distributed Control System (DCS). Figure 1

Figure 1. Example PLC Application Layout

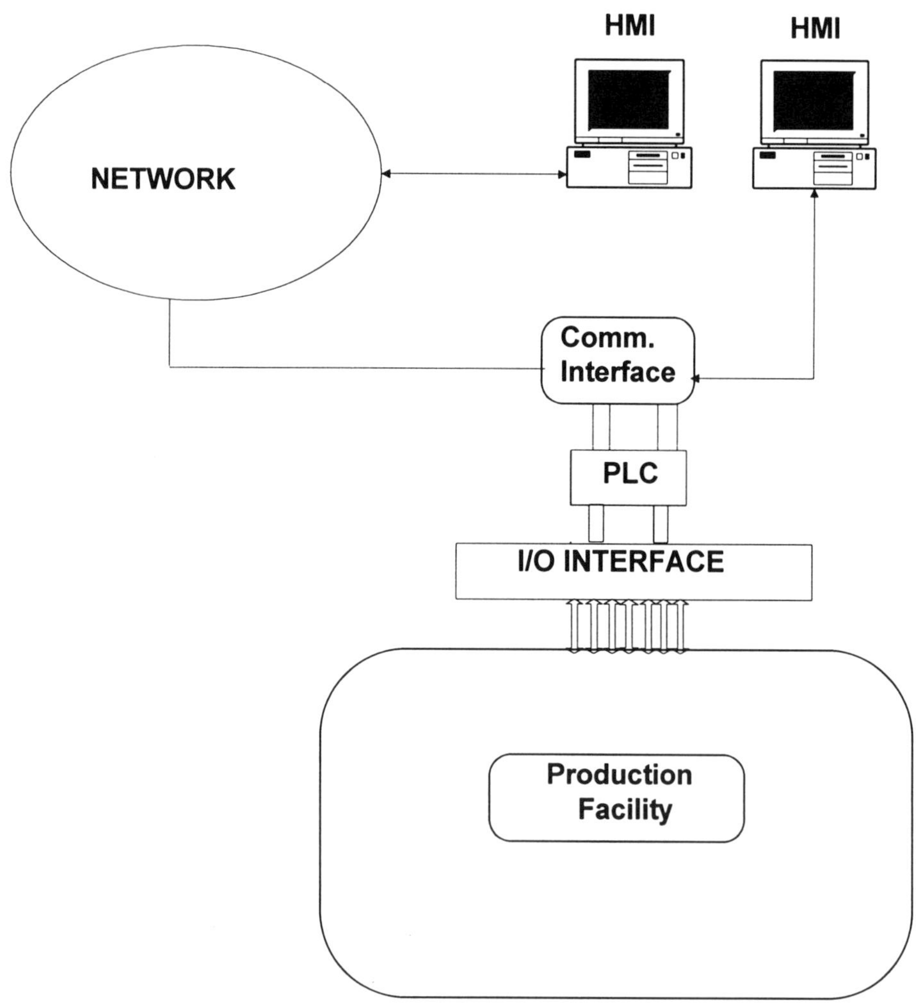

shows an example layout. Automation within the pharmaceutical industry is common and resources are required to develop, implement, validate, and maintain PLC–based systems.

WHY VALIDATE?

Validation of automation systems is now expected by the regulatory authorities governing the production of pharmaceuticals. It features extensively in articles in the literature and guidelines produced by both industry [2] and regulatory bodies [3,4,5]. The main reasons for validating PLCs are as follows:

- *Pharmaceutical regulatory compliance:* This is the main selling point for getting management to commit resources to what is an expensive overhead on automated systems. Allocation of resources to prospectively validate new PLC systems or a major modification to an existing PLC is easy to justify. It is much more difficult to justify the required resources to retrospectively validate a PLC that has, for many years, been controlling plant and equipment manufacturing product that meets its quality specifications. Regulatory compliance is really the only reason if the PLC is in a well-managed plant.
- *Other compliance:* The control of a production facility using PLCs also has ramifications for compliance with other statutory regulations, such as health and safety legislation and environmental regulations. Addressing all of these requirements in one validation study can help to focus effort and resources at the appropriate time. In addition, one set of documentation, properly written, approved, and controlled can minimise duplicative work. Some companies prefer to keep separate compliance documents for each regulatory body. This is a matter of choice.
- *Getting an application to work the first time:* This is the aim of most automation projects, and the validation process assists in fulfilling this objective. Failure can have significant cost penalties in lost production output, particularly if the project is on a tight implementation schedule.
- *Obtaining the full potential of a PLC system:* PLCs can easily be regarded as black boxes to those who are not familiar with their functionality and capabilities. Thus, they may not be used to their full potential. A team approach to validation can help all involved, particularly if a user is part of the team, leading to a better understanding of how the PLC controls their plant and indicating areas for improvement.
- *Continuous improvement:* PLC systems tend to be dynamic in that they are constantly being refined. Operating software is regularly

modified to cope with new processes, user requests, or changes to the hardware. Validation provides the documentation necessary for the process automation engineer to have the information he or she requires readily at hand to make the requested changes, or if the process engineer decides to leave the company, validation ensures that system documentation is available.

- *System maintenance:* Validation results in a well-documented system, which is a prerequisite for efficient planned maintenance schedules and in troubleshooting.

SELECTION OF A PLC

A lot of effort goes into selecting PLC platforms, as once selected, in-house experience is accumulated in utilising its capability and functionality. Once a particular system is in use, it takes a lot of justification to change. Much has been written about Supplier Audits [6,7] and we would concur with much of it. Practically, the main criteria that influence selection of a PLC are as follows:

- Pharmaceutical company–preferred suppliers
- Conformance to IEC 1131-3: structured design, standards for reuseable software, and interchange of software between different PLC products
- Hardware/software capabilities
- Supplier characteristics: durability, future-proofing, and cost
- In-house and contract programming knowledge availability
- Supplier has quality management systems in place and in use
- Cost

Supplier Audits should be used to obtain some of the knowledge required to assess the above criteria.

The selection of a PLC is critical to automation. The capabilities of the system will affect

- The degree of automation
- Performance of the equipment
- Benefits to efficiency
- Benefits to the user
- Maintainability
- Potential improvements

Customers are looking for confidence in the ability of a product to meet its business needs. Obtaining this confidence is usually an accumulation of evidence gained by the Supplier Audit and an intangible feeling of comfort with the way a supplier can justify its approach. Suppliers and customers must treat the Supplier Audit as a value-adding tool rather than an aspect of validation that must be completed.

VALIDATION OF A PLC

Prospective Validation

The methodology used to validate a PLC is very similar to that used to validate other automated systems that electronically communicate with external devices. Validation is generally viewed as a life cycle. There are many different types, but the current preference in the pharmaceutical industry is for the V-model [6]. It is important to recognise that a PLC must be validated in conjunction with its Human Machine Interface (HMI). If a PLC is being programmed to be connected to an existing networked system or to an existing SCADA or DCS HMI, then, unless some changes are required to the HMI, the PLC can be validated in isolation using the standard V model (Figure 2). Only the interaction between the PLC and the HMI need be validated. If, however, the application involves configuration of the HMI and programming of the PLC, then a variation of the V model is appropriate (Figure 3). This is the most likely situation that will be faced.

The difference between a DCS, where the HMI is usually an integral part of the system, and a PLC, which usually contains a controller and an HMI, is that separate software and hardware design specifications exist, and there will be separate build and Module Testing. Additionally, Integration Tests must take place to ensure that the individual systems communicate and interact in the correct manner. Any assessment of the potential hazards of such a system, such as a Computer HAZard and OPerability (CHAZOP) study, should cover the total system.

Retrospective Validation

In many automated plants, the use of PLCs predates the current emphasis on validation. Therefore, there is a requirement to retrospectively validate existing systems as well as to prospectively validate new systems or modifications to existing systems. Retrospective validation is often quite difficult as much of the information needed is difficult to locate, if it exists at all. It differs from prospective validation in ways that reflect the way information is put together in a documentation package and the amount of effort put into retrospective validation testing. The User Requirement Specification (URS) and

Figure 2. Validation Life Cycle

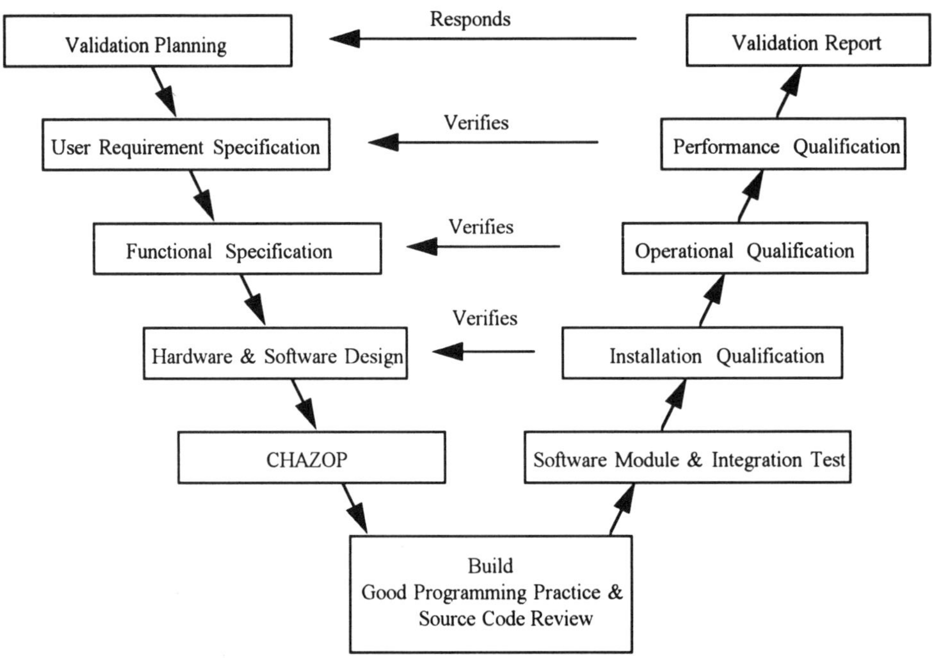

Functional Specification (FS) will be combined into one document. A Software Design Specification (SDS) and a Hardware Design Specification (HDS) are not necessary, but particular emphasis must be placed on Source Code Reviews. Installation Qualification (IQ) and Operational Qualification (OQ) are often repeated (or performed for the first time). This is often a good method for assessing the PLC in its current configuration. The documentation requirements for prospective and retrospective validation are summarised in Table 1. Retrospective validation requires a great deal of resources (time and money), and so the essential element of any retrospective programme is a risk assessment on the criticality of the computer system to determine how much validation will be completed, its priority in the programme, and the degree of resources to be allocated.

Prospective and retrospective validation requires a team approach for efficient execution. The key skill areas required are as follows:

- Production engineering—knowledge of the plant and equipment
- Automation engineering—knowledge of the PLC and the HMI
- Quality assurance and validation—knowledge of Good Manufacturing Practice (GMP) and documentation

Figure 3. Modified Validation Life Cycle for PLCs and Their HMIs

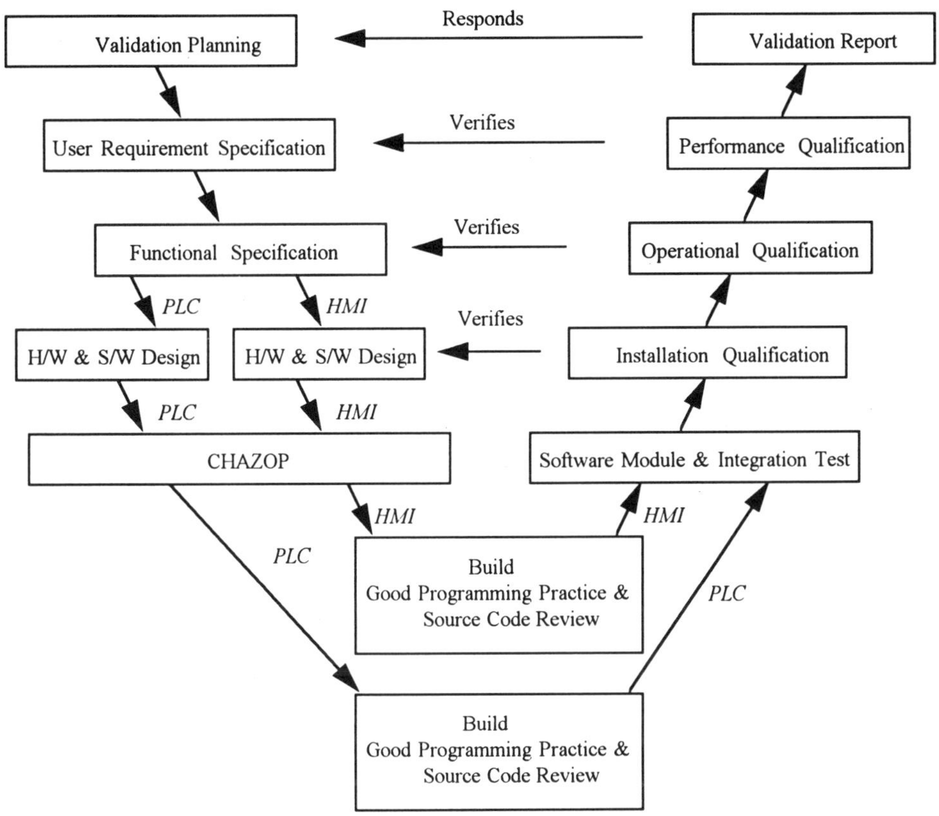

The representatives of these areas on the team have to work together and have to be committed to validation, otherwise conflicts and delays will inevitably follow.

THE VALIDATION PROCESS

The validation process can be divided into five sections. These five sections have distinct requirements but cannot be considered in isolation, as each has its own role in a validated system.

1. Planning
2. Specification

Table 1. Comparison of the Documentation Requirements for Prospective and Retrospective Validation

Document	Prospective Validation	Retrospective Validation
Validation Plan	yes	yes
User Requirements Specification	yes	} combined document
Functional Specification	yes	
Supplier Audit	yes	yes (if possible)
Software Design Specification	yes	no
Hardware Design Specification	yes	no
CHAZOP	yes	no
Source Code Review	yes	yes
Installation Qualification	yes	yes
Operational Qualification	yes	yes
Performance Qualification	yes	yes
Validation Report	yes	yes

3. Build
4. Testing
5. Maintenance

Planning

Putting some thought into how a PLC is going to be validated, in the form of a Validation Plan, is considered to be an integral element of the validation life cycle. A Validation Plan defines the strategy for establishing an appropriate level of documentation to demonstrate that a PLC functions in a manner consistent with its specification and does not in any way impair product safety, quality, and efficacy. A plan should be produced for all validation projects. The components of a plan for prospective and retrospective validation should include the following:

- Authority for the validation (e.g., Validation Policy, Validation Master Plan)
- Scope and purpose of the validation
- Overview of the process to be controlled
- Description of the environment in which the PLC is to function

- An historical summary of the PLC—if modifying or retrospectively validating an existing system
- GMP implications
- Background to the PLC installation
- Organisation and responsibilities
- Validation approach and the procedures to be used
- Results of any supplier selection process
- Ongoing operational requirements for GMP
- A milestone plan

A Validation Plan should be prepared by a validation specialist and approved by the process automation engineer and the plant manager. The main purposes of the Validation Plan are fourfold:

1. Get management to commit suitable resources to validation.
2. Make those involved in validating this PLC aware that their skills are required and when.
3. Define what documents need to be prepared and who is going to prepare them.
4. Demonstrate that validation is not an exercise at the end, but is integral throughout the project.

Validation Plans are produced at about the same time as the URS. The information in the URS is summarised in the Validation Plan with emphasis on GMP critical issues. This may be a critical temperature parameter or similar.

Specification

The critical step in any validation life cycle is the URS. This is ultimately the document against which any validation is assessed. Therefore, it is worth spending time and effort getting this document right. In our experience, users generally write incomplete URSs due to a lack of detailed knowledge of PLCs. This inevitably causes delays and problems getting validation right, as it is difficult to determine what is being validated against. However, users do know how they want their systems to operate, the features necessary for an efficient process, GMP, safety, and environmental constraints. We have instituted an Outline Specification (OS) in which they describe the critical parts of the system from a user perspective. It is an early warning that a PLC project is in the offing so that realistic plans can be made in busy work schedules. The OS is then developed into a URS by an engineer who is more familiar with the intricacies of PLCs. Care must be taken at this stage that the URS does not become an SDS. Our experience is that each project is different, people change and the content of various documents must be assessed during the life cycle of each project. The URS must highlight mandatory features and those that are desirable. Example sections of a URS are in Table 2.

This information is then used by the supplier/programmer to develop an FS. The FS describes the operational and performance criteria to be

Table 2. Some of the Elements of a URS

Section	Contents	Examples
Description of the automation project	Process description	Critical variables GMP implications Process limits
	PLC description	Contribution to production Degree of automation required Production considerations Engineering considerations
	Constraints	Timing Equipment availability Engineering constraints
	Operational environment	Zoning Cleanliness Potential electro-magnetic sources
Interfaces	Human interface equipment	Number and type of terminals Required displays in diagrammatic form Access security requirements and conformance with standards
	Process interface	I/O capacity Installed and future I/O spare capacity Communications interfaces
Control Requirements	Process control	Sequence control Continuous control Batch management

Continued on next page.

Continued from previous page.

Section	Contents	Examples
System Attributes	Alarms	Principle Method of viewing Method of acceptance
	Events	Change in status Trending of data
	Interlocks	Hardware Software
Other Requirements	Performance/ response time User training Maintenance Redundancy Intrinsic and operational safety Expansion philosophy Security and integrity	

provided by the PLC. It consists of the same sections as the URS, providing an overview of the PLC hardware and software required to fulfil the URS and notes any noncompliances.

Programming PLCs is becoming easier, and we have found spreadsheets invaluable in consolidating the I/O requirements requested in a URS. These spreadsheets can be built up, form part of the FS and detailed design, and then are used to generate the test sheets for IQ and OQ. Figure 4 illustrates this approach.

The FS is developed into a hardware design or a software design or both. The SDS provides the facility to break each functional requirement into appropriate subfunctions increasing in detail at each subsequent level, until eventually the design reaches a state where it can be translated into software code. The SDS should mimic the sections of the FS but be specific to software construction. Some examples are as follows:

- Design methodology (e.g., sequential function charts)
- Module design: inputs, functionality, and outputs
- Communications interface (data transfer protocols)
- Process interface (consideration of the signal from the instruments)

Figure 4. Spreadsheet Development

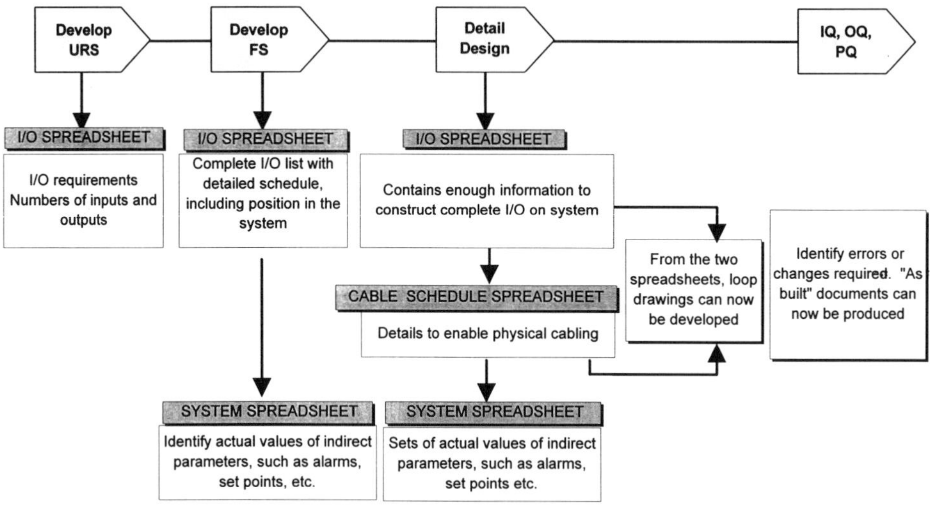

Hardware design defines the PLC platform that hosts the software, including the relationship with the HMI. It is often an overlooked part of PLC validation. Areas that need to be addressed include the following:

- PLC hardware
- Interfaces: human, process (analogue I/O, digital I/O, totalisers, interposing relays), and communications interface (hardware protocol, buffer capabilities, cable specifications, line drivers)
- Services (earthing, filtering, loading, surge protection)
- Maintenance procedures (spares, diagnostic checking, calibration)

The instrument supply industry is moving toward smart devices, with corresponding software to provide configuration, testing, and monitoring. Communication trends are starting to move away from the 4–20 mA analogue signal toward digital signals. The applicability of these developments to the project or staying with the tried and tested methods needs to be considered in the HDS.

In many applications, the SDS and the HDS are included in the FS. This is acceptable as long as this is defined in the Validation Plan.

Validation is no different to many processes, inasmuch that an inadequate specification will lead to extended project times, higher costs, and many frustrations. Our experience merely confirms the above. Get the specification right and the rest of the validation life cycle will be relatively plain sailing.

BUILD

Once the HDS and SDS have been completed, the supplier can get on with the science of building and programming. Putting sufficient time and effort into producing good specifications considerably eases programming. Testing begins during this phase.

TESTING

The testing of PLC software and hardware is in a number of different phases during the life cycle of the project and is designed to achieve different things. Some companies would not include CHAZOP as part of the computer system validation. However, the CHAZOP process can provide a formal mechanism for reviewing and assessing the design.

A CHAZOP provides a structured and documented process for evaluating the risks (failure modes) of a PLC that the standard Hazard Study (HAZOP) has identified as having an impact on plant safety. It should also explore countermeasures. It is not strictly a test, but a design review. It is the first formal step in assessing that the proposed automated system is fit for purpose. The process itself is similar to a HAZOP, in that it uses keywords and requires a team of people providing knowledge of the PLC, HMI, the process, the equipment being controlled, and an independent leader familiar with the study process. CHAZOP should be completed after design, but before programming or build has progressed too far so as to minimise abortive work. Our experience is no better than most as this approach is immature. We have learned that a CHAZOP must follow a HAZOP (where a HAZOP is required) and not vice versa, otherwise it becomes difficult to focus the CHAZOP on the automation system without exploring the consequences on the associated equipment. The best way to learn about the CHAZOP process is to do it in a controlled, planned manner.

Source Code Reviews are used to ensure that controlled development and a consistent programming style have been used. It also checks GMP critical features. Source Code Reviews need a standard against which to check, and programming practices for all programs should be documented. An audit of the supplier's compliance with their own quality management procedures should be carried out at this stage to ensure that appropriate quality is being built into the system. Programming details will vary according to the PLC manufacturer, but the overall style should be relatively constant. Areas that should be addressed are as follows:

- Directory structure
- Software construction
- File header and comments

- Version control
- File naming conventions
- Coding practice (e.g., naming conventions for ladder logic, special functions, subroutines, and loops)

Source Code Reviews of PLC software are not easy tasks as programs are constructed using low level code, such as ladder logic. It is not practical to review all code, as this would take considerable expertise, time, and associated cost. There is no guarantee that all errors would be identified. Effort should be directed to critical areas of the code and high level coding conventions to assure that software has been constructed in a structured manner.

The next phase of testing begins to investigate whether the implemented design conforms to the requirements of the design specifications and Functional Specification. This process starts with Module and Integration Testing conducted by the supplier. Completion of this is otherwise known as Factory Acceptance Testing or off-line testing. Module Testing of functional routines verifies the components of the design in isolation. Integration Testing assembles the various functional routines and tests the system as a whole. These tests provide the best opportunity to challenge the system in ways that are unlikely to be faced in operational use, and, as such, they should be carefully designed to test:

- Databases used to develop the design have been implemented correctly
- Devices
- Loops
- Fault trees
- Sequences
- Interface with HMI
- Invalid inputs

What we need to do, as previously stated, is to validate the PLC, the HMI, and the connection. We can use the HMI to help us do Integration Testing. The sequence is as follows:

I/O on PLC ﬁ devices on PLC ﬁ I/O via database on HMI ﬁ
devices on HMI ﬁ sequences

The careful design of tests can ensure that unlikely conditions can be assessed and their impact on the system evaluated. It also checks for errors in system construction. Comprehensive testing builds confidence into a system and can help reduce subsequent OQ testing (Site Acceptance Testing or on-line testing). This can often produce savings in time, particularly in plant downtime if modifications are being made to an existing system.

It is not feasible to test every aspect of the programs. Tests must be directed towards critical features. Coordination between the customer and supplier can help to minimise superfluous tests. The trend toward incorporating the programming standard of IEC 1131-3 means that validation becomes easier for each new system for which a PLC is used. There are only so many devices a PLC will support, most of which will be common to each system. We have found that the use of generic descriptions of how to test a device and automatic generation of specific test sheets from a database saves a considerable amount of time when testing new systems. There are some software tools available, such as simulation software, that can aid testing. However, this software must be validated before use.

Since Module and Integration Testing is done in isolation from the process and equipment, confirmatory tests are required, and this forms part of the OQ. Before this can be completed, proof is required that hardware and software is installed correctly. This is IQ, which ensures that all the PLC components are present and installed correctly in accordance with design specifications. Some tests are included in Table 3.

OQ ensures that each function of a PLC performs in accordance with its FS throughout representative or anticipated ranges. The boundaries of the system should have been tested in the Module and Integration Tests, but a proportion of these tests must be repeated in OQ now that real devices are attached. Vagaries in the devices can have effects on the operation of the software and these need to be evaluated. OQ tests include the following:

Table 3. Example Installation Qualification Tests

Item	Tests
PLC	Confirm all parts are present and correct. Confirm power supply voltages and quality are adequate. Confirm earthing meets manufacturer's requirements. Confirm correct versions of software have been supplied and installed. Confirm hard-wired interlocks have been correctly installed.
I/O cards	Identify serial numbers and model numbers of cards (where possible, this is not always easy for PLCs). Identify calibration certificates.
I/O Tests	Confirm signal continuity between field termination and PLC. Confirm signal continuity between HMI and PLC.
Documentation	Check that all required documentation is present and useable (e.g., correct language).

- Hardware/software startup and operation
- Operation of devices
- System timing
- Critical fault trees
- Security features, such as password protection
- Control sequences
- Ensuring GMP critical parameters have been implemented correctly
- Field I/O is correctly calibrated
- HMI interacts with the PLC in the desired way
- Backup and restoration

We have used a database not only to populate PLC and SCADA values, but also to generate forms used in the testing. These forms, referenced by each protocol, can help to minimise documentation, but, more importantly show at a glance the continuity of completed tests.

Other GMP issues that need to be addressed during IQ and OQ include the following:

- Training
- Standard Operating Procedures (SOPs)
- Calibration schedules
- Maintenance schedules

The final phase of validation is Performance Qualification (PQ), which ensures that the PLC performs its functional requirement, as specified in the URS, within the manufacturing environment. In reality, what this means is using the PLC to control the process while product is being manufactured. PQ tests include the following:

- Batch startup
- Monitoring of GMP crucial parameters
- Monitoring of alarms and messages
- Confirm security access procedures
- Confirm HMI is fully functional
- Confirm batch recording is correct

A final Validation Report is useful to summarise the results of testing and compare them against functionality defined in the URS and FS. This is usually performed by a validation specialist, who may have been a witness to some of the tests but is impartial. This is to provide a knowledgeable but independent summary of the validation exercise. A validation certificate is sometimes used to demonstrate that a PLC has been successfully validated and when the periodic review or validation assessment activity must be undertaken.

Validation Support

Validation does not stop when the Validation Report is completed and the PLC is on-line. A number of support procedures must be implemented to maintain the PLC in a validated state. Change control is the most important and ensures that future modifications to the PLC can be managed in a controlled way without impacting GMP, safety, or environmental considerations and to maintain the system in a validated state. Change control should have started before PQ, and revision control should have been implemented at the initial programming stage.

Contingency planning defines the plans and procedures that are required to ensure that system failure (hardware or software) can be recovered with no or minimal (quantifiable) impact on the validated state and without risk to safety, the environment, or product quality. Automation strategies incur the penalty that most if not all the eggs are in one basket—if a PLC goes down, there can be serious consequences for a number of different controlled or monitored areas. If there are serious consequences, then the URS should have specified some sort of backup system. Even if the plant can cope if the PLC goes down for a short period of time, procedures identifying equipment that are still operable, those that are in a safe condition, and areas with the highest risk (on whatever grounds this is assessed) are essential. The availability of recovery procedures and the location of the backup copy of the software is necessary in the event of an unplanned system failure.

Maintenance Plans can help to minimise the need for contingency procedures by having planned service outages to maximise the time between failures of the PLC. The strategy we have adopted is to carry a spare PLC and one of each of the I/O cards. This is not an expensive option as the spare PLC doubles up as a development machine.

Finally, a system should be in place to allow the user to record any observations, problems, or suggestions for improvement. These should be reviewed along with change control records, a selection of production records, and training records in a regular review of the PLC application. Periodic reviews are an important element of a continuous improvement programme. Periodic reviews are sometimes termed *revalidation,* with the emphasis that this terminology implies. The PLC cannot be used past the date set for revalidation. A topical issue at present is being able to demonstrate that source code has not changed. The use of PLC software tools that enable detailed comparison between software is a useful check during the periodic review, and an inspection of change control records, Contingency Plans,

Maintenance Plans, logbooks, and security measures demonstrate that the automated system is under control.

PLCs AS PART OF A SYSTEM

The validation of a PLC cannot be viewed as a stand-alone operation. PLCs are there for a purpose—to provide automotive functionality. An overall validation plan that details what other validation (equipment qualification, validation of other automated systems) is required. A timetable must be devised to ensure that validation of the PLC is not delaying qualification of equipment or validation of an automated system is not delaying validation of a PLC. The latter case is particularly relevant if the PLC is to communicate with another PLC embedded into an item of equipment. This link must be validated as must the individual PLCs, but the link cannot be validated until the software processing the information from the particular I/O point is validated. The definition of the boundaries of each validation prevents unnecessary duplication. For PLCs, it is best to use the I/O cards as the boundary. A final check from HMI to the device can then be performed to ensure the system works in its entirety.

EMBEDDED PLCS

Embedded PLCs tend to be standard packages. It is now nearly impossible to dictate to proprietary equipment manufacturers about the type of PLC to be used, so you are looking for a system built to a good quality management standard. Supplier Audits are used to determine whether the implemented system is appropriate for your validation needs and what, if any, corrective action is required. The focus of testing shifts from Module and Integration Testing to OQ. Design and justification for the tests must be included in the OQ protocol as, although the purchaser must have access to the supplier's test plans and results, they must be repeated in the OQ to assure that the PLC functions as required in your manufacturing environment.

Equipment suppliers may not be accredited PLC suppliers. The approach to validation will not change, but there may be increased emphasis on particular elements, such as functional testing, and less on others, such as Supplier Audits. This is very much a customer decision based on their own experiences.

The amount of testing depends on three factors:

1. Conclusions from the vendor assessment
2. Criticality of the PLC to controlling the equipment
3. Criticality of the equipment in your process

Unnecessary tests cost time and money.

Some PLCs can carry on functioning if the HMI is unavailable. More sophisticated PLCs are dependent on the HMI. It is important to validate this.

The current trend is to purchase a PLC and bolt on a SCADA system. The SCADA system tends to be written by a third party and must be configured for the application. Validation is not totally integrated and must be carefully considered during the validation life cycle.

SUMMARY DISCUSSION AND CONCLUSION

In an ideal world, validation would be an integral part of the development of every PLC application that has an effect on product quality. Over the past five to six years, awareness of validation has increased in both supplier and purchaser organisations. Validation is still being paid for either in direct monetary terms for increased documentation or indirectly by lengthening project times. Validation should be no more than documenting what happens now from planning to delivery, but the word *documentation* sends shivers down the spine of many a supplier and purchaser. This has tended to give validation, and those working in the area, a bad name.

The benefits of validation tend to go unnoticed as, by definition, the PLC is working according to its design, in the manufacturing environment contributing to consistent product meeting its quality parameters and is relatively trouble free.

The role of the Quality Assurance department in ensuring that the documentation produced is appropriate, required, and not excessive cannot be understated. Emphasis on the positive benefits of validation other than the ultimate benefit of regulatory compliance, which is often used like a stick rather than a carrot, helps to encourage efficient validation. The pharmaceutical industry must not lose sight of the fact that they are ultimately responsible for validation.

A structured approach to validation will ensure that quality will be built into a PLC system. For the automation of a production plant, we believe that the selection of the appropriate PLC platform and using in-house expertise to develop the control application gives us the confidence that the software has been constructed and tested in the appropriate way and that changing production demands can be addressed efficiently.

ACKNOWLEDGMENTS

The authors gratefully acknowledge the contribution of Paul Benson, Keith Brown, Hugh Langston, and Eric Wells of Pfizer Limited.

REFERENCES

1. *Control and Instrumentation* (1996), 28 (3): 7.

2. *Good Manufacturing Practices for Active Ingredient Manufacturers,* Final Draft. (December 1995), Published Jointly by European Federation of Pharmaceutical Industries Association/CEFIC, the European Chemical Industry Council.

3. Tetzlaff, R.F. (1992), GMP Documentation Requirements for Automated Systems, Parts 1, 2, and 3. *Pharmaceutical Technology,* 16 (3): 112–124, 16 (4): 60–72, 16 (5): 70–82.

4. Trill, A.J. (1993), Computerised Systems and GMP—A UK Perspective: Part 1: Background, Standards and Methods; Part 2: Inspection Findings; Part 3: Best Practices and Topical Issues. *Pharmaceutical Technology International,* 5 (2): 12–26, 5 (3): 49–63, 5 (5): 17–30.

5. European Union Guide to Directive 91/356/EEC (1991), *European Commission Directive Laying Down the Principles of Good Manufacturing Practice for Medicinal Products for Human Use.*

6. UK Forum (1994, 1995, and 1996), *Supplier Guide for Validation of Automation Systems in Pharmaceutical Manufacture.* First Draft (1994), Second Draft (1995), Version 2.0 (1996). United Kingdom Pharmaceutical Industry Computer Systems Validation Forum.

7. Grigonis, G.J., Jr. and Wyrick, M.L. (1994), Computer System Validation: Auditing Computer Systems for Quality. Report on behalf of the PhRMA Computer Systems Validation Committee. *Pharmaceutical Technology Europe* 18 (9): 32–39.

Case Study C

Validating Industrial Personal Computers

Owen Salvage
Eutech Engineering Solutions Limited
Billingham, UK

Industrial Personal Computers (IPCs) offer the opportunity to provide operator information at the point where manufacturing operations take place. At the factory floor or in the clean room, IPCs take computer technology to the local point of control, where there is often a harsh operating environment. Typically, IPCs must contend with the following:

- Sterilisation procedures within a clean room
- High temperatures, humidity, and long running times
- Dust buildup and chemical attack
- Vibration and mechanical shock
- Power disruptions and Electro-Magnetic Interference (EMI)

For small-scale control applications and the presentation of data to operating staff, IPCs represent a highly effective means of supporting production operations. Typical applications include the following:

- Control of intelligent instrumentation
- Control of analysis equipment
- Control of small-scale production units
- Presentation of operating guidance information

IPC technology is currently being applied in the pharmaceutical industry for these types of applications, taking full advantage of current rapid development tools and Man-Machine Interface (MMI) presentation software. IPC technology is readily available; indeed, virtually everyone now has some experience with office or home Personal Computers (PCs).

WHY VALIDATE IPCs?

Regulators have the power to prevent the sale of goods that are considered to have been produced without the application of Good Manufacturing Practice (GMP). IPCs by their nature are used to monitor and control manufacturing operations and are, therefore, subject to GMP validation.

The use of IPCs to support manufacturing processes means this technology has a major bearing on the quality, safety, and efficacy of the products manufactured. The GMP regulators, such as the U.S. Food and Drug Administration (FDA) and the UK Medicines Control Agency (MCA), are concerned about the hazards software can introduce in the manufacturing process [1]. IPCs are, therefore, required to be validated in compliance with the current regulatory standards.

THE VALIDATION LIFE CYCLE

Good Automated Manufacturing Practice (GAMP) is now well established as the means by which Quality Assurance is built in the development of automated systems. IPCs fall into the category of automated systems and are subject to the Quality Assurance methodologies supporting GAMP.

The validation of an IPC proceeds under the authority of a Validation Master Plan (VMP) and follows the V-model, leading from specification through to implementation and finally to qualification. The phases of the validation life cycle for an IPC and the sequence of activities are listed below [3,4]:

- Validation Plan
- User Requirements Specification (URS)
- Supplier Audit
- Supplier Quality Plan

- Functional Design Specification (FDS)
- Hardware and Software Design
- Design Qualification (DQ)
- Programming and Construction
- Supplier Testing
- Installation Qualification (IQ)
- Operational Qualification (OQ)
- Performance Qualification (PQ)
- Validation Report
- Ongoing Support

The IPC validation life cycle, shown in Figure 1, shows the relationship of the design and qualification documents as the project moves through the validation exercise.

Validation Plan

The Validation Plan defines the scope, organisation, and timetable of the validation programme. Supplier organisations may not be known at this stage and may be generically identified within the Validation Plan. Change control procedures during and following the validation exercise are defined and any necessary Standard Operating Procedures (SOPs) are identified.

The Validation Plan also outlines the general and specific acceptance criteria for validation, establishes the responsibilities for performing the validation, and specifies the documentation requirements for defining and controlling test protocols, results recording, and reporting.

User Requirements Specification

The URS is a statement of the system requirements in terms of how the IPC application is to operate in the intended environment. The URS should clearly identify the following:

- Process to be controlled
- Key environmental challenges for the IPC
- Power supply conditions on-site
- List the number and types of signals used in the control system
- System size including spare capacity (e.g., number of workstations)
- Requirements for data presentation, records, and reports

Figure 1. IPC Validation Life Cycle

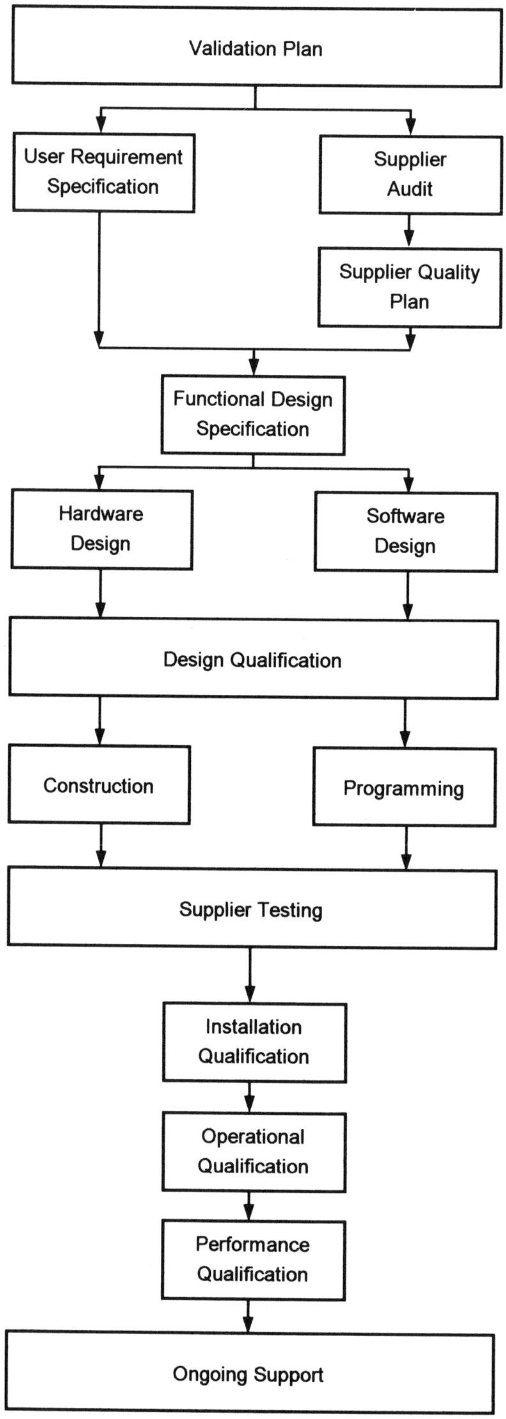

- Communications with intelligent devices
- Management Information System (MIS) networking requirements
- Availability target for the system (i.e., acceptable downtime)
- Maintenance requirements
- Documentation requirements

End user involvement in the development of the URS is strongly recommended to ensure good understanding of the operating environment of the IPC and the functionality required of the installed system. Examples of reports required from the system, engineering drawings, graphics, and location sketches greatly assist the IPC designer.

Supplier Audit

Few suppliers comply with the requirements of validated systems, even if the supplier is accredited to ISO 9000 or ISO 9000-3 (TickIT). The manufacturer is obliged by the regulators to ensure that proposed suppliers are suitable to handle the project, and this is generally carried out by a Supplier Audit [5].

Supplier Quality Plan

The Supplier Quality Plan identifies the organisation, standards, software tools, and timetables proposed by the supplier in the execution of the project. Any inconsistencies between the standards and timetables required by the VMP and those stated in the Supplier Quality Plan must be identified and resolved, to support the validation case of the IPC.

Functional Design Specification

The FDS translates the requirements of the URS into the technical solution proposed to fulfil the project requirements. Operational and performance criteria for the IPC are stated in such a way as to facilitate testing of the installed system. The FDS should specify the following:

- Functional requirements to facilitate software development
- System performance (e.g., timing, memory storage, and spare capacity)
- Communications and network protocols (e.g., RS232, TCP/IP, Ethernet)
- Method of storing and retrieving data
- Maintenance requirements for hardware, software, and system parameters

- Performance of the IPC under the environmental conditions on-site
- Signal conditioning, signal noise reduction, and power supply methods
- Availability data for the IPC
- IPC hardware architecture including backplane and memory (Winchester, EPROM)
- Peripheral devices (e.g., printers and backup devices)
- Number of users and response time required from the IPC
- System and application software configuration and the design methodology
- Functional descriptions of the control system operations
- Start-up and shutdown procedures
- New or novel technology used—hardware or software
- Security and access control methods
- State the date and time setting method for the IPC
- Screen layout

A typical architecture of an IPC system is shown in Figure 2. At this stage in the specification, the design of the IPC screens confirms that the IPC supplier has correctly interpreted the URS.

With Rapid Development Software (RDS) tools, the screen layout and "look and feel" of the screens can be quickly built and used as the basis for discussion. Screen input, output, and display requirements are also clarified, along with definition of the database [1].

Hardware Design

The Hardware Design for the IPC control system identifies the components and connections required to support the functionality demanded by the FDS. Table 1 can be viewed as a checklist of items the Hardware Design must address [6].

The Hardware Design includes lists of equipment, instruments, cables and cable identification, label schedules, and instrument loop drawings of the signal installations. General arrangement drawings identify the location of the IPC displays, keyboards, cable routes, and marshalling cabinets. Instrument certification and calibration certificates are included, along with the stated environmental conditions the equipment can tolerate.

Figure 2. Typical Architecture of a Networked IPC System

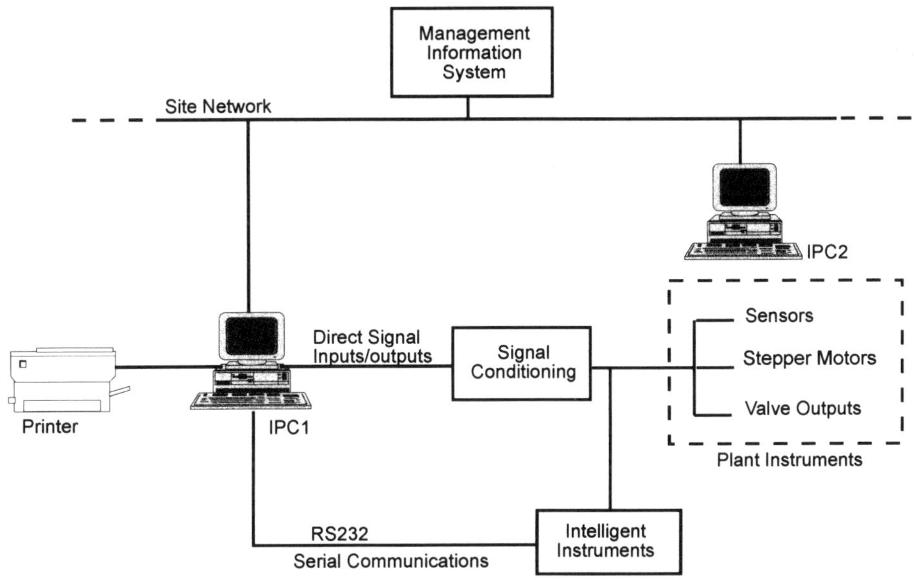

Software Design

The software design of the project covers system software and application software required to fulfil the project [3]. An IPC system software model is shown in Figure 3.

A typical standard operating system for IPCs is Windows. The control system operating system provided by the manufacturer supports software building blocks. For a specific project, customised building blocks may benefit the project (e.g., the control of motor drives). These project software standards would be included in the software design.

Application-related configurations are parameters chosen to meet the needs of the project (e.g., for a specific hardware platform, communications protocols, or printers chosen for the project). Application-specific programming refers to the project-specific code, designed in modules that, when integrated, provide the full functionality required by the FDS.

With RDS tools, the tool itself is not installed in the final IPC. This ensures that any changes to the functionality must be carried out away from the target IPC, and under controlled conditions.

The Software Design should include the following:

- Software modules and application configuration
- Interrelationships between modules

Table 1. Hardware Design Checklist

Signal Types	Stepper motor, analogue inputs and outputs (4–20 mA), digital inputs and outputs
Earthing	Instrument and factory earths Comms earthing
Power Supply Units (PSUs)	Redundancy, supply filters, fed from different transformers, PSU alarms Uninterruptible power supply (UPS) support time UPS bypass for maintenance purposes Scope of UPS support (e.g., IPC terminals including measurements)
Measurement Instruments	Capable of sterilisation Accurate, accessible, and maintainable
Cable Routes	Secure route in factory Sealed entries into clean rooms Marshalling arrangements
Hardware Failure Modes	State of signal outputs on power fail and power up
Signal Isolation	Opto-isolation Galvanic isolation Barriers
IPC Location	MMI location and ergonomics of the IPC Purging of the IPC display and keyboard, size considerations IPC cooling fans, air filters Sealed keyboards, IP65 Mechanical vibration protection
I/O Card Channel Allocation	Segregate critical signals to avoid common failures due to a single card
Communications	Comms channels and interfaces IPC port allocation

- Alarms and operator messages, including out of range data input messages
- Calculations
- MMI graphic design and hierarchy
- Software module design specifications

Figure 3. IPC System Software Model

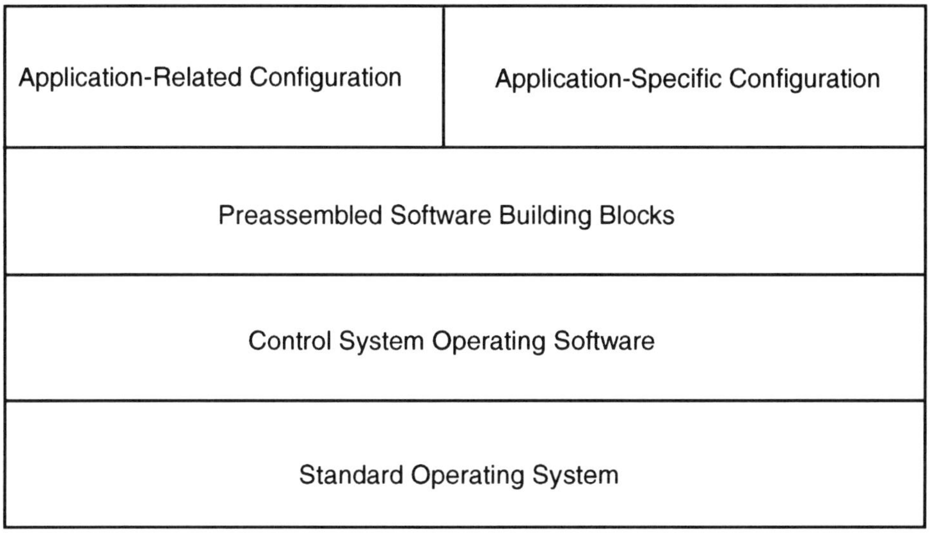

- I/O database structure design and signal parameters
- Communications driver design and interface with the database
- Signal diagnostics and maintenance
- Control functions, interlocks, and permissives
- Hierarchy of module interactions
- Storage of batch record data and reports
- Security: password and protection from network introduced problems
- Data key-in checks (e.g., range checks, "Are you sure?", validation of inputs)

Design Qualification

The DQ checks the design documentation and accurately describes the IPC system and operation [3]. Engineering drawings, operating and maintenance procedures, parts lists, and system descriptions are included in the DQ. The DQ offers the opportunity to ensure specified components are compatible with the target environment and meet electro-magnetic compatibility (EMC) regulations.

Programming and Construction

Implementation of the software design proceeds once the design has been approved. Development facilities may need to be purchased or rented to enable the programming to take place. The software produced must be capable of execution on the hardware platform used for supplier testing and the IPC installed on-site.

Programming

IPC applications benefit from the existence of inexpensive RDS tools that greatly increase the speed of software production. The tools currently available allow flexibility of graphic design, use of standard programming blocks, and testing routines.

Each module should be uniquely identified with an author, version number, data, and change history [1]. Extensive comments within the code assist debugging and maintenance.

The following phases apply to the programming element of the project and result in a hard-copy paper listing of the final system, required by the GMP regulators:

- Graphic development
- Module development
- Database development
- System integration

Construction

Construction of the IPC system includes the building of cabinets to house the IPC hardware, wiring marshalling cabinets and junction boxes, and cable and instrument installation. Much of this work is carried out on-site.

- Marshalling cabinet build
- Cable installation on-site from the instrumentation to the IPC
- Cleanroom integrity considerations
- Communications links installation
- Handover documentation (e.g., as-built drawings, electrical safety checks)

Supplier Testing

Supplier testing carried out at the factory includes hardware and software tests. Successful completion of the tests allows the shipment of the IPC to the site.

- Hardware tests: earth continuity, high voltage tests
- Radio Frequency Interference (RFI) immunity
- Calibration certificates for instruments
- Loop testing for all inputs and outputs, including spare channels
- Graphics checks
- Source Code Review
- Calculation verification
- Power-up/power-down tests
- Integration Tests
- Functional checks
- Communication driver tests
- Security testing

Installation Qualification

IQ consists of documented checks that all equipment, parts, services, and documents have been supplied and installed as agreed. The equipment supplier is responsible for all construction and installation activities, which will be performed to the satisfaction of the project manager.

Operational Qualification

OQ is a series of tests to demonstrate that all GMP critical functions of the equipment operate as designed. With the OQ, typically, a large number of functional test scripts test each of the functions identified in the FDS. Careful sequencing of the tests can greatly improve the efficiency of the testing.

Performance Qualification

PQ is the documented evidence that the process performs effectively and reproducibly to produce a product meeting its specification and quality attributes specified in the URS.

SPECIAL TESTS FOR THE INDUSTRIAL ENVIRONMENT

The extent of IPC testing depends on the severity of the target environment. A range of tests for the industrial environment may be identified to simulate closely the conditions the IPC will be expected to withstand [3]. These tests include the following:

- Loop testing of sensors. Test the sensor input up to the screen displays (diagnostic and operating displays).
- Visual inspection of signal shielding and earthing arrangements to eliminate noisy signals. Continuity checks on earth bonding.
- Inspection of seals on components in sterile conditions. Confirmation of positive pressure within purged cabinets.
- Heat soak tests for the IPC system. Under controlled conditions in the factory, monitor the performance of the IPC under high temperature. A warm, poorly ventilated room at a temperature of approximately 25°C, not unduly uncomfortable to humans, can cause PC–based systems to fail.

SUPPLIER ISSUES

Many companies offer technical services in providing IPC systems to companies. In very few cases are these services complemented with the necessary validation skills [7]. The responsibilities of the supplier, Engineering departments, Quality Assurance, and Manufacturing are all important in achieving the aim of a fully validated system on handover of the project.

It is the responsibility of the Quality Assurance and Manufacturing groups to manage the validation exercise on behalf of the client company. The responsibility for producing the VMP, PQ, and Validation Report rests with these groups.

Engineering departments can specify what is required by the IPC system and select a suitable supplier. Coordination with the Quality Assurance group is advisable during a Supplier Audit in order to assess the validation capability of the supplier.

Once the supplier is selected, the interface between the supplier and the Engineering department is vital to the delivery of a well-engineered, validated system. Completion of the OQ represents the handover of the system to the Manufacturing group to carry out the PQ. Representatives of the client company need to be present at Supplier Testing, IQ, and OQ to witness testing.

Close cooperation between all groups is essential to ensure that the expectations of the IPC match those intended by the URS and the demands of the validation process. Following handover, the validated status of the IPC application must be maintained through change control and the training of operating and maintenance personnel.

SUPPORT ISSUES

Once the choice has been made to utilise an IPC, there are certain inherent support issues associated with these systems.

Maintaining the Validating Status of the IPC

The ease with which IPCs may be implemented implies that change is also straightforward. Control of the application software resident on a machine may be ensured by removing the software development tool.

Changes are carried out on a separate development system and are subject to the normal validation testing and documentation updates of the IPC. Changes to hardware are assessed for compatibility with the intent of the control system prior to implementation. The System Specification is updated and the new equipment tested prior to return to service.

It is recommended to avoid installing software other than that required for the intended purpose of the IPC. Avoid using the IPC for operator word processing or any other administration purpose.

Upgrading IPC Software

Implicit with IPC systems is the rate of change of the available hardware and software. Current PC hardware and software has a life cycle of approximately two years.

Upgrade paths must be controlled to ensure the IPC is maintainable into the future. There is a classic story of control systems implemented only several years ago and now the hardware is no longer available, let alone the relevant software skills.

Management of the IPC upgrade path is a key skill in protecting the company from threats to the IPC's validated status and serious maintenance problems in the future. Potentially costly fast-track projects can be avoided with managed upgrades.

IPC Security

Defeat of an IPC password security system is possible, particularly if the IPC is based on DOS. More recent developments in operating systems have improved the security features in this area. IPC security may be enhanced by disabling floppy disc drives. In this case, the IPC may boot off a networked server.

Networked IPC systems may be subject to interference from connected systems. Careful checks on the system security arrangements, through a Threats and Controls Analysis, can prevent unwarranted access to the IPC system [1,2]. System security can be enhanced by allowing read only access at the terminals of a networked system.

Date & Time for Year 2000

The clocks of many IPCs installed prior to 1995 have an inherent flaw in the date and time mechanism. When the year 2000 is reached, most machines will recognise this time change and set the year to 1900. Care is required in choosing IPC hardware and operating systems to ensure this flaw is not unwittingly installed.

Training of Operating and Maintenance Personnel

Operating and maintenance personnel must have documented training in how to use and maintain the IPC system [3]. In addition to the functional and engineering aspects of the system, training is advisable in how to maintain the validated status of the IPC.

CONCLUSIONS/SUMMARY

IPCs are increasingly attractive to manufacturers and offer the opportunity to provide operator information at the point where manufacturing operations take place. The ease with which IPC systems may be implemented makes them ideal for small-scale control systems that may be increased in size in a modular way.

Networking gives possibilities of integrating information flow from the factory to business systems. On the other hand, greater security issues arise when linking systems; it is certainly not desirable for control systems to be accessed via the network.

Delivery of a total package of hardware, software, and documentation for validated IPC systems is not yet available from all suppliers. Client companies must be careful in choosing suppliers and must make clear the validation requirements for any installation with an impact on product quality.

The maintenance of systems, once installed, is a key area of concern for organisations, particularly if a large number of installations are not yet "year 2000 friendly". Change control and upgrade paths for IPCs are particular areas of concern with rapidly developing technology and a typical product life cycle of two years.

Despite these issues, IPCs are here to stay as they provide an effective, low-cost means to implement small-scale control systems that fit into most companies' existing IT hardware and network arrangements.

REFERENCES

1. Kreuger, J.E. and Kreuger, J. (1993), Computer Systems Validation. In *Pharmaceutical Process Validation,* 2nd ed., edited by I.R. Berry and R.A. Nash. New York: Marcel Dekker, Inc.

2. European Union Directive 91/356/EEC and U.S. Code of Federal Regulations Title 21, Parts 210 and 211, detailing Good Manufacturing Practice for Pharmaceuticals.

3. Dannapel, B. et al. (1995), Qualification of Control Systems, Joint GMA and NAMUR committee on validation. *ATP Journal* 37 (10): 64–67.

4. UK GAMP Forum (1996), *Supplier Guide for Validation of Automation Systems in Pharmaceutical Manufacture,* 2nd version. United Kingdom Pharmaceutical Industry Computer Systems Validation Forum. International Society for Pharmaceutical Engineering, Tampa, Florida.

5. Wingate, G.A.S, Smith, M., and Lucas, P.R. (1995), *Assuring Confidence in Pharmaceutical Software,* 1st Annual ENCRESS Conference, 12–15 September, Bruges, Belgium.

6. Booty, F. (1996), Industry Gets Hard on Computers, *Manufacturing Computing Solutions.*

7. Wingate, G.A.S. (1994), *Life Cycle Methodology for Computer Systems Validation,* ISPE European Computer Validation Seminar, November, Stuttgart, Germany.

Case Study D

Validation of SCADA Systems

Chris Reid
Imperial Chemicals Industries plc
Billingham, UK

Validation is an extremely emotive subject, with vastly differing perspectives of its requirements existing throughout the pharmaceutical industry. This, coupled with the almost incessant desire of the pharmaceutical industry to introduce new terminology for concepts that existed long before the arrival of validation in the 1970s, often obscures what is simply good practice. Good practice ensures that computer systems are specified, designed, implemented, installed, commissioned, and tested in a thorough, unambiguous manner that satisfies the specified requirements and expectations of our customers. Suppliers who fail to appreciate the subtle difference between specified requirements and customer expectations will inevitably be doomed to failure.

PHARMACEUTICAL REGULATIONS

Regulatory compliance within the U.S. and UK markets is policed by the Food and Drug Administration (FDA) and Medicines Control Agency (MCA), respectively. These regulatory bodies inspect manufacturing facilities to verify compliance with Good Manufacturing Practice (GMP) legislation and guidelines prior to the issue of a manufacturing licence. This licence provides the authority to market drug product in the governing nation and can be suspended or withdrawn should subsequent periodic inspections uncover serious noncompliance.

Table 1 identifies the main regulatory legislation and guidelines prevailing on the use of computer systems in the pharmaceutical industry. As guidelines often present the regulators' perspective of the requirements of GMP, it is advisable to take them seriously and apply them with as much vigour as statutory legislation.

SCADA SYSTEM ARCHITECTURE

Before discussing specific validation issues, we must first understand the Supervisory Control and Data Aquisition (SCADA) system architecture. SCADA systems do not provide direct control of plant equipment and instrumentation, rather they offer a suite of custom-built communication interfaces to third-party devices. These devices range from large Distributed Control Systems (DCSs) to Programmable Logic Controllers (PLCs) and intelligent instrumentation. The SCADA system provides the platform for the development of the overall process control philosophy, leaving the mechanics of the low-level plant equipment and instrumentation to the developers of such third-party devices. The SCADA system further provides a window through

Table 1. Good Manufacturing Practice Legislation and Guidelines

Title	Legislation	Guidelines	Country of Origin
Code of Federal Regulations—Title 21, Part 210: *Current Good Manufacturing Practice in Manufacturing, Processing, Packing or Holding of Drugs* [2]	✓		U.S.
Code of Federal Regulations—Title 21, Part 211: *Current Good Manufacturing Practice for Finished Pharmaceuticals* [2]	✓		U.S.
Rules and Guidance for Pharmaceutical Manufacturers 1993 (Orange Guide) [4]	✓		UK
GMP Directive 91/356/EEC *Medicinal Products for Human Use* (Incorporated in Orange Guide)	✓		Europe
UK GAMP Forum, *Suppliers Guide for Validation of Automation Systems in Pharmaceutical Manufacture, Version 2* [3]		✓	UK

which plant operators, maintenance engineers, and production managers control and monitor processes (see Figure 1).

SOFTWARE ARCHITECTURE

The software architecture of the SCADA system typically comprises a number of modular blocks or packages collectively providing the system functionality (Figure 2). A robust, modular design ensures that the SCADA system can be continually developed to meet constantly evolving customer requirements and expectations. Poorly designed systems, constructed from monolithic software programs serving unrelated functions, are not easily maintained and inevitably lead to sleepless nights deciphering faults or, in many cases, the early demise of the product.

Database

The core of any SCADA system is the database. A typical database is partitioned into three discrete areas for maintenance of continuous, historical, and networked data. Invariably, three discrete databases are provided, each constructed to reflect the specific characteristics of the incoming data (e.g., analogue, digital, pulsed signals).

Continuous Database

The continuous database maintains records of continuously updating data. The source of continuous data is application dependent, but generally comprises external communication interfaces to third-party devices, internally derived data, such as calculations, or data generated by user programs. The database is refreshed with incoming data at configured intervals that are then immediately available for utilisation by the various SCADA system functions for control, display, or recording purposes.

Historical Database

The historical database provides medium- to long-term storage of continuous data, batch data, and reports for subsequent interrogation. Constraints on on-line disk capacity or short logging intervals may necessitate archive or automatic transfer of historical data to mass storage Management Information Systems (MISs). Historical data are of particular importance to GMP as it provides the mechanism by which batch compliance is demonstrated.

Network Database

The network database provides a buffer between third-party communication interfaces and continuous or historical databases. Raw values from field devices are validated in the network database before being deposited in either

Figure 1. SCADA System Architecture

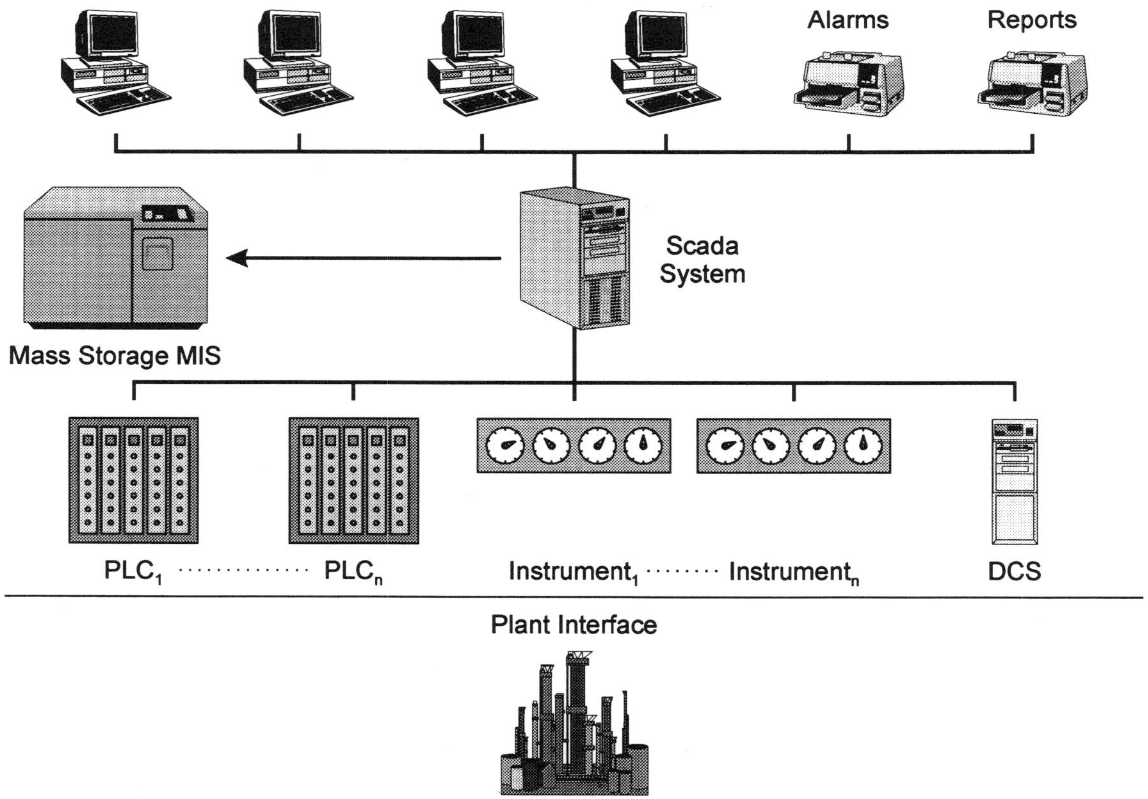

Figure 2. SCADA System Software Architecture

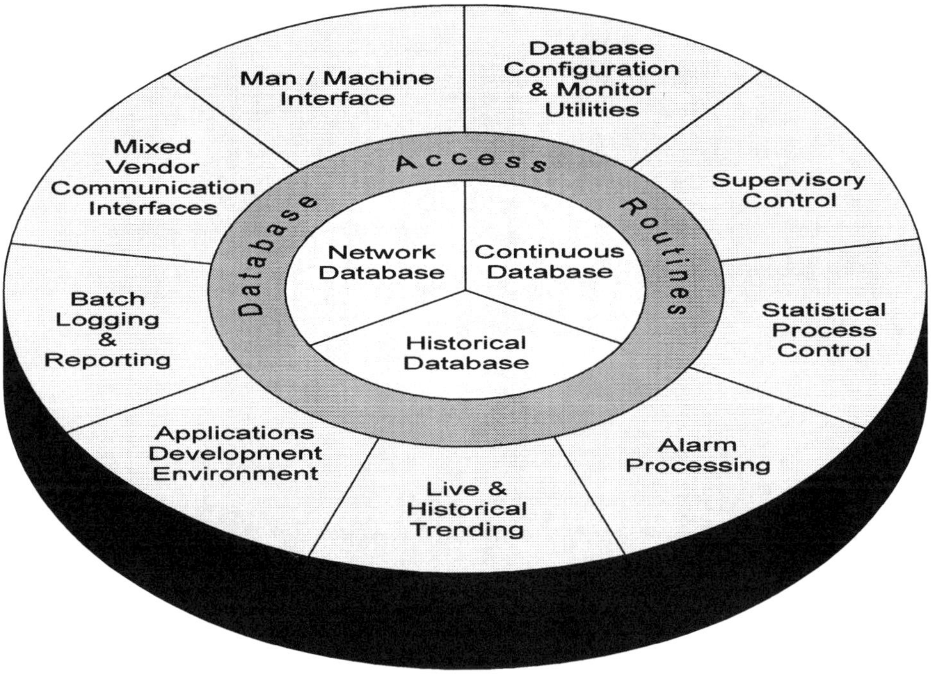

the continuous or historical database. Invalid data can be detected, processed, or discarded as appropriate without jeopardising the integrity of critical compliance reports, calculations, logs, or trends.

Man-Machine Interface

The Man-Machine Interface (MMI) provides a common interface to process control and monitoring functions for plant operators, maintenance engineers, and production managers. The ergonomics of the MMI will determine system acceptability. Users invariably judge a system by the ease with which new displays and functions can be accessed and updated and by the presentation format of critical data. I have experienced systems where excellent underlying functionality is rendered redundant simply because the system is difficult to navigate and response times are slow.

A major consideration of all systems employed within the pharmaceutical industry is security. The MMI provides access to critical functions and data that control and demonstrate process compliance. Consequently, safeguards must be integrated into the MMI to protect against inadvertent or malicious access.

Database Configuration

Database configuration tools enable on-line and off-line creation and modification of database records. Configuration tool design must recognise relationships between database records to avoid duplication or creation of partially configured records. Database configuration tools must also provide an environment that is easy to interpret by system administrators to minimise the risk of erroneous configuration.

Database Access Controls

The majority of SCADA system functions require access to continuous, historical, or network databases. Data are often manipulated or compressed prior to transfer to the database. It is important that such data manipulation and compression is transparent to the software developer. This is achieved through access routines that provide a secure buffer between SCADA system functions and the various databases. Data are validated and access authorisation is verified before reading from or writing to the database, thus maintaining data integrity.

Supervisory Control

SCADA systems by their nature do not provide direct control of plant equipment and instrumentation, rather they offer a suite of communication interfaces to third-party field devices ranging from DCSs to PLCs. As such, the SCADA system developer is able to concentrate on high-level control philosophy design rather than the actual mechanics of individual field devices.

Statistical Process Control

Statistical Process Control (SPC) is an integral function of modern SCADA systems. SPC functions control processes by means of mathematical relationships between process events. Current and historical data enable advanced prediction of future process performance, thus allowing early compensation to maintain process control and compliance.

Alarm Processing

Detection of malfunctions or divergence from critical process parameters is a fundamental GMP requirement. Effective alarm processing packages enable monitoring against multiple alarm levels. Alarms can then be configured to warn of pending failures, enabling compensation to be made before total failure or process noncompliance. Prioritisation of alarms is also important to enable differentiation between compliance failures and less critical events.

Live and Historical Trending

Plant operators, supervisors, and production managers utilise trending functions to monitor process variables against predetermined set points and alarm limits. Live trends enable detection of process deviations before they impact on product quality. Historical trends facilitate analysis of previous batches to verify compliance with process specifications.

Applications Development Environment

Application Development Environments (ADEs) allow the development of bespoke software to suit specific process requirements. Bespoke software usually takes the form of sequential or batch control programs. As application software is specific to each manufacturing process, extensive validation is required to ensure adherence to a formal software development life cycle. Applications software, however, is often written by site engineers who have neither the experience nor formal training in software development. To minimise the risk of database corruption, therefore, the ADE must provide database access controls, as discussed earlier, to inhibit unauthorised or invalid database access.

Batch Data Report and Storage

Process variables, events, calculations, times, and trends are logged to document batch manufacture. Reports are retained on-line in the medium term and subsequently archived to mass storage media for retention as dictated by the various GMP legislation and guidelines. Completeness and integrity of batch data is a fundamental GMP requirement. The SCADA system must, therefore, provide robust controls to avoid inadvertent or malicious modification or deletion of batch records. Verification of data forming the batch record is an essential component of system testing.

Mixed Vendor Communications Interfaces

Mixed vendor communication interfaces constitute the greatest development effort of the SCADA system. As SCADA systems do not directly control the plant and equipment, they must rely on interfaces to third-party systems that do. Marketing potential invariably increases proportionately to the number of communication interfaces provided. Even with the advent of standard communication protocols, such as Fieldbus™, many manufacturers continue to utilise in-house bespoke protocols to maintain competitive position or due to high redevelopment costs.

Serious validation issues arise when developing and maintaining communications interfaces. During initial development, third-party equipment will generally be available to facilitate testing. However, this equipment is often a deliverable of the project, and consequently will not be available to the supplier after the project. Even if equipment is retained by the supplier, it will generally only provide a subset of what is required to carry out full functional testing. This poses a major problem when implementing subsequent modifications, this is often overcome by the development of test harnesses. Test harnesses are software programs developed to simulate the behaviour of third-party equipment. This raises a further issue as to whether test harnesses themselves should be developed and tested in accordance with a formal development life cycle. The answer is simply yes; it is essential that the supplier demonstrates that the test harness issues the commands and responses in accordance with the defined communication protocol.

LIFE–CYCLE APPROACH TO SCADA DEVELOPMENT

I am a great advocate of practical, value-added validation. I do not subscribe to the production of documentation for its own sake. Although, validation does increase the burden of documentation, it should only be produced if benefits can be quantified.

Figure 3 helps visualise the level of documentation required to demonstrate robust design and verify implementation in accordance with regulatory

Figure 3. Documentation Levels

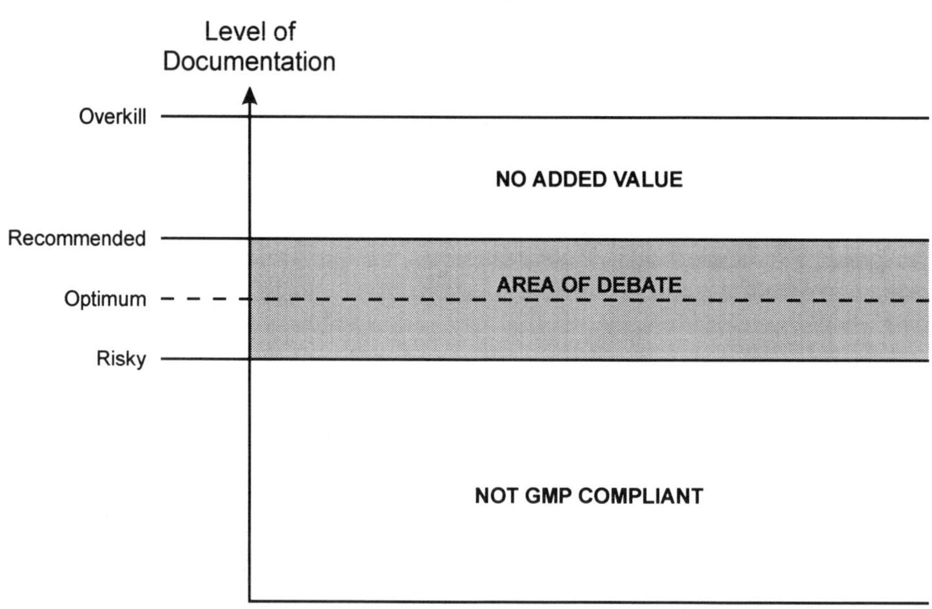

requirements and good practice guidelines. Documentation in excess of the "recommended level" rarely adds value to the SCADA product and, in many instances, obscures critical information. Documentation below the "risky level" is not sufficient to demonstrate that the system is adequately specified, designed, implemented, and tested. The shaded region identifies the area of great debate. Whilst documentation anywhere above the "risky level" will often satisfy regulatory inspections, the cost of delivering to the "recommended level" is rarely greater than the cost of wasted time in debating the issues arising from the shaded region.

I cannot offer statistics in support of this theory; however, by critically reviewing documentation requirements at the start of the project and subsequently reviewing the content of documentation at each phase of the software development, it is possible to discard superfluous information or demand further clarification of GMP critical functions where appropriate.

SCADA systems evolve over a number of years from initial conception, providing basic functionality to a market-leading product, benefiting from years of experience and customer feedback. A good Quality Management System (QMS) enables large-scale development in parallel with practical implementation of minor modifications. Too often, documentation is produced as a mandatory requirement of the QMS rather than to add value to the product.

System Development Life Cycle

The system development life cycle is an iterative process as indicated in Figure 4. Constraints or enhancements at any phase of the life cycle may necessitate rework at one or more preceding phases. Volumes of documented case studies stand as testimony to the need to overcome constraints and correct defects as early in the life cycle as possible. Problems that manifest themselves during acceptance testing or operational phases are significantly more expensive to rectify than those found during specification and early design.

User Requirements Specification

Suppliers of any computer system will seldom be involved in the production of a User Requirements Specification (URS). In some companies, systems analysts may provide a separate function to system designers, implementers and, as such, may produce a URS. Similarly, marketing departments may produce a URS based on their knowledge of industry expectations and competitive products. Both, in my experience, are rare occurrences with the responsibility for production of the URS firmly attributed to the supplier.

It is important, however, that SCADA system suppliers have a sound understanding of the objectives of the URS. The URS defines a customer's desired functionality and performance expectations. The supplier must have a

Figure 4. Life-Cycle Model

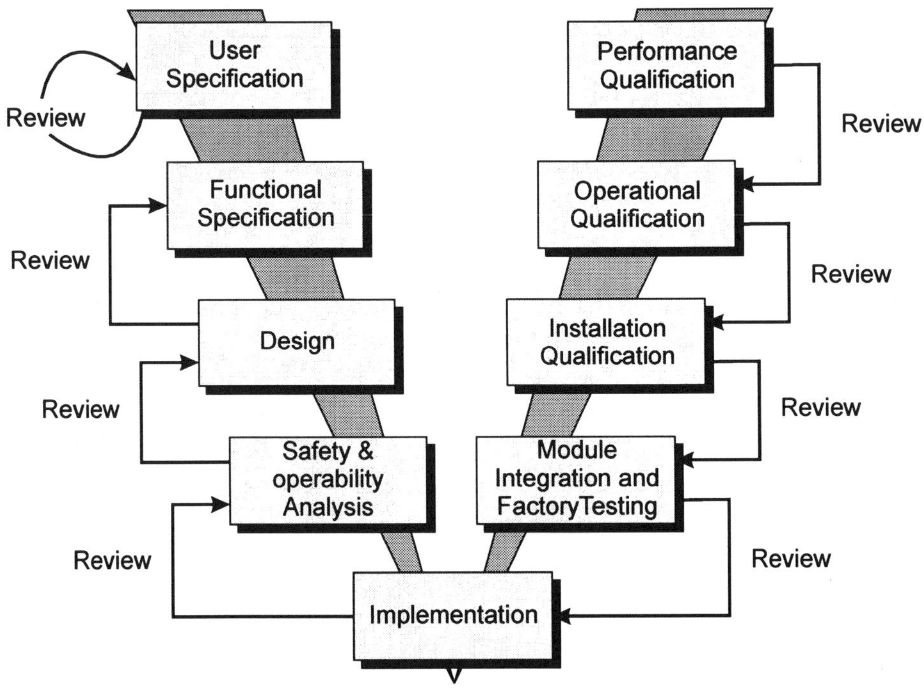

clear understanding of the URS in order that requirements can be clarified and ambiguities and inaccuracies challenged. Validation aside, a lack of understanding of the URS can lead to contractual difficulties when the delivered system fails to meet customer expectations. Tables 2 and 3 define typical hardware and software specifications that should be included in the URS.

Project/Quality Plan

Project and Quality Plans define the milestones, deliverables, responsibilities, organisations, and systems that shall be employed to develop the SCADA system to a satisfactory quality standard. Too often, the QMS dictates the production of separate Project and Quality Plans. The need for separate documents should be dictated by the size of the project, not the QMS. The QMS however, should dictate the contents. It is very easy to develop a Project and Quality Plan that defines unrealistic objectives that can never be achieved. These documents should be referenced on a daily basis to ensure that quality standards and project timetables are being met. The Quality Plan is a contractual document that the supplier must adhere to in order to fulfil his or her project commitment.

Table 2. Typical Hardware User Requirements

Man-Machine Interface	Type and number of operator, supervisor, and manager consoles
	Safety ratings of consoles (e.g., IP [ingress protection] rating)
	Other console attributes (colour/monochrome, location, antiglare devices, connection details)
	Data entry/selection medium (keyboard, mouse, etc.)
	Physical security (e.g., key switches)
Data Storage	Medium (hard disk, floppy disk, optical disk, tape, etc.)
	Capacities
	Access Speed
Communication Interfaces	Type (serial/parallel, LAN/WAN [Local Area Network/Wide Area Network], optical fibre, single/multidrop
	Connection configuration requirements (RS 232, RS 443, coaxial, etc.)
	Hand-shaking requirements
	Data transfer rates
	Cable lengths (line drivers)
System Performance	Processing power (CPU speed, data transfer rate, coprocessors, etc.)
	Memory (on-board, cache, secondary, etc.)
Expansion Philosophy	Future system loading
	Future storage requirements
	Future communications interfaces
	Future MMI requirements

Functional Specification

The Functional Specification (FS) forms the supplier's response to the customer's URS. A weakness of many QMSs is that they dictate the format of the FS rather than the content. I subscribe to a common document structure as it aids review; however, I am prepared to sacrifice this passion in favour of an FS that responds directly, clause for clause, to the URS. The FS is a statement of what is to be delivered in response to the URS. It is not a direct copy of the URS, as systems rarely offer functionality that exactly satisfies the URS. If the QMS does dictate a document structure, then an FS-to-URS cross-reference matrix will more than satisfy this objective. For each clause in the URS, a response clause within the FS is listed. This is the simplest, yet most infrequently adopted, method of ensuring that all requirements of the URS are addressed by the FS.

Table 3. Software User Requirements

Database	Number of continuous, historical, and networked database points
	Device specifications (analogue inputs/outputs, digital inputs/outputs, pulsed inputs, totalisers, valve control, motor control, etc.)
	Instrument ranges
	Alarm limits
	Scan frequency
	Source of data
	Logging frequency
	Batch data formats
	Current and future expansion capacity
	Security
Man-Machine Interface	Display hierarchy
	Plant overview graphics
	Interlock graphics
	Alarm graphics
	Control points
	Function key definition
	Refresh and response rates
	Security
Supervisory Control	Detailed definition of process control philosophy
	Security
Statistical Process Control	Detailed definition of SPC philosophy
	Mathematical models and formulae
	Security
Alarm Processing	Alarm priorities
	Limits
	Cause and effect
	Scan rate
	Logging and printing requirements
	Suppression and enabling
Live and Historical Data Trending	Trend groups
	Data points

Continued on next page.

Continued from previous page.

	Log and refresh rates Retention period Alarm bands Security
Applications Development	Definition of application software requirements in the form of structures design methodology, flowcharts, state transition diagrams, etc. Security
Batch Data Reporting and Storage	Report format Data points Retention period Manual entry requirements Calculations Batch trending requirements Security
Mixed Vendor Communications Interfaces	Data transfer protocol Unidirectional/bidirectional Software hand-shaking Data transfer rate Data points Security

Having developed the FS, test planning can commence. I am not a great advocate of proceeding prematurely with test procedure definition. The system development life cycle is an iterative process and early test procedure definition could result in unnecessary rework. Acceptance criteria, however, can be set forward as the FS should have clearly defined the inputs and outputs of each function. Obviously, it is impractical to assume that no changes to functional requirements will occur.

Hardware and Software Design Specification

Hardware and Software Design (HDS and SDS) follows FS approval. Bespoke hardware will rarely be developed; consequently, hardware design generally entails construction of standard components to meet performance, capacity, and safety requirements.

Software design starts with a high-level architectural design that can be progressively decomposed into smaller, detailed design components. The QMS should not dictate the level of decomposition required, as this will be determined by the complexity of the development. The QMS, however, should define areas to be considered in the design. Similarly, the QMS should not impose a design methodology; rather it should insist that an appropriate design methodology is utilised and that all development engineers are adequately versed in the chosen methodology. Justification for the selection of the methodology should be documented.

Both the HDS and SDS are response documents to the FS. As such, they should directly cross-reference the FS either by parallel structure or by cross-reference matrix.

Implementation

Time constraints, commercial pressures, inexperience, incompetence, and laziness are typical examples of why unstructured, unreadable, untraceable, and unmaintainable software continues to be developed, well into the 1990s. Software coding standards are required to guard against such failings and should ensure a common approach to software implementation without stifling creativity. The objectives of software coding standards are to increase

- Readability
- Consistency
- Maintainability
- Traceability
- Fault reduction

In order to achieve these objectives, software coding standards should address

- Module layout
- Module size (procedures per module)
- Naming conventions
- Modification histories
- Use of documenting comments
- Data transfer rules
- Use of global and local data
- Use of hard-coded values

- Indentation of control blocks (including maximum number of levels)
- Violation of control structures

Configuration Management

Configuration management (Figure 5) controls access to the SCADA system software. Multiple releases of system software will be in use on many customer sites at any given time. Even if suppliers only warrant to support, say, the three most recent releases of the software, it is probable that in excess of two years spans the most recent and oldest releases. Therefore, it is vital that new system software releases are not simply constructed by direct modification of master software modules. Once released to market, system software must be frozen and archived. System software remaining resident on development systems for support activities must be protected against modification.

Subsequent developments are derived from a copy of the current system software release maintained within a separate development area. Carte blanche access, however, is not provided to the development area. Development software must be protected against ad hoc uncontrolled modification,

Figure 5. Software Configuration Management

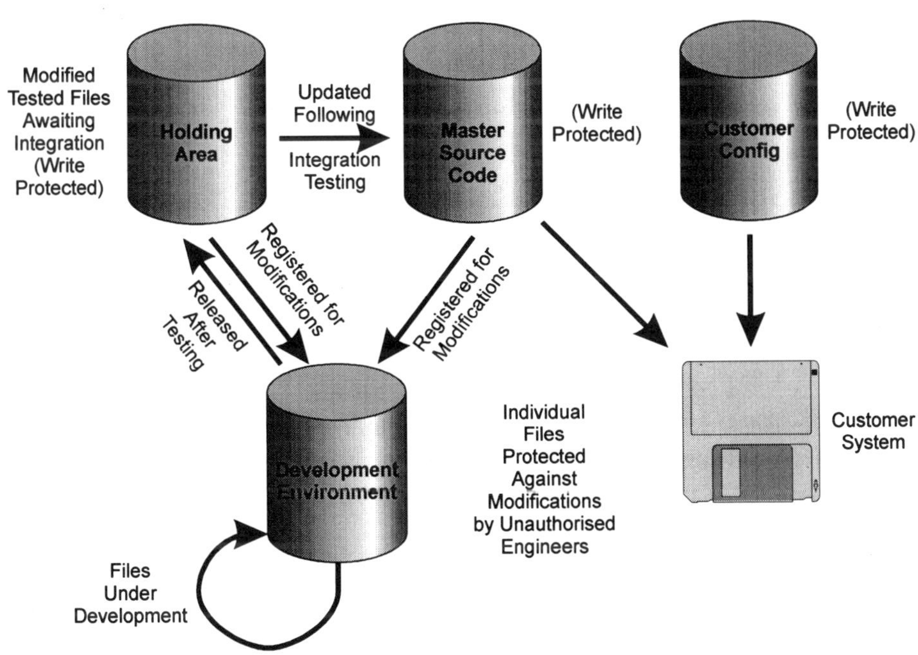

preferably on write-protected storage media. Files requiring modification must be formally registered before modification commences. Appropriate change control must be raised and development engineers authorised before the release of any files to the development area.

Having registered a file for modification, the development engineer has exclusive access to files until the modification is complete. This avoids loss of modifications arising from multiple engineers accessing the same file. Once a modification is complete and satisfactorily tested, it can be released to a holding area to await subsequent modification or integration into the system.

Several partial integrations may occur before the final system integration to enable phased testing of modifications. Files contained in the holding area are reviewed prior to integration to ensure that they have been implemented in accordance with software coding standards and have been adequately tested.

The benefits of configuration management include the following:

- Protection against integration of partially complete modifications
- Exclusive access to files undergoing modification
- Automatic record of modifications
- Automatic record of authorising change controls
- Verification of test data prior to integration
- Controlled recovery from defective modifications

Control of System Build Environment

Many problems arise due to the lack of control of the system build environment. The system build environment comprises the linkers, compilers, assemblers, and command files that translate implementation into an integrated executable system.

Compilers, assemblers, and linkers are the least cause for concern, as they infrequently change. This does not, however, mean that they never change; therefore, they must be strictly controlled as with any other software configuration.

Command files, however, present the greatest concern for product development managers and engineers alike. Engineers treat command files with far less respect than they do system software. Command files are modified ad hoc in the absence of change control, new command files are generated, and master system build command files are modified on a temporary basis to meet short-term needs.

This lack of control inevitably leads to disaster, which, at best, results in a loss of valuable time due to failed system builds. At worst, untested software is integrated into the system undetected, increasing the risk of subsequent costly batch failures and investigations. Modifications to any system command file must be subject to the same degree of change control as all other software.

System Testing

As we will witness during the following discussions, system testing contributes several phases to the system development life cycle. However, the underlying objective of all testing is the same—it must be

- Specific in its objectives
- Clear in its method
- Repeatable

These three objectives are satisfied by the definition of detailed step-by-step test procedures that set forward clear acceptance criteria. Test procedures should enable controlled progression through the test and should identify key milestones on route to demonstrating the final objective. I do not subscribe to the school of thought that suggests test procedures can be executed without prior knowledge of the system, although this may be true of test witnesses.

Unambiguous and appropriate acceptance criteria should be stated for all tests. Acceptance criteria should cater for current and anticipated process parameters, not necessarily total system capability. I have witnessed test failures arising from acceptance criteria that are more demanding than anticipated process parameters. I have further reviewed many regulatory citations against acceptance criteria that do not adequately demonstrate control within defined operating parameters. It is worth remembering that justifying failed tests in validation reports is a time-consuming activity.

Raw Data

Raw data are those items that support test results from Module Testing to Performance Qualification (PQ). Raw data take the form of written results, printouts, screen dumps, error logs, calibration certificates, and so on. A measure of the adequacy of raw data is that it should be possible for a colleague unconnected with the project to review the test results and confidently conclude whether the test has satisfied its predetermined acceptance criteria. Raw data should be referenced to the relevant test procedure and retained for subsequent inspection by regulatory authorities.

Module Testing

The extent of Module Testing is determined by the level of decomposition within the detailed design. If only minimal decomposition is required, then it may be practical simply to proceed to Integration Testing. Module Testing avoids the "Big Bang" approach and simplifies the testing process to build confidence that discrete module functionality and module interfaces conform to specification. The QMS should not impose Module Testing but should provide practical guidelines to the level of decomposition before Module Testing becomes essential.

Integration Testing

Integration Testing demonstrates that the system as a whole functions in accordance with the specification. Integration Testing is often referred to as in-house checks and is the process by which the supplier gains confidence in the software prior to inviting the customer to approve the system formally. Integration Testing demonstrates that new software has been satisfactorily woven into the system, modified software functions as specified, and existing software remains unaffected by the integration. As a rule, at least 10 percent of all existing functionality should be revisited following system integration.

Factory Acceptance Testing

Factory Acceptance Testing (FAT) provides the opportunity to demonstrate satisfactory operation of the SCADA system to customers prior to site installation. FAT, as with Integration Testing, utilises hardware and software simulation to demonstrate that all functions operate across current and anticipated operating boundaries. FAT may provide the only opportunity to demonstrate correct or safe operation of certain functions such as failure mode recovery. Satisfactory completion of FAT will authorise delivery of the system to the customer's site. Although a number of tests will be revisited during Installation Qualification (IQ) and Operational Qualification (OQ), FAT should satisfy a significant percentage of the customer's validation requirements.

Good Manufacturing Practice Review

The level of on-site testing is determined by a GMP Review (sometimes referred to as a GMP Assessment). The GMP Review identifies those functions of the SCADA system that directly or indirectly impact on product quality. All GMP functions, unless exhaustively tested during FAT, will form the basis of on-site testing or qualification, as it is referred to within the pharmaceutical industry. In reality, the majority of functions provided by the SCADA system or any other control system are GMP critical. In order to limit testing, a customer may review the system to identify functions that will not be utilised. However, in such circumstances, procedures or physical inhibitions must be put in place to prevent use of unvalidated functionality.

Installation Qualification

IQ verifies the installation of hardware and software components against the FS. For subsequent system upgrades, the IQ will, in addition to verifying hardware and software against the FS, ensure that existing configuration has not been adversely affected. Common examples of upgrade failures include the following:

- Batch data corruption/loss
- Historical data corruption/loss
- System configuration corruption/loss
- Incompatibility of configuration tools with existing data structures

Common sense dictates that a system backup or archive is taken prior to commencing the upgrade. System restoration is then a relatively simple task in the event of upgrade failure. Controlled recovery from failure is a fundamental requirement of GMP.

It is essential that both the supplier and the customer maintain accurate records of software and hardware configuration. Generally, suppliers maintain records of system software configuration and customers maintain records of application configuration. The customer may, however, outsource this responsibility to the SCADA system supplier or another third party under the control of a Service Level Agreement.

Operational Qualification

OQ demonstrates conformity of all GMP functionality against the FS. OQ testing must verify operation across current and anticipated operating ranges and must challenge all operating boundaries. OQ tests may be a subset of FAT; however, where it is possible to further challenge functionality under operational conditions, it should be done. For instance, the testing of security features will not change from FAT to OQ. However, FAT of control loop operation will demonstrate that the control loop output operates in the correct direction in accordance with a step change in the process variable. The OQ will extend this test to ensure that the process variable is returned to the set point within a defined period and that control loop parameters have been tuned to provide a controlled reaction to the set point deviation.

Performance Qualification

PQ monitors and records the operation of the system over a prolonged period, ensuring that the system consistently performs in accordance with the FS. Customers will normally be responsible for PQ.

System Support and Maintaining the Validated Status

GMP dictates that appropriate provision is made for ongoing maintenance of computer systems utilised in the manufacture, processing, packing, or holding of pharmaceutical products [1]. As a supplier of SCADA systems to the pharmaceutical industry, it is important to understand the problems associated with implementing modifications on a validated system.

First consider fault rectification. In the absence of unlimited time and resources, it is virtually impossible to guarantee fault-free software. Validation simply provides a high degree of assurance that the software will meet its predetermined specification. Depending on complexity, faults either can be rectified on site or must await full design, implementation, and integration into the next release of the product.

Site Modifications

Site modifications enable the prompt rectification of problems, thus returning the manufacturing process to a controlled state as early as possible. However, there are fundamental problems that must be addressed when implementing site modifications. The main issues arising from site modifications include the following:

- Traceability of the system configuration
- Availability of a compatible development and system build environment
- Testing on on-line systems
- Controlling integration of site modifications into master system software
- Impact on other functionality
- Recovery in the event of a test failure

Traceability

Site modifications must be traceable, that is, a record of all modifications implemented on a site system must be maintained by the supplier. Further, it must be possible to identify all modified files. To this end, unique references must be assigned to each site modification and a register of site modifications maintained. Appropriate change authority must be obtained for all modifications, site modifications being no exception. The site modification register must identify the change authority for each site modification. This provides traceability and ensures that the site modification is integrated into the next release of the product.

Compatible Development and System Build Environment

When developing site modifications, it is essential to ensure that the modification is implemented within an identical development environment to the site system. Archives of all site systems are, therefore, taken following each upgrade. As application configuration modifications are controlled and implemented by the customer, it is important that the latest database configuration is transferred from the site system to the development environment prior to implementing the modification.

Testing

Site modifications, as for all modifications, must be tested prior to becoming operable, preferably before installation. In some instances, however, site modifications can only be tested on the on-line system. This should be avoided wherever practically possible. However, if testing can be conducted only on the on-line system, every effort should be made to avoid testing whilst batch manufacture is in progress.

Integration into Core System Software

The integration of site modifications into the master system software must be controlled. All site modifications must be reviewed prior to integration to determine whether a direct copy of the site modification is appropriate or whether further design of a more comprehensive solution is warranted. More comprehensive solutions usually arise when the site modification comprises an intermediate solution to the problem. Following the upgrade, all site modifications must be removed from the site system.

Impact on Other Functionality

It is often difficult to assess the impact of modifications on other system functionality when implemented as a site modification. Prior to implementing any site modification, a review of the potential impact must be conducted and recorded. This activity normally forms part of the change control review. Where potential impact on other system functionality is identified, the scope of testing must be extended to include affected areas.

Controlled Recovery from Failure

It is difficult to guarantee defect-free software. Accepting that we are all human and as a result fallible, recovery plans must be put in place prior to the implementation of site modifications. Recovery plans will, as a minimum, ensure that application configuration is backed up and system software archived prior to the implementation of the modification. Further, existing files should never be overwritten by their modified counterparts, thus enabling speedy recovery in the event of a failure.

SUMMARY

I am a great advocate of a QMS that delivers a practical, yet robust, approach to system development and verification. We must always remember that it is the quality, not the quantity, of documentation that is important.

Conformance to quality standards, such as ISO 9001, does not automatically guarantee delivery of a quality system. The QMS must be continuously reviewed in order to optimise the development process and improve standards.

The Suppliers Guide for Validation of Automated Systems in Pharmaceuticals Manufacture [3] provides guidance for suppliers of systems to the pharmaceutical industry based on a life-cycle approach. The GAMP guidelines are of particular importance to those suppliers who do not currently adhere to a formal QMS.

System validation provides only the baseline by which a supplier can demonstrate conformance to specification. Ongoing maintenance can rapidly jeopardise the validated state of the system if not conducted in a controlled, documented manner.

All too often, validation documentation is filed in dusty cupboards for review by regulators during their periodic inspections. Validation documentation provides the evidence and confidence that the SCADA system has been documented and verified against the customer's specification. If validation documentation is not referenced and updated during subsequent maintenance, the SCADA system will soon become noncompliant and the validation exercise will be rendered useless.

Finally, great emphasis is placed on the special needs of the pharmaceuticals industry. It is clear why these special needs exist; however, all customers have a right to expect systems that are adequately specified, designed, implemented, and tested, regardless of the industry in which they operate. To achieve this apparently simple desire, however, customers must realise that there is an associated up-front cost with delivering quality systems, a cost that should be recovered several times over through a reduction in the number of faults detected during the operational life of the system and through more effective, efficient, controlled maintenance.

REFERENCES

1. European Union Guide to Directive 91/356/EEC (1991), *Directive Laying Down the Principles of Good Manufacturing Practice for Medicinal Products for Human Use, European Commission.*

2. U.S. Code of Federal Regulations Title 21, Part 210: *Current Good Manufacturing Practice in Manufacturing, Processing, Packaging, or Holding of Drugs (General);* Part 211: *Current Good Manufacturing Practice for Finished Pharmaceuticals,* The Office of the Federal Register National Archives and Records Administration.

3. UK GAMP Forum (1996), *Suppliers Guide for Validation of Automated Systems in Pharmaceuticals Manufacture,* Version 2, International Society of Pharmaceutical Engineers.

4. *Rules and Guidance for Pharmaceutical Manufacturers 1993,* Her Majesties Standards Office (UK).

Case Study E

Validating Distributed Control Systems

Christopher Evans
Eutech Engineering Solutions Limited
Billingham, UK

Mark Whitehouse
Yokogawa UK Limited
Runcorn, UK

The Distributed Control System (DCS) has been developed to address the automation control needs of diverse processes within a wide range of industries, including bulk chemicals, utilities, food, and pharmaceuticals. This case study is deliberately generic to allow the reader to gain an overall appreciation of the DCS validation life cycle rather than to concentrate on a specific supplier's DCS. The validation approach described is compliant with current Good Automated Manufacturing Practice (cGAMP).

DISTRIBUTED CONTROL SYSTEMS

DCS Concept

The concept of a DCS is to provide *distributed* control of a process. This is achieved by using Input/Output (I/O) modules located in the vicinity of plant equipment and operator interface equipment located in a central control room. This distributed equipment is connected by means of a system network.

DCS Usage

DCSs are used to control and monitor a variety of different processes, ranging from small batch plants with 250 I/O points to large-scale (bulk) continuous processes with 100,000 plus I/O points. Typically, they are used to provide

- PID control of analogue feedback loops
- Control of complex loops (e.g., cascade and feed-forward)
- Sequence control for startup, shutdown, or batch operations
- Software trip and interlock handling for valves, pumps, and motors
- Operator mimic displays for process monitoring and control
- Historical data storage (e.g., trending)
- Management information—process reports
- Facilities for communications with other computers (e.g., SCADA systems or PLCs)
- Alarm and event management

Core DCS

One very useful feature of the DCS is the ability to install a minimal solution to automation requirements. This minimal DCS contains the standard system "core" functionality and will provide the option of simple expansion at minimal extra cost. The core DCS will normally consist of

- Control/applications processor
- Network
- Media storage
- Operator interface
- I/O module

DCS Expansion

Following initial installation, expansion will generally mean the installation of new I/O cards or modular subsystems that are then configured within the existing core DCS. For an existing validated DCS, any changes must be assessed and any revalidation must be conducted to ensure that the existing validation status is not compromised.

PROJECT LIFE CYCLE

DCS projects should follow a repeatable life cycle to ensure a consistent, reliable, and efficient validation approach. The project life cycle also allows the supplier to demonstrate that a suitable approach has been taken to the design and testing in line with cGAMP (see Figure 1) [1].

VALIDATION PLAN (PLANNING)

The Validation Plan for a DCS project will normally be produced by the manufacturer, information relevant to the supplier in the Validation Plan should include the following:

- Scope of the validation to be performed by the supplier.
- Documentation the supplier is to provide as evidence of validation.
- References to any procedures to which the supplier must adhere. These procedures may, in some cases, override the supplier's quality procedures (e.g., change control, security practices, contingency planning, etc.).
- Résumés of supplier staff demonstrating their validation competency.

It is essential that the supplier be specifically informed, prior to the contract being awarded, what is expected by the manufacturer in terms of DCS validation. This does not necessitate the supplier being given a copy of the Validation Plan; however, this information will form the basis of the Supplier Quality Plan.

USER REQUIREMENTS SPECIFICATION (PLANNING)

A User Requirements Specification (URS) is usually produced in addition to the Validation Plan to define the operational requirements of the DCS. The supplier will design and develop the DCS and produce the associated project and validation documentation in response to the requirements set out in these documents.

The URS is normally the first document seen by the supplier in a project (usually a draft version). The final agreed-on version of the URS will be the

Figure 1. DCS Layout

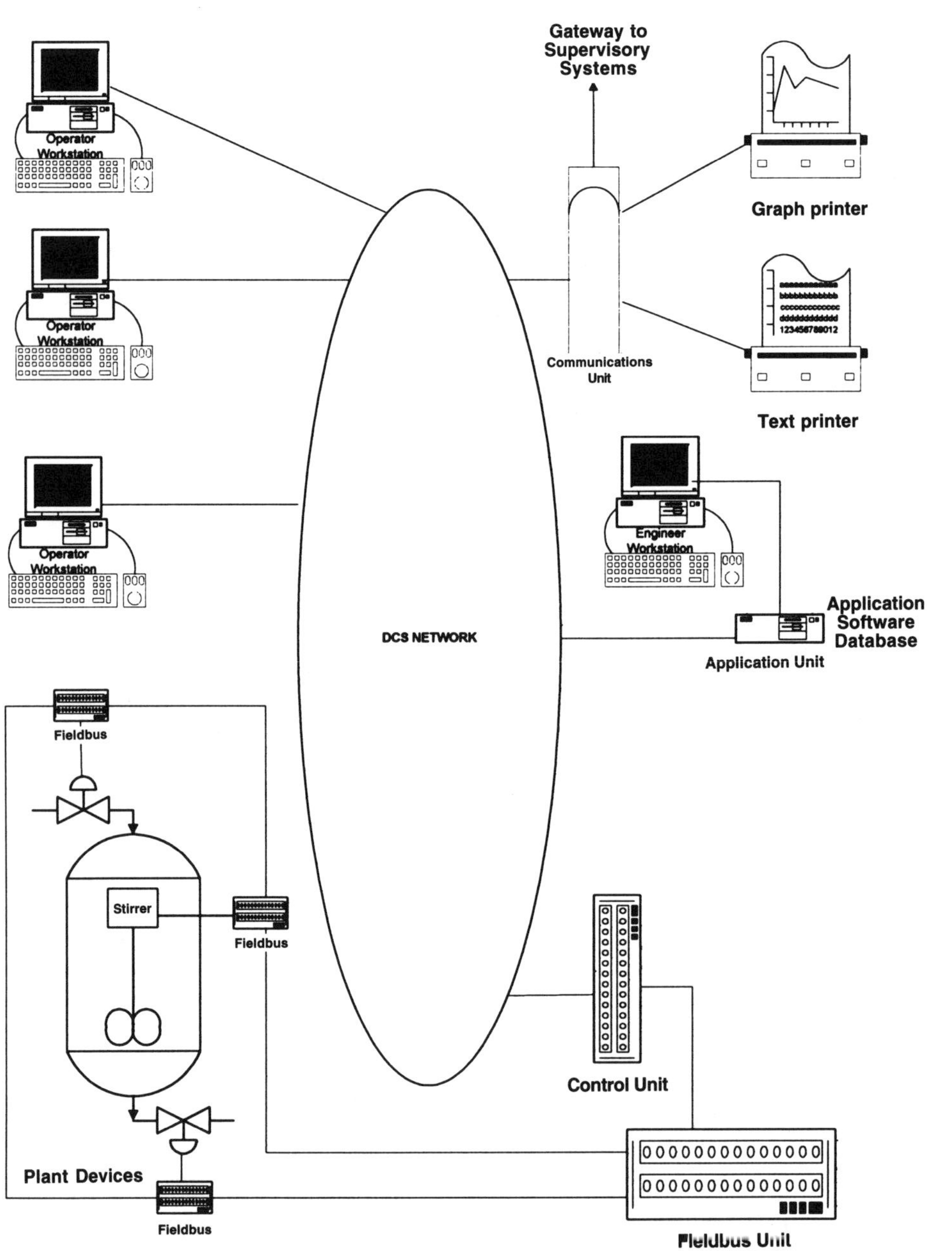

document against which the installed DCS will be ultimately validated (see Figure 2). It is essential that the manufacturer spends sufficient time in the detailed production of the URS, as a clear, well-thought URS is crucial for project success.

Project pressures on the manufacturer could lead to the design of the DCS being based on inadequately defined requirements. If more time is spent

Figure 2. DCS Validation Project Documentation

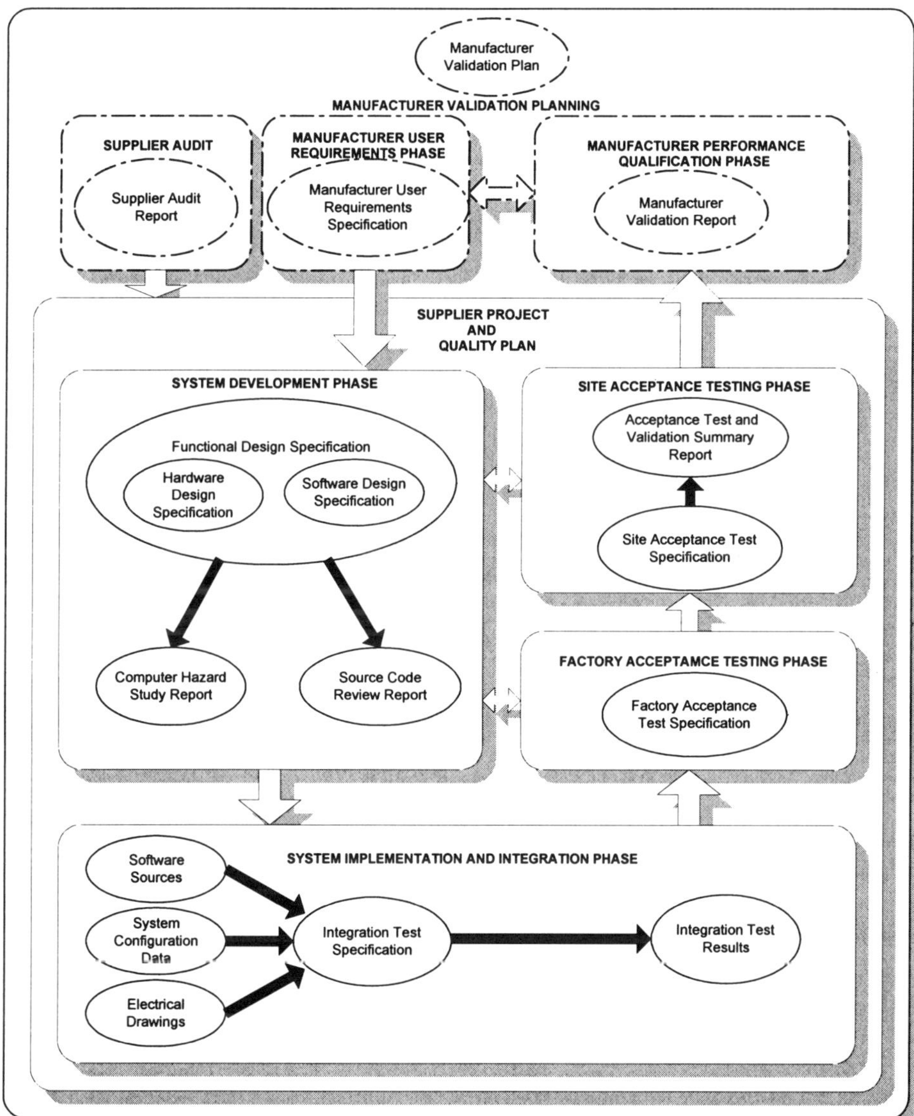

ensuring that the URS is fully detailed and fully understood prior to the beginning of design, the extra time taken will invariably be rewarded by the project pull-through.

URS Purpose

The URS is a means of converting operational requirements into a form that can be understood in DCS terms by the supplier. If this conversion is not successful or is not in sufficient detail and logically laid out, there is a high risk of project failure. The design and development of the DCS should not begin until the supplier is absolutely clear of these requirements.

The URS may take more than one form:

- *Basic URS:* Contains minimal information (e.g., I/O counts, controller counts) that will allow the manufacturer to gain a general idea of basic costs and functionality from the supplier. This is likely to be a draft version of the URS presented at the enquiry stage of the project.
- *Detailed URS:* Contains full details of the requirements of the user in non-DCS specific terminology. This level of the URS will require the supplier to discuss in detail the technical aspects of the user requirements in order to produce a suitable functional design.
- *Designer URS:* Contains full details of the user requirements in specific design terminology. This level of the URS will normally provide the supplier with details of required DCS functionality (normally in the form of flowcharts, transition diagrams, etc.). The design and development of the DCS will be directly based on this information. There is, however, still room for misunderstanding to occur, as each party will have their own understanding of what is being represented by the information.

The initial stage of the project is to rationalise the manufacturer's requirements for functionality against the cost and capabilities of the DCS. This will result in a frozen version of the URS against which the supplier will design and build the DCS.

SUPPLIER AUDIT AND SELECTION (PLANNING)

Audit Purpose

An integral part of the current best practice approach to validation is for the manufacturer to ensure that the supplier is competent to supply a validated DCS. This is achieved by subjecting the supplier to an audit by an independent experienced auditor, in accordance with ISO 10011. The audit will cover the quality attributes of the DCS, the manner in which projects are handled, and the support service available for the future maintenance of the installed DCS.

Audit Types

The audit may take two forms: the supplier may be subject to a visit by the auditor or it may be appropriate to conduct a postal audit that may or may not require a follow-up visit to the supplier's premises. The type of audit that is appropriate should be assessed on a case-by-case basis and will also include all subcontractors to be used in the project. The supplier normally runs his or her own internal quality audits to provide ongoing confirmation that the project is being conducted in line with cGAMP.

Audit Report

As a result of an audit, the supplier will receive a report from the auditor indicating which areas of the supplier's operation do not satisfy the requirements of cGAMP as appropriate to the DCS. The report will contain advice on the resolution of any deficiencies in the supplier's current operation. When the supplier is chosen for the project, part of the acceptance of the contract will be the resolution of any deficiencies highlighted in the audit report.

SUPPLIER QUALITY PLAN AND PROJECT PLAN (SYSTEM SPECIFICATION)

The production of the Supplier Project Plan and Quality Plan is the response of the supplier to the Validation Plan. The Quality Plan document will detail how the supplier will conduct the project. The Project Plan will provide details of proposed timetables and resource usage.

Quality Plan: Contents

The supplier will detail the following in the Quality Plan:

- Deliverables (documentation and electronic media)
- Procedures to be used (both supplier and manufacturer, e.g., change control, etc.)
- Tools to be used in project development (software design, project control, etc.)
- Responsibilities/roles/accountabilities
- Description of the project life cycle to be followed by the supplier

Quality Plan: Documentation as Validation Evidence

The Quality Plan will detail the written evidence of DCS development that is essential in supporting DCS validation.

- Functional Design Specification (FDS) (based on the URS)
- Hardware Design Specification (based on or included in the FDS)
- Software Design Specification (SDS) (based on or included in the FDS)
- Computer HAZard and OPerability Study (CHAZOP) (based on the FDS)
- Source Code Review and Report (based on Software Design Specification)
- Integration Test Report (report on success of integration of hardware and software)
- Factory Acceptance Test Specification (based on the contents of the FDS)
- Site Acceptance Test Specification (based on the contents of the FDS)
- End of project report (supplier response to his or her Quality Plan)

The procedures to be followed may be the supplier's own, if deemed satisfactory by the manufacturer, the manufacturer's, or a mixture of the two. The final decision regarding which procedures are to be used must lie with the manufacturer, as he is ultimately responsible for the validation of the DCS.

Project Plan: Gantt Chart

As a means of diagramatically displaying the timetables for a project and the interdependencies of tasks, it is common to provide project information on a Gantt chart (see Figure 3). The Gantt chart shows the status of the various project tasks to be performed by the supplier, and "at a glance", the current status of the project can be estimated. The number of tasks shown on a Gantt chart should be limited to allow the plan to be readable; however, it may be appropriate to produce more detailed Gantt charts for individual project phases. This Gantt chart should be produced using an automated software tool for ease of updating and held under document change control. The Gantt chart will be updated and reissued on a regular basis to ensure that the persons responsible for the project are provided with up-to-date project progress.

Figure 3. DCS Validation Project Gantt Chart

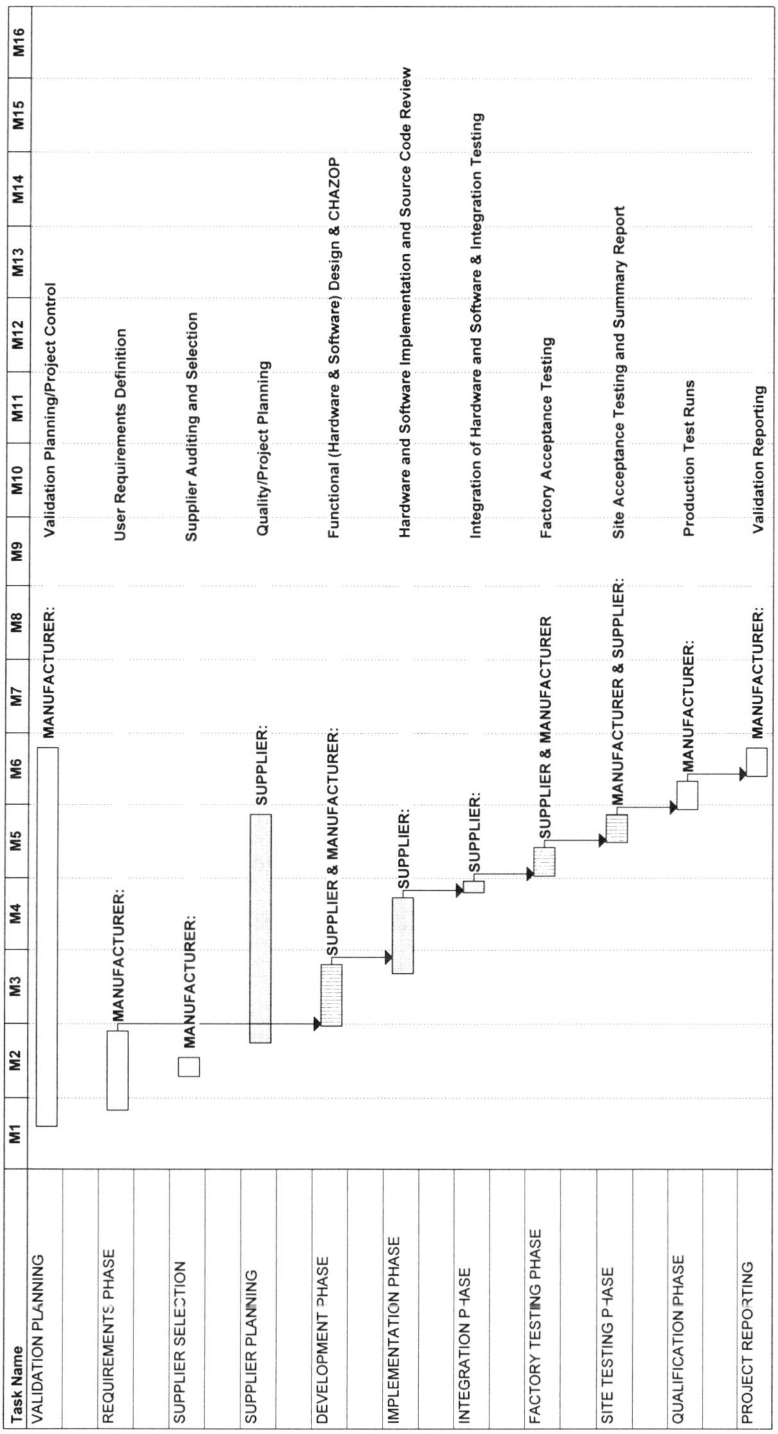

Quality Plan and Project Plan: Contract Status

The Quality Plan and Project Plan will act as the contract between the supplier and the manufacturer. Therefore, it is essential that these documents be formally agreed on at the beginning of the project and be put under documentation control. This agreement is normally demonstrated by both the manufacturer and the supplier signing the documents.

DCS DEVELOPMENT (DESIGN AND DEVELOPMENT)

The development of the DCS begins following the formal agreement of the URS by the supplier as the agreed-to user requirements for the DCS. During any DCS project, it is accepted that there may be a requirement to revise the URS. There are occasional errors and statements open to misinterpretation. It is crucial that these problems are highlighted as early as possible in the project to limit the effect they will have on the project. Any modifications required to the DCS design that were not agreed on in the final URS will normally be agreed to, with the supplier, as amendments to the FDS and associated design documentation.

Functional Design Specification

The FDS is where the supplier converts the URS into a form that may be implemented on the supplier DCS. The typical contents are as follows:

- Introduction—author, purpose, contractual status of document
- Overview—key benefits and high-level description of system
- Functions—description of objective, performance, safety/security of individual functions
- Data—definition, access method, capacity, and retention time for data
- Interfaces—with users, other systems (e.g., PLC/SCADA systems and plant equipment)
- Nonfunctional attributes—availability and maintenance information
- Glossary—terms that may be unfamiliar to the reader
- Appendices—other supporting information, hardware/software design (for small systems)

Where the implementation will only require standard hardware and software supplied by the supplier, there may be no requirement for detailed documents for hardware and software design. In this case, the Source Code Review and software implementation will be based directly on the details held within the FDS. As part of the design process, the operability of the computer system software and failure modes of the hardware and software must be assessed. This is often performed as a separate study, with the results of the study influencing the hardware and software design.

Software Design Specification

Where there is a requirement for bespoke software or complex software configuration, it may be appropriate to detail the software in a SDS. This specification will normally take the form of a text description and some form of pictorial (e.g., Yourdon, Grafset, flowcharts, etc.) representation of the software. This document will act as the basis for the software Source Code Review and software module testing. The typical contents are as follows:

- Introduction—author, purpose, relationship to other documents
- Overview—high-level description of system and system diagram
- System description—description of individual system modules, external interfaces
- System data—database, file structure definitions
- Module description—operation, interfaces, timing, error/data handling for each module
- Module data—which system data is accessed by each module
- Glossary—terms that may be unfamiliar to the reader

Hardware Design Specification

Hardware design documentation will be produced to show wiring layouts, terminals, general arrangements, and so on. This document will act as the "as-built" documentation for the future maintenance of the DCS and will form the basis for hardware inspections for Factory Acceptance Testing. The typical contents are as follows:

- Introduction—author, purpose, relationship to other documents
- Overview—high-level description of hardware and interfaces, hardware system diagram
- Computer system
- Main computer—CPU, memory, bus, clock description
- Storage—disks, tapes, backups, and capacity

- Peripherals—printers, displays, keyboards, and housing/mounting details
- Interconnections—cable/network/connector specifications and screening
- Input/output—digital and analogue I/O circuitry: accuracy, isolation, range, timing
- Environment—temperature, humidity, external interface, physical security, electrical interference
- Electrical supplies—filtering, loading, earthing, uninterruptible power supply
- Glossary—terms that may be unfamiliar to the reader

DCS IMPLEMENTATION AND INTEGRATION (SYSTEM BUILD)

During the implementation and integration phase of the project, the supplier will construct the hardware and generate the software to create a complete DCS. Hardware and software implementation are generally performed as parallel tasks, with the software being developed on Personal Computers (PCs) using appropriate supplier software. This means that the software implementation in line with the Software Design Specification can begin independently of the state of the hardware design.

Hardware Implementation

The hardware implementation for a DCS should be quite straightforward. The DCS will be made up of a standard set of interconnecting parts, designed and manufactured specifically for the supplier, which plug together in the designed configuration. The DCS hardware will typically consist of the following:

- *System cabinet:* Central processor cards, application processor cards, and power supply cards
- *I/O cabinets:* For communication with plant instrumentation and devices, a set of I/O cabinets will be located separately from the system cabinet (usually in the plant rack room) containing analogue I/O, digital I/O, pulse inputs, relays, and power supplies. The cabinets are normally of standard 19-inch rack mounting construction interconnected with the system cabinet via DCS network cabling.
- *Peripherals:* The operator interface for the DCS will be via peripherals that normally consist of screen/mouse/keyboard units, printers, and annunciator panels. The engineer's interface, used for

development/configuration, consists of a screen/mouse/keyboard and printer.

- *Panels and consoles:* The parts of the hardware that may not be provided directly by the supplier are panels and console housings; these items will be purchased from an approved local subcontractor.

Software Implementation

Software implementation may be made up of a number of areas, depending on the complexity and availability of features on the DCS that will require appropriate testing to demonstrate acceptability (see Figure 4).

Operating System

The operating system requires no special implementation; it will be loaded directly onto the DCS hardware during the integration phase.

DCS Configuration

The configuration of the DCS covers a number of areas, all of which may be processed on a separate machine to the DCS. It is normal to use a PC to perform this work.

- Database implementation
- Software loop implementation
- Standard software package implementation (e.g., historical database, standard logs)
- Display creation
- Message implementation

Bespoke Software

Where there is a requirement for bespoke software to be provided as a supplement to the supplier standard DCS, this will normally be developed in a high-level language. In some cases, the supplier will provide a software shell within which the manufacturer can implement software functionality using standard building blocks or lines of code. In both of these cases, there is a need to ensure that the design of the software and the manner in which it has been implemented is in line with Good Programming Practice. For validation, this is often achieved via the use of a Source Code Review.

Source Code Review

To ensure that any bespoke software used in the DCS is written in line with Good Programming Practice, it is useful to perform a Source Code Review on

Figure 4. DCS Software Testing

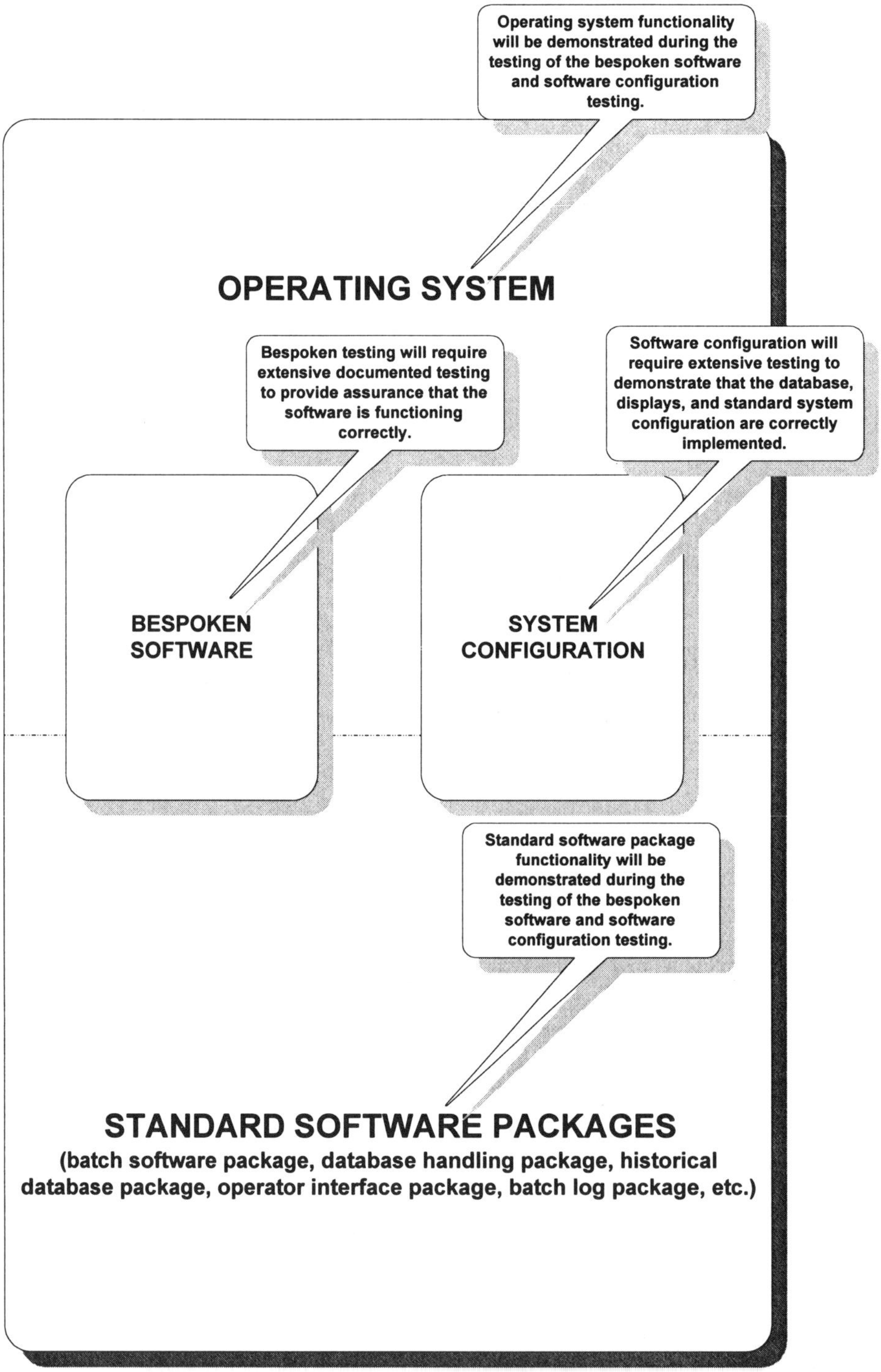

a representative sample of the supplier software. The amount of software inspected will be assessed on a case-by-case basis and is based on the experience of the assessor. In the event that serious errors are found during the course of the Source Code Review, a more detailed assessment of the code may prove to be appropriate. The software should be compared to the supplier procedure for programming and the software design documentation. A Source Code Review report will be produced as part of this review, detailing any exceptions found and recommendations for actions to resolve the exceptions.

Computer System Hazard and Operability Study

In order to assess the threats and hazards that are associated with the use of a DCS as a solution to an automation requirement, there should be a hazard study of the proposed computer system hardware and software. This CHAZOP study should cover failure modes, reliability, computer system operation, and so on.

Hardware and Software Integration

Following the construction of the hardware, the integration process may commence. This will begin with the implementation of the operating system and standard software product to create the base DCS. Where validation projects are concerned, it is essential that the hardware implemented at this stage is the same as that which will ultimately be installed on the manufacturer's site (i.e., the target system).

Basic Integration Testing

The base DCS will be subject to a series of diagnostic tests that will test the hardware and all interconnections between the component parts of the DCS. This testing will also demonstrate that the DCS operating system and standard software have been implemented correctly. During the testing of the base DCS, records of test success and failure should be recorded as evidence in the supplier integration test specification. The Integration Test specification should be a standard document used by the supplier as an initial check of the basic system. Any failures in the testing must then be rectified, and appropriate retesting must be performed. When testing is successfully completed, the supplier may then move on to integrate the configured part of the DCS and any bespoke software.

Configuration and Bespoke Software Testing

It may be appropriate that Integration Testing follows a similar line of inspection and testing to be used in Factory Acceptance Testing (FAT). When testing is performed on the configured software, this is normally a laborious check that the database and displays are fully implemented in line with the design documentation. Appropriate test harnesses (simulation software) may be produced to test the bespoke software if it is not possible to demonstrate correct functionality via simpler methods. The use of test harnesses should, however, be avoided whenever possible as, in effect, the simulation software will require to be validated before it may be used and also maintained with the running system in case of system modification.

Integration Testing Completion

The end of the integration phase will be the acceptance by the supplier's internal quality system that the DCS is fit for customer inspection and testing; this will be supported by the supplier's Integration Test results. It should be noted that the time spent by the supplier in ensuring that DCS functionality is correct at this stage will increase the likelihood of successful Factory Acceptance Testing.

FACTORY ACCEPTANCE TESTING (PREDELIVERY TESTING)

The testing performed by the supplier in the presence of the manufacturer or its representative is normally called FAT. The document used by the supplier for this phase is the Factory Acceptance Test Specification.

Factory Acceptance Test Specification

In order to provide documentary evidence of comprehensive DCS testing, the supplier will produce a Factory Acceptance Test Specification, based on the design documentation. It is accepted that there may be tests that cannot be performed in this phase due to the lack of external plant hardware; these tests will be agreed on with the manufacturer and will become part of the Site Acceptance Test Specification.

Each test should specifically relate to a design document—this should not be an opportunity for allowing ad hoc tests, such as "cycle computer power and see what happens". The results of all tests should be predictable and repeatable based on previous design work.

Due to the time required to produce a suitable Factory Acceptance Test Specification, the supplier should begin the production of this document as early as possible in a DCS project, although this cannot start in earnest until all design documentation is complete.

FAT should cover the following areas:

- *Hardware inspection* will concentrate on demonstrating that the installation is correct as per the hardware design. This testing will take the form of inspections of the physical hardware (i.e., peripherals, computers, wiring, terminations, earthing connections, cabinets, and consoles that are to be installed on the manufacturer's site.

- *System and standard software inspection* will cover the inspection of the standard software packages to be installed on the DCS (i.e., operating system, batch software, database handling, historical database, operator interface, reporting, communications). Unique descriptors and version numbers of the software packages will then be recorded as evidence.
- *Operating system and standard software testing:* It is not practical to comprehensively test this software, as it is far too complex. The correct functionality of this software is demonstrated, in effect, by testing of the configuration and bespoke software. This approach to testing is acceptable provided that overall functionality testing is comprehensive and that the system software has had a considerable amount of usage on existing systems.
- *Software configuration testing* will concentrate on demonstrating that the standard software and operating system on the DCS has been correctly configured. This testing will include database to I/O point-to-point testing, database to screen displays point-to-point testing, timers, messages, historical database points, display configuration, internal variables, and printouts.
- *Bespoke software testing:* The testing of bespoke software will be project specific, as this software is by definition providing a specific functionality that is not available in the standard system software. With bespoke software, the testing must ensure that there is a full test of functionality, including normal program flow, interface with database, links with other systems, complex control loops, correct error handling, links to human interface (printouts, alarm handling, displays, keyboards, etc.), trips and interlocks, and special calculations.

Factory Acceptance Test Results

As each agreed-on test is performed, the tester and an independent witness will be responsible for assessing whether or not the result meets the specified acceptance criteria. This decision should, whenever possible, be backed up by documentary evidence supplied by the DCS (e.g., printouts and screen dumps). In the case of failure, it may be deemed by the tester and witness that there was an error in the test sheet, or misinterpretation of the functionality of the DCS by the test sheet author, in which case the test may be rerun and comments written on the results sheet by the tester. The dated signatures of the tester and witness on the test sheet will then close out the test.

At the end of FAT, the supplier will have generated a set of test sheets containing details of the success or failure of the tests performed. For any tests that have failed, a retest must be performed, following the correction of the reason for the failure, or acceptance of the failed test must be justified. It is important to perform a thorough review before any retesting to identify any previously successful tests that may be affected by subsequent corrections. In the worst case, it may be necessary to rerun all tests.

SITE ACCEPTANCE TESTING (ON-SITE TESTING)

Prior to the commencement of the Site Acceptance Testing phase of the project, the DCS hardware and software will be transported to site and installed. This activity is normally the responsibility of the supplier and the installation contractor. Following the installation of the DCS, the supplier will expect to have only a small amount of involvement in on-site testing. Most of the site inspection work for the purpose of validation is associated with environment and loop testing (i.e., 100 percent point-to-point checks for continuity) performed by the manufacturer. Following this installation, a percentage of the tests performed in FAT will be repeated—a figure of 10 percent is often used—and also any tests that could not be performed during FAT. This testing will usually be performed by the manufacturers with assistance from the supplier.

SUPPLIER END-OF-PROJECT REPORT (REPORTING)

In order to complete the DCS project life cycle, the supplier should produce an end-of-project report. The report will contain reference to all validation documentation produced and detail the status of all activities performed by the supplier in support of validation (e.g., Source Code Review, Integration Tests, Factory/Site Acceptance Test). Any exceptions to the testing process will be highlighted in the report for action by the manufacturer. This report will provide the manufacturer with a valuable reference for the production of his Validation Report.

PERFORMANCE QUALIFICATION (ON-SITE TESTING)

Following Site Acceptance Testing, the manufacturer will perform a number of trial batch runs to confirm that the DCS and associated plant can consistently produce product within specification. This phase is normally conducted without the direct involvement of the supplier.

VALIDATION REPORT (REPORTING)

The manufacturer will complete the validation life cycle by producing a Validation Report. The Validation Report will cover all aspects of plant validation and will detail the actions taken to clear any issues raised in the supplier end-of-project report associated with the DCS.

MAINTENANCE PHASE (ONGOING VALIDATION)

Following the satisfactory completion of the initial validation process, the manufacturer will enter the maintenance phase for the DCS. The manufacturer will now be required to monitor any modifications to the DCS (e.g., upgrades to operating system, application software modifications, replacement of faulty hardware) and determine if it has compromised the existing system validation. If this is the case, supplementary documentary evidence must be generated to revalidate the part of the system affected by the modification.

RETROSPECTIVE VALIDATION

For each nonvalidated DCS used for pharmaceutical production, the manufacturer will need to consider the cGAMP validation requirements. Where adequate documentary evidence for the installation and operation of the DCS is not available, the manufacturer will be required to arrange for retrospective validation on the system. Retrospective validation will take a similar form as for the above described prospective DCS validation, except that there may already be documentation available. The system is, of course, already designed and, therefore, original design documentation and evidence from DCS operation may be used as evidence in the validation process.

REFERENCES

1. UK GAMP Forum (1995), *Validation of Automation Systems in Pharmaceutical Manufacture,* Second Draft United Kingdom Pharmaceutical Industry Computer Systems Validation Forum.
2. Wingate, G.A.S. and Evans, C. (1995), *Computer Systems Validation: Hitting the Mark.* Computer and Process Validation '95, 24–25 April, Manchester Conference Centre, England.

Case Study F

Validating Manufacturing Execution Systems

Martin Smith
Zeneca Pharma France
Reims, France

A Manufacturing Execution System (MES) enables real-time monitoring and control of production processes. It effectively networks systems together, so it must be able to pass data from often widely different operating environments. This aspect brings a range of challenges for validation.

The MES system used in this case study is a pharmaceutical plant manufacturing granular product for compression into tablets. The system is shown in schematic form in Figure 1.

There is a supervisory computer connected via an industry standard interface to six Programmable Logic Controllers (PLCs), each controlling a process package, for example, a dryer or a mixer. The flow of the process is from left to right across the diagram.

The six PLCs are linked to a data concentrator that acts as the interface between the network and the supervisory computer. It acts as a master controller on the network. The data concentrator manages the network, polling each PLC in turn on a cyclical basis. This reduces the risk of "data overload"

Figure 1. Tablet Granulation Plant—Computer-Based Systems

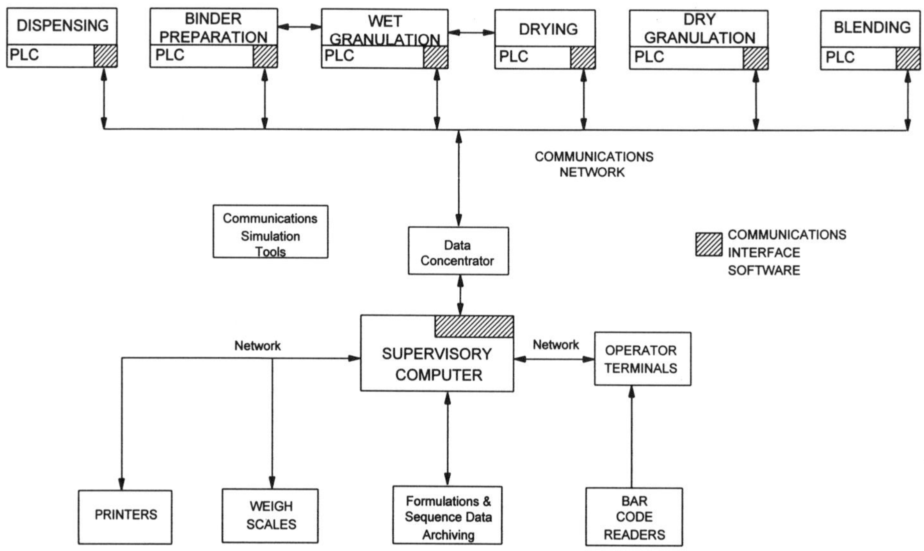

that might occur if all the PLCs were to communicate to the supervisory computer directly.

The communications between the supervisory computer and the data concentrator are via a standard serial communication link. Product formulation and sequence data are held on a separate system that transfers data to the supervisory computer to create an empty batch record.

At the end of the production of a batch of granules, the supervisory computer can generate a complete "hard copy" batch record. This comprises data collected from the PLC systems during the production process that have been transmitted through the communications network. Archiving of the batch record back to the formulations and sequence storage system completes the process.

The purpose of the system is to

- Manage the creation of batch records of pharmaceutical product using predefined formulations and sequences.
- Report events on a batch log.
- Control sequence of operation and manage starting and stopping of process equipment.

PLANNING

Much thought must be given to the kind of integrated system desired. A number of questions must be asked that must be based on the functionality required:

- What are the needs of the system?
- Has it been done before?
- How complex does it need to be?
- What expansion possibilities do there need to be?

The emphasis should be on providing a system as simple as possible, as the problem of control rises exponentially as complexity increases. Focussing on the needs of a system rather than on the "nice to haves" will tend to produce a better controlled and robust solution. The system that promises all but delivers less than needed will not be welcomed in any factory.

The overall project planning must integrate all the tasks involved with the definition and control of an MES and its validation. The person responsible for this should be part of the project team and play an active part.

There is a necessity for a coherent, well-integrated overview plan that considers the validation of each piece of equipment separately as well as focussing on the interfaces, especially the common data that pass between systems. By careful scoping, a good definition of what is included (and excluded) should be part of the plan with justification.

The use of diagrams to explain this clearly is very useful, and it should be possible to draw boxes to define the limits of each Validation Plan that divide up the whole task into manageable pieces. There should be no gaps between systems. Examine what crosses the interface between Validation Plans and make sure each references all the other Validation Plans that butt up against it.

Think about how the build will take place. Is all equipment to be installed together? Probably not, as delivery times will vary between suppliers and the physical constraints of equipment installation prevent the construction of communications at the same time as everything else. Because of this, consideration should be given to the testing of the interfaces if the adjoining systems are not there.

The easiest way is to develop test software is to simulate the interface of other systems. If they cannot be simulated in any way, it may be essential to plan to install together or have an irate supplier who has not been paid because another is late. Considering this at the precontract stage and weighing the alternatives may save expensive rethinking later. Ask questions like the following:

- Who will define the test software?
- What will it simulate (which protocols will be used)?
- What data will be used?
- How to validate (specification, design, test, control)?

The common data to be transferred between the systems are the basis of the communication and must be carefully defined in terms of

- What data?
- When will it be transferred?
- Acceptable ranges of data and any thresholds for transfer.

All of this information will very much determine the size and type of hardware and software needed, and the evaluation of this is best done prior to the sanction of capital. This information must be shared between suppliers in order to adopt

- A standard format for the common data
- One make of PLC for all process equipment

The standardisation of one manufacturer will reduce the complexity of support later, even though a premium may need to be paid for a particular brand of PLC with some suppliers. "Standard" supplier software may need to be modified to install the same interface in all machines, but the effort spent in this area will provide paybacks in ease of maintenance long after the project is completed.

In the case study considered, there were also some simple handshake communications between process equipment to enable the transfer of product automatically between machines. This also needs to be defined with the suppliers concerned. Responsibilities and roles within and outside the company also need to be part of the plan that benefits from wide circulation in spite of it being a basically internal document.

As part of the wider planning with other activities, a handover from phase to phase must be planned. This does not have to be a drawn out affair, but it allows all those involved to appreciate and accept all the problems that can pass between one phase and another.

Typical phases are those of the different stages of test in

- Precommissioning
- Commissioning
- Computer validation
- Process validation
- Production

There must be an evaluation of the willingness of suppliers to cooperate in what in simple terms is a collaborative affair for an MES. Because problems can occur in one system as a result of problems in another, intersupplier relationships must be discussed and developed in order to solve these problems when they occur in an efficient and amicable manner. Supplier Audits used as part of negotiating information prior to order placement are useful to assess the capability of suppliers to cooperate as well as their ability to control what they do.

The use of the Good Automated Manufacturing Practice (GAMP) standards in discussions is valuable as a baseline from which to work, as a manufacturer may not have a framework of procedures for documentation; a common approach with all suppliers will be less confusing for future change and support.

The use of Quality Plans is valuable to prompt suppliers to plan documentation delivery and standards for their systems. Ensure there is enough time to do two to three reviews of documents, and do not forget to include a "turn round" time for correcting and resubmitting amended documentation. Although it is possible to manage incomplete late documentation and still keep control, the best solution is not to have the problem in the first place.

Depending on the organisation, the use of an engineering contractor is fairly common on a large project. As well as the more traditional skills of project management and civil and mechanical construction, contractors could be involved in the validation process. There are a number of risks and benefits:

- Suitable (specialist) skills are required.
- They can bring expertise not on the project team.
- Do they understand computer validation?
- Do they understand company standards?
- What is their role exactly?
- How is documentation to be managed?

Stage payments based on the receipt of acceptable documentation as well as system delivery is a good idea to reinforce the importance of timely documentation delivery. This will be more critical on an integrated plant, such as an MES. Being specific on documentation requirements will enable the project documentation to fit into existing site documentation systems after the project is complete. The definition of standards where possible will help this.

Factory testing is an important stage for a piece of stand-alone equipment; for networked equipment it is only as good as the quality of the test tool that simulates the interfaces with other equipment. Include this issue in the planning and discussions with suppliers.

There is no accident that this section is one of the biggest in this case study as it is important to emphasise that MESs, more than other systems, require significant amounts of planning and forethought to work on time, on budget, and in control.

SYSTEM SPECIFICATION

A User Requirement Specification (URS) covering the integrated MES at a plant level is very valuable in the early stages of a project to help define with the project team exactly what is needed. For an integrated system like an MES, it is useful to have this high level of definition to test against when all is connected. The detail at this very high level should be limited to the key interactions proving that all can work together. Lower levels of the URS and functional definition follow just as for an individual system.

Functional Specifications for each piece of equipment and the communications are essential. The definition of the common information that passes between systems is useful to include in each equipment specification that interfaces so the integration can be checked on paper at least. Do not forget ancillary software, such as operator panels, that have mimic software or message displays. In the case study used, all the PLCs were the same, but the message displays and operator consoles were as the supplier chose to supply. However, all this needs to be defined somewhere and controlled. A detailed definition of interfaces will minimise the possibility of errors later.

Simulation software should be specified like any other code and managed using a Validation Plan. It could form part of the communications validation as it is related. This area should be defined relatively early in the project to enable each of the equipment suppliers to use the information in their documents for the interfaces.

DESIGN AND DEVELOPMENT

A formal assessment of the threats specific to an MES together with associated controls is useful to address the special features of this kind of system before this phase begins. Issues to consider include the following:

- Loss of communications
- Timing of data transfer
- Power up problems of equipment and communication
- Range checking of data passing between systems
- Operation of the plant if the system fails

For an MES, the interface software at either end of communications network, as well as the data concentrator, are elements that must be designed and tested earlier than the other equipment. The related simulation software to be used to test the individual process equipment code also must be done earlier so it can be used in the development stage of the process equipment code.

The Source Code Review is an important stage to assess the quality of the interface code between systems as well as its more normal use of

- Checking code structure
- A detailed examination of critical areas of the code
- Checking the quality of the design documentation

The amount of design documentation to expect for a given system is difficult to define because of the possible wide range of systems involved in an MES. For a piece of process equipment as in this case study, equipment software is based on existing code and designs that are perhaps 10 years old, and the quality of documentation of that code will be very variable between suppliers. Although it is something that must be managed system by system, this issue is worth discussing at the Supplier Audit so consideration can be given to the potential problems that may arise.

BUILD

The build phase can proceed for the separate pieces of equipment as if they were stand-alone. The earlier planning and definition stages should have considered the integration issues peculiar to an MES. Progress meetings are useful, especially when dealing with an unknown supplier. It will be much easier to correct problems in the early stages, and there will be much more resistance later as the cost and control problems of change increase.

PREDELIVERY TESTING

Different views related to Predelivery Testing can be taken:

- Test formally at the equipment suppliers and then take a copy of code after testing, doing random or "critical" sample retesting on-site, loading the version taken after supplier site Factory Acceptance Testing (FAT).
- Test informally at suppliers to give confidence, leaving formal testing until later.

There are risks and benefits for each option, but experience shows it is often very difficult to have confidence in factory testing unless the machine really is self-contained. Certainly, the FAT must include the test of the communications interface software using the simulation tool. As with other problems, the earlier in the process they can be discovered, the cheaper they are to fix. Version control of software is good to start in FAT to ensure that a good level of control is maintained for any modifications needed.

ACCEPTANCE TESTING

Acceptance Testing is one of the most important levels of testing and must be carefully controlled. For an MES, it has the the added complexity of interfacing systems. As with stand-alone systems, documentation approvals are important to complete before testing starts.

Both static and dynamic testing is useful to build confidence. A formal static comparison of computer-generated data from interfacing systems is a valuable double-check to ensure suppliers have defined exactly what is required before carrying out dynamic interface checking as part of Acceptance Testing.

Because of the likelihood of having systems commissioned at different times, the communications simulation software tool is very important to use as early as possible to build confidence in the correctness of the communications code. Similarly, the communications system itself should be testable without having the live system attached, requiring a simulator both ways.

A strategy of layered testing to build confidence is very valuable, ranging from simulating communications on individual equipment to connecting the live equipment together. The use of formal test specifications, results recording, and reviews at each stage will give a structured approach and assist in the tracing of problems later. This could also be shown to a regulatory inspector, if required, to demonstrate the process followed.

It is possible to approve documents with documented reservations for inclusion later, providing that the missing information is considered during testing and subsequent review. There will inevitably be small amendments to make on the documentation as testing progresses, and the technique of marking up document copies as errors are noticed makes later changes easy. The working copies can be reviewed at the end of testing and used to update documentation under change control.

Keeping close to testing to ensure standards are maintained is essential in the early stages. One or more training sessions are useful to define expectations to the test teams. This should include examples of form completion using test problems.

Formal results reviews should accompany each stage of testing including action lists where needed. Doing this immediately after testing captures all of the issues, as some may not be as well documented as perhaps they should have been. Added tests should be evaluated and their value determined. The review does not have to be a long process, but needs to capture issues and the state of completion. This gives confidence to hand over to the next stage as well as maintaining a documented and, therefore, traceable level of control. Being realistic on testing times is beneficial for everyone concerned. Working all hours is not effective as things can be missed and control lost.

REPORTING

At the end of the process, the Validation Reports provide a summary of all that took place. It is valuable to obtain approval for this as early as possible so the organisation can acknowledge the state of validation and progress into the ongoing evaluation phase of the life cycle. Often, there are minor issues that can be outstanding for a period of time after all of the main activities have been completed. Seeking a provisional or interim approval of the validation plan clearly defining the outstanding minor actions achieves the acceptance of the organisation to validation and also indicates the things left to do. By defining a date for the completion of outstanding actions in the document, a time limit is defined for final approval.

The levels of the Validation Report should match exactly with the Validation Plans created. The Validation Master Report written against the Validation Master Plan is the highest level and should confirm the philosophy followed during the project or define with justification any deviations from it.

Including tables of metrics in Validation Reports can give a clear and quantitive summary of what happened. Examples of useful metrics are as follows:

- Change requests—up until end of acceptance phase
- Review actions from stages of test and software review
- Testing—how many tests, how long, number failed, passed, and so on

The amount of detail to include will vary, but as for the highest level of the Validation Report, there should be a summary of activities and a highlighting and justification of any deviations from the plan. At the end of each Validation Report, there is a need for a statement to say that the system is validated.

OTHER ISSUES

Ongoing Validation

Because of the interaction between systems in an MES, the aspects of interface and impact of change on communicating systems must be considered in the change control system adopted. Communications, being a separate "system" without a user interface, is not likely to change its functionality unless interfacing equipment changes. Therefore, it must be included in any evaluation of change between systems. The ownership of communications is decided perhaps arbitrarily, as it is connected to all equipment, but probably best rests with the ownership of the supervisory system. Using a comprehensive checklist to support change requests will help the evaluation process consider system interfaces.

Management of Problems

The tracing of problems in an integrated system can be especially difficult and requires a higher level of knowledge to solve than stand-alone systems. It is very easy for a supplier to blame another supplier's machine for a problem occurring on linked systems. Unfortunately, the MES plant manager is left with the problem if both suppliers cannot resolve their differences on where the problem is. Maintaining good supplier relationships can be difficult in these situations, and there really is no substitute for maintaining several highly trained individuals to solve problems. This is one of the disadvantages of this kind of system. It is important not to forget that the training itself must be validated.

Security

There are issues of security for each of the PLC systems and the supervisory system where direct user access to create, modify, or delete data must be controlled by the use of a password or some other kind of protection. The communications network may or may not have similar access routes. In the case study concerned, access to communications software was only via specialist interface units that were removed and stored in the maintenance section. Use of these units is limited by procedure to qualified technicians.

Introduction of New Products

It is probably best to develop another Validation Plan to coordinate the changes needed for new product introduction, as potentially the whole MES could be affected with the need to alter common data passing between systems.

Retrospective Validation

As with other systems, the quality of retrospective validation depends on the amount of information on the system already existing from the original design and commissioning. It is, therefore, difficult to give advice, but a number of issues would benefit from some thought:

- Use of simulation software
- Documented evidence of successful operation and records of faults
- Level of interest and expertise existing in supplier companies of the equipment supplied

The planning of test programmes will be a sensitive issue for existing MESs, as a large number of networked systems may be involved, leading to extensive and costly downtime.

Supplier Audits

Supplier Audits can give valuable information in the early evaluation stages of a project on how manufacturers manage their work. By visiting and formally assessing suppliers, it is much easier to assess the level of control they have and the way quality is viewed in the organisation. Even if there is little choice in the selection of suppliers, this information can be used to help them raise their standards to a more acceptable level.

Working in Several Languages

Language poses a number of problems that can be made more complex with an integrated system. Agreeing on one language for all key documentation, especially for communications, is important to avoid the confusion of misinterpretations in translations. System messages should, of course, be in the native language of the client country. Unfortunately, this is not always completely possible, as some operating system messages are not language configurable. Documents are best produced in one language and approved as master copies, then translations approved into other local languages if needed. This can be costly and should only be done where necessary, for example, documentation used by the maintenance personnel.

Copying Plants

Doing it all again is not as simple as it may seem, even if the installation is on a green field site the same as the original. Advantages are easy to appreciate as one change can be applied to other plants without revalidation if they are *truly* identical. Perhaps country differences on standards will make differences. Certainly there may be organisational differences and preferences. Great care is needed to avoid complete revalidation and, therefore, loss of potential advantages. Keeping plants identical, even if built the same, requires the commitment of often disparate management teams to do so. It only takes one organisation to decide that they do not wish to implement the changes of the sister plant to lead to a divergence of the plants. The most pragmatic solution is to maintain ties between the plants to manage the differences that are likely to occur over time, keeping the same functionality, if not the detailed design.

CONCLUSION

The process of validating an MES requires a level of overview focussing on the interactions between equipment that makes it unique from most other validation exercises. Because of this, emphasis must be placed on early and detailed planning. This should include the consideration of the following:

- Validation planning—levels and grouping of plans
- Definition of communications protocols
- Agreement of shared data
- Supplier relationships
- Simulation testing of interfaces—development of test software
- Integrated approach to definition and test considering interfaces

Given that these points are fully explored, the route to validation and successful, well-managed operation can be achieved in a timely and cost-effective way.

SUGGESTED READING

1. U.S. Code of Federal Regulations Title 21, Part 211 (last amended 1995), *Current Good Manufacturing Practice for Finished Pharmaceuticals.*
2. FDA (1983), *Guide to Inspection of Computerised Systems in Drug Processing,* Technical Report, Reference Materials and Training Aids for Inverstigators, Rockville, MD: Food and Drug Administration.
3. European Union Guide to Directive 91/356/EEC (1993), *European Commission Directive Laying Down the Principles of Good Manufacturing Practice for Medicinal Products for Human Use,* Annex 11.
4. UK GAMP Forum (1996), *Supplier Guide for Validation of Automated Systems in Pharmaceutical Manufacture,* Second Draft, The Hague, Netherlands: International Society for Pharmaceutical Engineering.

Case Study G

Validating an Electronic Batch Recording System

Peter Bosshard, Thomas Hefti, and Hans O. Sucker
Hoffmann-La Roche
Basel, Switzerland

The pharmaceutical industry is obliged to document carefully every single step in the drug manufacturing process. This is one of the mandatory activities in order to ensure that a drug is safe for use. An Electronic Batch Recording System (EBRS) allows efficient documenting, making good use of the possibilities offered by today's Information Technology (IT). The following case study gives an insight into the business needs leading to the introduction of an EBRS. Furthermore, it describes the system and the realization concept, the system specification, and the approach used for computer system validation (CSV).

HISTORY

In 1992, the decision was taken to introduce an EBRS in the galenical production of the pharmaceuticals division of F. Hoffmann-La Roche Ltd. in

Basel, Switzerland. The project was launched as "PK System," in August 1994. By mid 1996, a major part of the system was in operation and working as intended.

BUSINESS NEEDS

The functions of the planned computer system had to satisfy the current requirements of Good Manufacturing Practices (GMP). Regulations, such as the GMPs in the European Union (EC GMP) or the Code of Federal Regulations (CFR) by the U.S. health authorities, require the recording of batch-specific information during the production stages (EC GMP 4.17 [1] and 21 CFR 211.188 [2]). These records must be properly reviewed before the batch is released for further processing (e.g., packaging [21 CFR 21 211.192 {2}]). At the point of decision, the galenical production process, from active ingredient to the galenical dosage form, led to 4,000–5,000 batch records per year, consisting, on average, of 10 pages each. These records were reviewed manually by the responsible pharmacists, the plant supervisor, and other pharmacists.

PROJECT OBJECTIVES

The main objective of the project "PK System" was to develop a computer-aided batch recording system. This system should deliver the benefits described below.

Time Savings

- Batch record review is performed immediately, not delaying the following production steps (e.g., packaging).
- The review process of the electronic batch records becomes much easier, with all data available in an orderly and structured form.
- Deviations (if any) are easier to analyse if they are all listed automatically by the computer.
- Recording the entire process and control data allows the easy performance of investigations for failure analysis and production optimisation.
- Batch records can easily be sent by electronic mail, provided that this function is validated and secure (no changes possible to the record). This is important in case product batches are exported to other countries.

Improvement of Process Control

- The completion of every production step, the corresponding results, and procedure parameters can be checked immediately.
- The sequence of the production steps can be defined by the EBRS, thus managing the manufacturing process (if necessary).
- The state of the production equipment is controlled. This means, for example, that a production vessel can be used only if it is clean, and a balance can be used only if it is calibrated.
- The successful process validation or preventive maintenance is monitored.

Improvement of Security

- Boundary checking of process parameters is performed automatically. This means that whenever manufacturing data are outside the specified limits (alert and in-process control), the application reports this deviation (on screen or by electronic mail). This increases the certainty that any irregularities are detected properly. Thus, it gives management the possibility for immediate reaction, so that timely and cost-saving corrective actions can be taken.
- The automatic data capture of the relevant process reduces input errors.
- Every batch record must be accessible at least for the shelf life of the drug (21 CFR 211.198 [2]). The introduction of the new system gives the possibility to store the batch records electronically on various storing devices, such as optical disks. Compared to paper-based batch records, electronically stored records need much less room and increase the safety of the data.

SYSTEM DESCRIPTION

System Concept

A batch record, as it is stored in the database, is represented by a collection of different data on the actual production procedure and the current production environment. Back in 1994, at the point of decision, the data available electronically were stored in several databases. Database update was time-consuming and difficult; data analysis even needed different program interfaces. Therefore, the database for the new system had to be a central, uniform database for the whole production plant. This central database should then store all data on the production procedure, product controlling, the production environment, equipment, and production personnel, allowing reporting across the whole database. To achieve this, a database-oriented application was needed for the collection and analysis of the data. The system was realised as a custom-built software, instead of using a standard software package for electronic batch recording. The reasons for this decision were the following:

- An evaluation of the standard software packages for electronic batch recording (available in 1994) showed that essential user requirements could not be satisfied. Add-on software would have been needed to provide the missing functionality. With that, the overall expenditure for the system would have been similar or even higher than the custom-built solution, satisfying all requirements.
- The combination of standard and custom-built software would have led to higher maintenance expenditure and higher cost for license fees.
- Implementing only those user requirements covered by standard software not addressing the unsatisfied requirements would have reduced the user acceptance of the new computer system.
- To be efficient, a computer-aided batch review system needs software that covers at least 90 percent of the requirements. If the pharmacist still has to check a part of every batch record manually, there is no significant time reduction for the batch record review.

Realization Concept

The project was divided into two phases to ensure management control of cost, time, and resources.

Phase 1.

- Administration of the general data
- EBRS for bulk production (granulation, ointment, syrup, and sterile solution manufacturing)
- Data processing of the in-process control and the environmental monitoring tests results

Phase 2.

- EBRS for the sterile filling plants, the capsule filling plant, and the tablet compressing plant
- Administration and controlling of the maintenance data of the production equipment

- Administration of the personnel education data
- Automatic data capture from production and measurement equipment
- Controlling of the filter test procedure

SYSTEM SPECIFICATION

User Requirements Specification

Figure 1 gives a data flow schematic to show the interrelationships between each system.

General Requirements

- Definition of authorizations for the specific functions of the system to ensure the appropriate workflow at the production line
- Reporting system for fast information regarding encountered deviations from the specified limits
- Identification of the materials used with unique identifiers (such as raw material, intermediates, filters, spare parts)

Figure 1. Schematic Data Flow

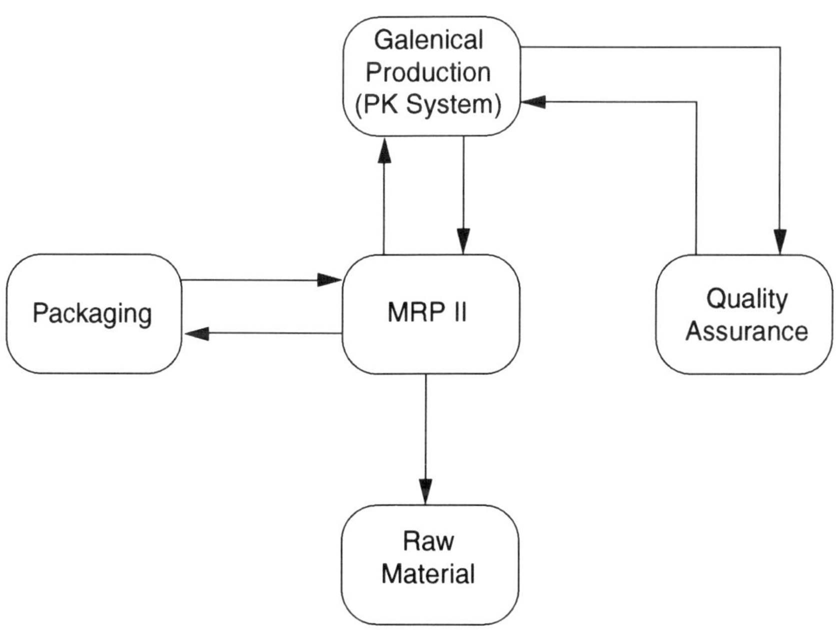

- Interface to the production planning system (MRP II)
- Identification of the production staff (attributes, resources, and training)
- Identification of the production equipment (status, cleaning, calibration)
- Identification of the types of production rooms used (cleaning, sterile, control, etc.)
- Identification of the desktop workspace (workstation, printer, screen, bar code reader, etc.)

Bulk Production

- Definition of master production protocols (21 CFR 211.186 [2]), through which the operator is instructed (through individual operating procedures) how the various production steps must be carried out.
- Creation of the master production record, by copying the valid master production protocol, before production is started.
- Filling in data by workers turns the master production record into the batch production record.

In-Process Control/Environmental Monitoring Test

The following parameters must be documented by the system:

- Environmental monitoring tests
- Final product control
- In-process control
- Validations and calibrations

VALIDATION

The validation was performed according to the "Roche Computerized System Validation Policy and Guidelines" [3,4]. This comprised the definition of a Validation Plan, the performance of the planned activities, and the creation of a Validation Report. In addition, the project was accompanied by external consultants, providing know-how regarding the validation-specific aspects of the development, including the management and auditing of the software developer. The scope of the validation activities was defined by GMP Analysis (also known as a GMP Assessment) [5]. The system requirements were analyzed regarding their GMP relevance. The network functionality was beyond the scope of this validation.

Prequalification Phase

The prequalification phase consists of the following:

- The analysis and definition of user requirements
- The definition of the system delivery specification
- The technical system design [6]

Qualification Phase

In the qualification phase, the programming was performed according to the user requirements and the system delivery specification. The finished program was tested by the developer, using unit and integration tests. In addition, Installation Qualification (IQ) of the hardware and the Operational Qualification (OQ) of the complete system (hardware and program) was performed on-site. The qualification activities included the following:

- Definition of the programming standards
- Ensuring the independent functioning of each individual software module
- Vendor Audits (Supplier Audit)
- Program description (source code)
- Source Code Review
- Ensuring the proper integration of software and hardware
- Definition of the necessary installation procedures
- Definition of the hardware components used

Test Phase

In the test phase, the user acceptance tests were performed. The goal of these tests was to verify whether the completed system was performing according to the user requirements defined in the prequalification phase. The successful test completion was documented in the Validation Report, confirming that the system had been validated for use in daily business. Also included in this phase was the development of various operating procedures. The activities carried out are summarized below.

GMP Analysis

The user requirements must be analysed regarding their risk potential and GMP relevance. The analysis, as defined by Hambloch [4], determines if a function:

- Has influence on the pharmaceutical technical quality
- Affects the medical safety of the drug
- Has influence on the data that become part of the registration documents
- Is critical for another important reason

Test Strategy

A precondition for any testing is the availability of a document that correctly specifies the functions of the system. It is the basis for the verification test specification. In the case of the PK System, this was the User Requirement Specification (URS). The major testing was done as black box testing. White box testing was limited to the modules ranked as most critical in the GMP Analysis. This included the formulas of active ingredient strength and the verification of algorithms in the source code [7].

Verification Test Procedure

A first step toward the validation of the system was the development of a testing procedure to be used for the different software modules and future revalidation. This procedure defines how test plans must be specified, how the tests are performed, and how they are documented. The goal of the testing is to establish documented evidence that the system is performing according to the specifications.

Defining the Verification Test Specification

Once the functions to be tested had been completely identified based on their GMP relevance, they were added to the verification test specification. For each test case, the following information was added:

- Verbal description of the goals that a specific test must achieve
- Detailed description of the test procedure
- Definition of the required test data and the expected results
- Definition of the test protocol
- Listing of any related documents referred to in the tests

The following areas and functions were tested during the validation of phase 1 of the PK System:

- *Daily usage of the system,* including authorizations and security, Windows™ menu control, error reporting, and communication with other devices (e.g., peripherals)
- *Characterization and handling of materials,* including the definition of raw materials, products, and auxiliary material (e.g., packaging)
- *Workflow at the production line,* including production steps, line type, line status, and line schedule
- *Production equipment and locations,* including definition and current state of buildings, production areas, and individual workstations
- *User specifications,* including the definition of user characteristics, groups, responsibilities and privileges, training, and scheduling
- *Control of auxiliary materials and equipment,* including characteristics and calibration of computers, containers, scales, and so on
- *Supplier management,* including the analysis of the vendor's Quality Management System (QMS) and its ability to deliver the requested system
- *Lot data control,* including the identification and maintenance (corrections, deletions, restrictions) of the lot data and content/ingredients calculations
- *Further testing,* including areas such as material storage, MRP II, cleaning protocols, product content, and archiving

Corrective Actions

Any deviation from the expected results that were encountered during the testing had to be analysed for their relevance and documented. Problems that prevented GMP–conformed usage of the system had to be corrected immediately.

Special Testing

Stress Testing. A stress test regarding the data volume was performed by expanding the database to the possible volume of a half year's production records. The acceptance criterion was that it would still be possible to use the system with reasonable response times.

Client Interrupt Testing. It was tested to determine what happens in the case of a sudden breakdown of a client's Personal Computer (PC). The acceptance criterion was that the database would not be corrupted. Data not saved properly should, thus, be rolled back automatically to the latest secure version of the data.

Automated Testing

Splitting the project into two phases made it necessary to integrate several modules sequentially. This process led to frequent revalidation activities. To reduce the testing time and to prevent typing errors during test execution, an automated test tool was used. However, this tool did not deliver all the benefits initially expected, because manual editing (programming) of the generated scripts for the testing tool could not be avoided completely and proved to be very time consuming. Such editing was necessary because

- Windows™ objects (e.g., buttons, menus) reacted differently than the testing tool expected.
- Test execution was influenced by synchronisation problems arising from response time differences.
- Scripts had to be commented to ease later editing, such as the insertion of additional test cases.
- Date- and time-related functions, which are quite frequent in batch recording systems, led to problems during testing. For example, running a test script on a Friday, creating a production order for the following day, triggered the "unexpected" question of whether the production order really should be started on a Saturday or the next Monday. Such questions would not arise Sunday through Thursday.

Furthermore, the execution of the test scripts was halted due to Microsoft Windows™ problems. Finally, maintenance became difficult once the system had been handed over to the business, since the know-how required to maintain and rerun the test scripts was no longer available.

Example

The following example (Table 1) describes how testing was done for a specific function of the system. The situation described in the example is such that within the PK System, menus can be specified for the combination of

- Organization (plant, production line, etc.)
- Workplace type (weighing, drying, sterile conditions, etc.)
- User group (= access level), where each user group has access rights for its own or all lower access levels

In the validation database, person 1 was set up with user name = *TESTP1*, belonging to user group 1 with the access level *level1*. The PC on which the validation testing was run was set up as workstation *WS0001*, belonging to the organization *B1* with the workplace type *AT2*. There is no menu prepared for organization *B1* with workplace type *AT2* and user group *level1*.

Table 1. Example Test Case

Function	Log-in of person 1 on the workplace defined by organization (plant) = *B1* and workplace type 2 = AT2
Test procedure	1. Fill out log-in mask using the test data. 2. Fill out workplace-identification mask *(log-in2)* using the test data (see Figure 2). 3. Check if the menu displayed corresponds with the expected result (see Figure 3).
Test data	4. Log-in mask: User name = *TESTP1,* password = *XXXX00* 5. Log-in2 mask: workplace type = *AT2,* organization = *B1*
Expected result	No menu should be displayed, because there is no menu defined for user group 1 at the workplace *B1/AT2* (see Figure 3).
Test documentation	Printout of the workplace-identification mask and printout of the main menu mask (sign-off with initials plus date)

Figure 2. PK System Workplace Identification Mask

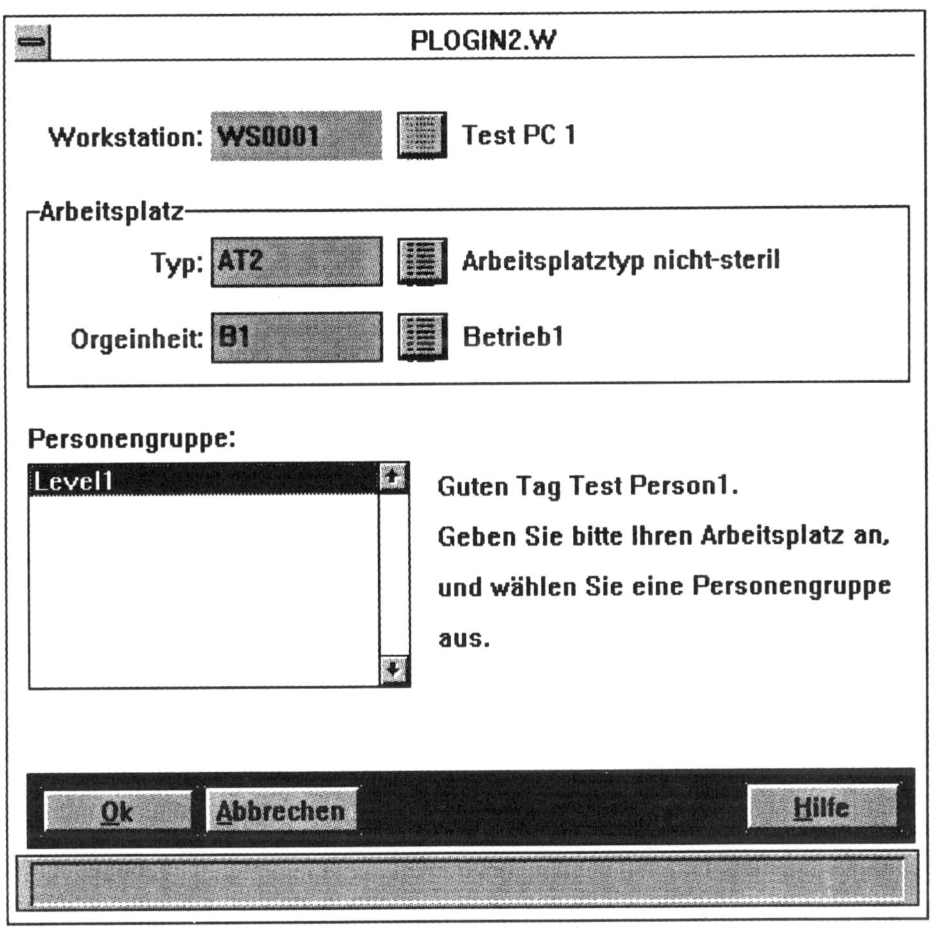

Figure 3. PK System Main Menu Mask

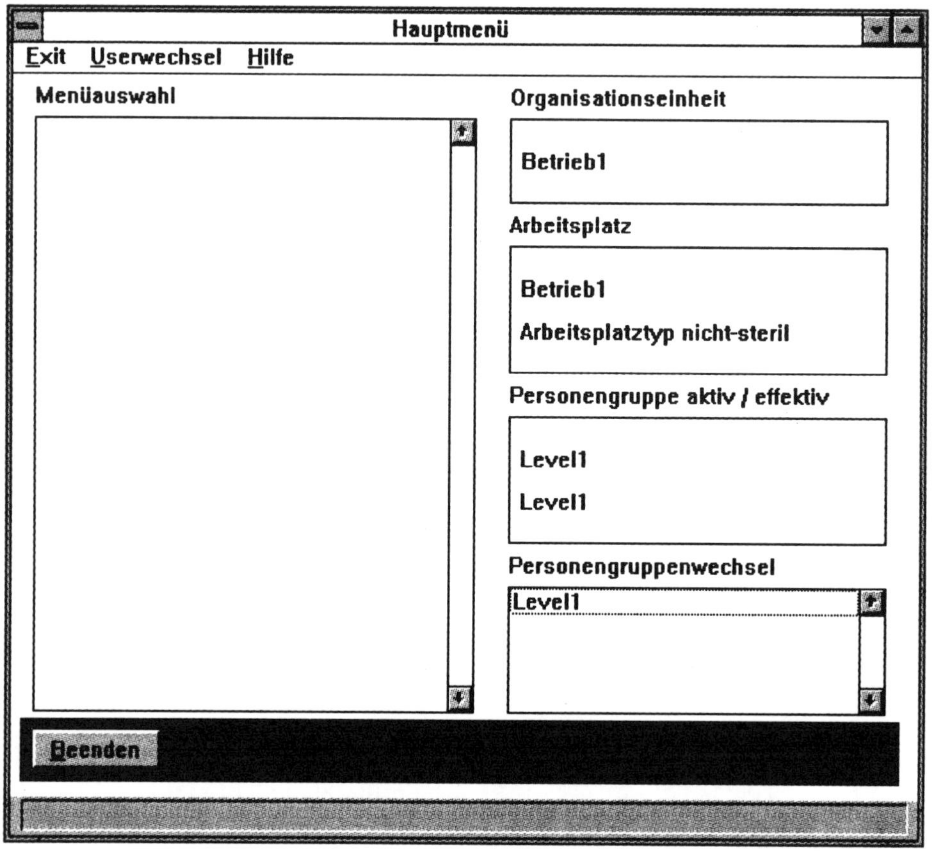

Ongoing Evaluation

Once the system was successfully implemented and now is partly in operation in the daily business, the validated status of the system is maintained, using the necessary technical and organizational procedures.

- Periodic system reviews are performed to verify that the system is operating as specified (performance, disk space), that it is properly administered (e.g., authorisations), and that the documentation is accurate.
- Change and configuration management involves procedures that control and report the implementation of changes that may affect the validation status of a system. This includes the tracking of problem handling, resulting from fault reports or change requests, to their solution. Change management ensures that the configuration of the system is identifiable and reproducible [3].

Currently, the system is still under implementation and revalidation is done frequently—each time a system module is handed over to operations. Experience with ongoing validation of the system has yet to be gained.

CONCLUSIONS

Realization of the Expected Benefits

High Degree of Automation Required

To be efficient, electronic batch recording must eliminate more than half of all manual collection, analysis, and review work. Otherwise, there will not be any significant time reduction.

Creation of a Central, Uniform Database

To ensure the efficiency and effectiveness of the system, all data required for batch review and release should be stored in one central database, eliminating the necessity of interfaces between different databases.

Efficient Validation

Availability of a Company Policy on Computer System Validation

Validation was performed according to the Roche company policy on CSV [3]. A Validation Plan was established, the activities were performed and documented according to this plan, and the results were entered in the Validation Report. As a result, the product (drug) manufacturing process is better documented and analyzed, thus contributing to the safety of a product.

Analysis of GMP Relevance

The validation approach should be based on the analysis of the GMP relevance for each function of the system. The results should then be used to define the test strategy and the corresponding test cases.

Proper Vendor Selection

It is important to select a vendor who is capable of delivering the system in compliance with the requirements of the CSV policy [3]. This ability should be verified by proper vendor selection and auditing.

Ensuring Ongoing Validation

Once the system is in a validated state and handed over to operation, it is important to ensure that the system remains in such a state. The available operating procedures must take into account that the unit operating the system does not have profound system knowledge, which the project team had.

REFERENCES

1. European Union Guide to Directive 91/356/EEC (1991), *European Commission Directive Laying Down the Principles of Good Manufacturing Practices for Human Use.*

2. U.S. Code of Federal Regulations Title 21, Part 211 (last amended 1995), *Good Manufacturing Practices for Finished Pharmaceuticals.*

3. *Roche CSV Policy and Guidelines,* Version 1.0 (1993). Basel, Switzerland: Hoffmann-La Roche Ltd.

4. FDA (1983), *Guide to Inspection of Computerized Systems in Drug Processing.* Rockville, MD: Food and Drug Administration, Department of Health and Human Services.

5. Hambloch, H. (1994), Existing Computer Systems: A Practical Approach to Retrospective Validation. In *Good Computer Validation Practices: Common Sense Implementation,* edited by T. Stokes, R.C. Branning, K.G. Chapman, H. Hambloch, and A.J. Trill. Buffalo Grove, IL: Interpharm Press.

6. Summit-D Handbook (1994), Version 2.6. Coopers & Lybrand Associates Ltd.

7. FDA (1987), *Software Development Activities,* Technical Report, Reference Materials and Training Aids for Investigators. Rockville, MD: Food and Drug Administration.

Case Study H

Validating Electronic Document Management Systems

Rob Almond
Glaxo Wellcome Operations
Barnard Castle, UK

Guy Wingate
Eutech Engineering Solutions Ltd.
Billingham, UK

Electronic Document Management Systems (EDMSs) manage the creation, modification, use, and retention of documentation, which accelerates the process of review, approval, and distribution across an organisation. Figure 1 provides a summary overview of EDMS functionality. Examples of documentation that can be managed by an EDMS include the following: policies, Standard Operating Procedures (SOPs), reports, batch records, and project documents. Maintaining the security and integrity of these documents is paramount to the successful implementation of an EDMS.

Figure 1. Documentation Life Cycle

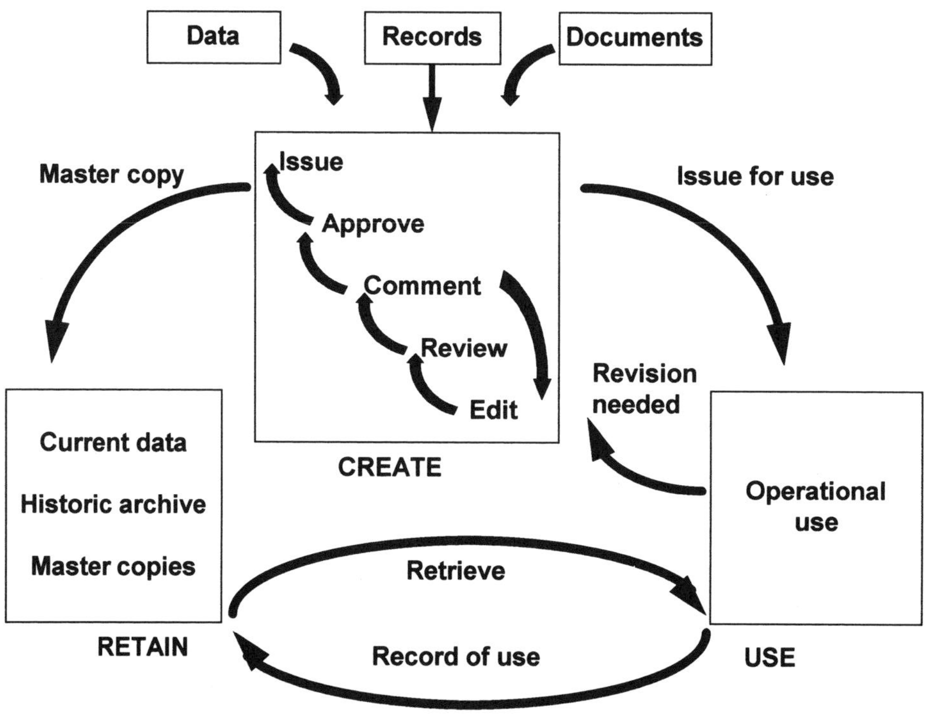

The architecture of a typical EDMS, consisting of application software and a document server connected via a network, is shown in Figure 2. The application software has three core features:

1. Office applications, providing functions such as edit and review to personnel preparing, reviewing, and authorising documentation ready for issue
2. Specialist applications, providing administration functions for use by the system manager and technical support staff
3. Viewing applications, for ordinary end users of the system to locate, view, and print copies of authorised documents

The EDMS may also be required to link with a Manufacturing Execution System (MES), a Manufacturing Resource Planning (MRP II) system, and a Laboratory Information Management System (LIMS) as part of the pharmaceutical manufacturer's integrated manufacturing strategy.

EDMSs are often based on standard configurable packages, providing a central or distributed depository of information (sometimes referred to as an

Figure 2. Example EDMS Architecture

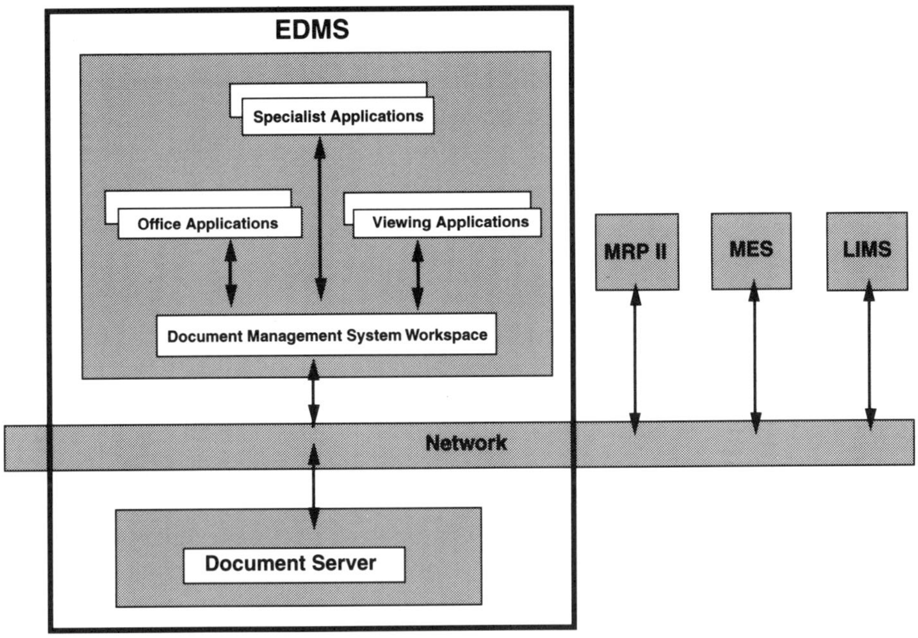

information warehouse) with local on-site or intersite access. Organisations implementing such systems will, therefore, need a suitable communications network, which may include a company's intranet. This case study examines the validation requirements for configurable EDMS.

An EDMS controlling critical Good Manufacturing Practice (GMP) documentation, such as SOPs, user instructions, master batch records, and quality control records, must be validated to comply with the regulatory requirements of the European Directive 91/356/EEC Chapter 4 [1] and the U.S. CFR 211 Subpart J [2]. Approximately two thirds of U.S. Food and Drug Administration's (FDA) citations for GMP noncompliance involve documentation. It is essential, therefore, that systems controlling such documentation are validated. Furthermore, the European Medicines Evaluation Agency (EMEA) and FDA are encouraging the pharmaceutical industry to think about electronic submissions of regulatory information. Currently, regulatory submissions are sent as a paper copy or on floppy disc rather than electronically via the Internet. The EDMS for this activity would require validation. Since retrospective validation can cost up to 20 times that for prospective validation, many firms may consider it prudent to validate their new EDMS for this reason alone.

LIFE–CYCLE VALIDATION

An EDMS represents a significant investment by pharmaceutical manufacturing companies and is often implemented following implementation of an MRP II system as part of an Enterprise Resource Planning (ERP) initiative.

The basic validation approach for an EDMS is shown in Figure 3 and is based on the validation life cycle presented by the GAMP Forum [3]. The life cycle is described below with emphasis on important issues affecting an EDMS. The fundamental principles of validation have not been altered, just the context of their application.

Concept and Feasibility Phase

The life cycle starts with a *concept phase,* during which a draft of the User Requirements is developed with an initial high-level Validation Plan. It is important to note that these documents do not form the final User Requirements Specification (URS), as this will evolve during prototyping. Indeed, the initial draft URS is likely to include a justification of the business case for the system with estimates for the lifetime ownership costs and the quantified benefits of improved efficiency of document management.

The *feasibility phase* is based on evaluating and selecting a supplier (system vendor and application integrator). This may involve gathering information using postal questionnaires and inviting the various suppliers to organise trial demonstrations of their proposed solutions. A formal visit to a supplier's premises to conduct a Supplier Audit might only be arranged by the pharmaceutical manufacturer for their preferred solution.

Criteria for consideration when selecting an EDMS include the following:

- Available word-processing formats for creating documents
- Distribution control for documents: read/write access rights
- Amendment, review, approval facilities (access rights)
- Printing facilities for document copies
- Expiry date management for master versions and printed copies
- Expiry date messages and actions for users
- Search and sorting facilities (including their speed) for documents
- Capacity (numbers and size of document archive, number of users)
- Access security and authorisation for individuals and user groups
- Network capability and hardware platform (are they open systems?)
- Data interchange compatibility with other interconnected systems
- Facilities for pilot (e.g., networked PCs)

Figure 3. Validation Concepts Applied to the Implementation of an EDMS

Development Activities		*Validation Activities*
Draft User Requirement	Concept	Initial (high level) Validation Plan
Evaluate suppliers Select supplier(s)	Feasibility	Supplier Audits
Prototyping - Refine User Requirements - Functional Specification (Both for core system and for customised software and interfaces)	Specification	Detailed Validation Plan Specification Review
- Design Specification - Software Specification - Hardware Specification	Design	Design Review
Build interfaces and customised software Unit and link test of interfaces and customised software	Construct Interfaces etc.	Monitor suppliers (Source Code Review)
Install hardware and software	Installation	IQ
Pilot - Integration testing - Load pilot data - Conference Room Pilot Cutover (go live) Live monitoring	} Acceptance Testing	OQ + PQ
System acceptance	}	Validation Report
Maintenance Change control	Operation	Ongoing operation

Supplier Audits

Supplier Audits are used to verify the capability of a system and its supplier. The UK GAMP Guide [3] provides a very useful checklist for conducting a supplier audit. The track record of the EDMS in the pharmaceutical industry with reference sites may prove a key factor in the assessment of the supplier's capability. Where such evidence is not available, confidence may have to be established through demonstrations. Whilst a product may be industry standard, the application it is intended for may have unique needs and, therefore, confidence required that the system is suitable. Other issues for the Supplier Audit may include how easy the system is to configure and use, as well as any planned developments, which could impact on the true cost of implementing the system. If the audit uncovers unrecoverable problems (technical capability or validation compliance) with the supplier, then an alternative solution should be selected as the preferred option and subjected to an audit.

Supplier Audits should not be considered a one-off activity, but rather as a mechanism for the ongoing monitoring of suppliers. Initial audits may be by postal questionnaires, with a follow-up visit to the supplier's premises for a more detailed assessment of their capabilities. Indeed, there may be further audits, either during or after project completion, to check any earlier corrective actions placed on the supplier or as part of an ongoing preferred supplier relationship for future projects.

Project Planning

After successfully justifying the purchase and implementation of an EDMS, and selecting the system vendor and application integrator, detailed project plans can be prepared. These will include the pharmaceutical manufacturer's Validation Plan for the project and Supplier's Quality Plan. It is important that resource requirements are identified and allocated. It is normal practice for the pharmaceutical manufacturer to supply staff to assist in the prototyping phase. An overview of potential project milestones is given in Figure 4.

Prototyping Development

The Prototyping Phase essentially takes the draft URS produced in the concept phase and extends it to cover functional and design specifications. Prototyping does not conform to the conventional distinct and sequential Functional Specification and Design activities, rather it consists of many iterative cycles of stepwise refinement.

The development environment and team structure must be carefully considered. Teams usually consist of staff from the pharmaceutical manufacturer and supplier organisations. The balance of team membership and the availability of suitably experienced staff will be key factors in organising

Figure 4. An Overview of Project Milestones

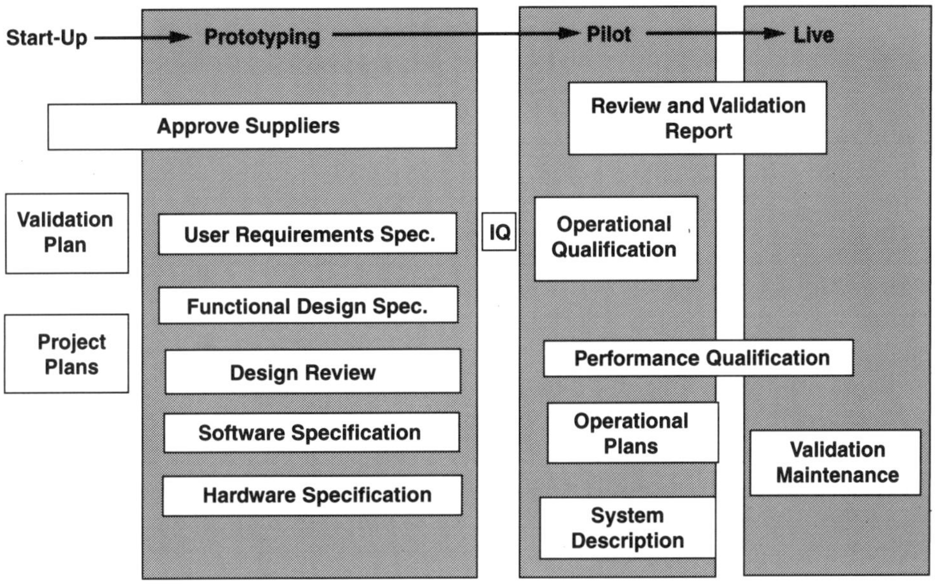

teams, as too the location and the available of rooms for prototyping. The pharmaceutical manufacturer must ensure sufficient Quality Assurance personnel are available to fulfil their duties and, if necessary, transfer internal staff or recruit new staff. The GMP regulatory authorities hold the pharmaceutical company, not the system vendor or application integrator, accountable for validation.

The development of bespoke interfaces to other systems (including operator screens and printers) and the customisation of existing facilities should be discouraged because of the added validation effort needed to deal with such work. Detailed Source Code Reviews and functional and structural testing will all be required. Industry standard EDMS products are normally subject to frequent upgrades by their originating vendors. Any customisation by the pharmaceutical manufacturer to the standard product may require rework to continue functioning correctly with these upgrades. Experience has shown that such rework can incur significant revalidation costs.

Wherever possible, it is recommended that prototyping be limited to configuration; bespoke interface developments and customisation should be minimised. If this approach is adopted, and assuming a satisfactory Supplier Audit outcome for the standard EDMS product, the remaining validation by the pharmaceutical manufacturer can be largely limited to functional testing.

At the end of the *prototyping phase,* it should be possible to define the "ways of working" in SOPs, user instructions, and so on. Only when the prototyping phase is complete can the *piloting phase* begin. Design and configuration details should be collated into formal documents, noting any additional hardware requirements (user licences, memory) for cutover of the EDMS to live operation. Entity-relationship diagrams can prove to be very effective means of describing a design, but must be accompanied by a narrative. Finally, there should be an independent health check to review GMP compliance and business benefits. Some organisations refer to this health-check review or an activity very similar to it as a Design Qualification.

Conference Room Pilot (Business Testing)

The piloting phase starts with an Installation Qualification (IQ) of the prescribed EDMS software on the hardware platform. The IQ should also include a check to see that user manuals, technical support manuals, user procedures, and so on are present and correct. Data sets for the pilot are then loaded, possibly taken as a subset of information from a current existing system or input specially from another source solely for the purpose of pilot testing. This activity is sometimes called *data migration* or *data population.*

Following these preparations, the Operational Qualification (OQ) then takes place. Testing at this stage will include the following:

- Correct document distribution
- Correct allocation of access rights (edit, view, etc.)
- User access and security challenges
- Hidden and visible comments facility
- Group review or named individuals
- Document status (draft for revision, awaiting review or approved)
- Worst-case impact analysis (fail-safe scenarios)
- Electronic signatures

The majority of tests should consider the worst-case impacts to document status and security. For instance, a scenario that uncovered a problem with one particular system concerned documents that could be inadvertently authorised, regardless of whether the person attempting to authorise the document had permission, if there was a communication failure during document authorisation processing. Gross errors will normally be readily identifiable; it is those more subtle error conditions that the impact analysis aims to discover.

The use of electronic signatures has been a topical issue for several years now. Many pharmaceutical companies must fulfil the requirements of a new U.S. CFR 11 concerning electronic signatures [4] before considering whether to incorporate this facility into their EDMS. Clarification from the GMP regulatory authorities on what they consider acceptable signatory mechanisms, which are practical for pharmaceutical manufacturers to implement, does not appear to be imminent. In the mean time, handwritten signatures are necessary for all GMP documentation, such as batch records and SOPs.

The aim of OQ is to establish confidence in the EDMS functionality ready for cutover. Some aspects of Performance Qualification (PQ) may be possible to test at this time, but most can only be tested after cutover.

Assuming the pilot has a successful outcome in its off-line test environment, preparations for cutover can begin. To cope with the increased number of licenced users and potential documents, an upgrade to the hardware platform is usually conducted, and hence, the IQ will normally have to be revisited. Further data migration from legacy systems to convert the entire live data scenario to the EDMS is also required. The integrity of data transferred must be checked. All GMP critical data must be included in this check. Once this has been achieved, the EDMS can go live. Qualification, however, is not yet complete. A period of "live" monitoring of key parameters is required to complete the PQ. Key parameters will include the following:

- Verify peak demand operability
- User acceptable document retrieval times
- Sustained computer room environment (e.g., temperature, humidity)
- Functionality of access control in live environment
- Trend analysis of document management lead times

A management summary report should be prepared at the end of IQ, OQ, and PQ. Any outstanding issues should be resolved before the next sequential phase of qualification begins. Concessions to proceed without problem resolution may be appropriate for some issues if they do not have a critical impact on GMP and corrective actions are planned and approved.

Validation Reporting

Once the project has been completed, the EDMS is supporting drug manufacturing, and PQ has demonstrated consistent operation, a report is produced by the pharmaceutical manufacturer summarising the validation outcome. This document, usually referred to as a Validation Report, reviews the Validation Plan, implementation and testing of the EDMS, and sets out plans for resolving any outstanding issues, together with an outline on how the validated status of the EDMS will be maintained. Whilst suppliers may be invited to submit material and information relevant to this document, the Validation Report itself usually remains confidential to the pharmaceutical manufacturer.

ONGOING SUPPORT

Once implemented, the EDMS requires ongoing support to maintain the validated compliance of the system. In particular, change and version control of the standard software product should be monitored, and documentation and testing revised as necessary with any upgrade. Regression testing may be used by the system vendor; the validity of the regression strategy and the validation of any automated testing tools should be checked. A formal system for change control must also be used for any modifications made by or on behalf of the pharmaceutical manufacturer to the system's configuration or bespoke elements.

Ongoing support must also ensure any hardware maintenance is recorded. A service agreement may exist for the system's hardware platform, and this should be reviewed to establish that maintenance and repair procedures and records are acceptable for operating within a GMP organisation.

Security access should be demonstrably managed. Lists of access rights and authorised users should be maintained. These lists should be updated when authorised users join or leave the company. Password access to user identification codes for personnel leaving the organisation must be denied. Unauthorised access attempts should be logged and investigated.

Training requirements for system managers, technical support staff, and end users should have been identified in the Validation Plan. It is vital that those needing training obtain it before the system goes live. Training may be given through formal courses or hands-on tutoring, perhaps during OQ. Ongoing training in the form of refresher courses, training for new upgrade functionality in the standard EDMS product, and introductory training for new personnel should all be planned, delivered in a timely fashion, and recorded. If training is not delivered in a timely fashion, then the competency of personnel to fulfil their duties may be compromised.

A Disaster Management Plan should prepared, authorised, and distributed to those who will potentially need it. The plan covers prescribed recovery actions, contact names and telephone numbers, and so on. A paper copy of the plan must be distributed because in the disaster, it is assumed that electronic access will have been lost. There are two basic disaster situations:

1. The document storage media becomes unretrievably corrupted.
2. The document storage media cannot be accessed.

Options for dealing with media integrity include mirrored disc images, fault-tolerant document servers, and duplicate archives. Options for dealing with document access include duplicate network cable highways, alternative access routes (e.g., more than one local workstation or PC with access to the EDMS), and driving a mobile command centre onto the pharmaceutical manufacturer's site to replace unavailable communication links (possibly via cable or satellite). Any contingency mechanism employed must be validated and regularly checked in conjunction with the plan. The level of investment made in making the EDMS infrastructure robust should be balanced against the consequences of the unavailability of the EDMS.

USER GROUPS

User groups consisting of a number of pharmaceutical companies can conduct shared audits and influence future developments of an EDMS. Many pharmaceutical companies actively encourage User Groups because EDMS suppliers may not rely on the pharmaceutical sector for a significant proportion of their sales, and User Groups can collectively bring compliance issues to the fore. Indeed, a partnership between users and suppliers should bring both benefits of cost-effective delivery and validation compliance.

CONCLUSION

Many pharmaceutical manufacturing organisations are considering the implementation of EDMSs. These systems offer the following advantages:

- Standard approach to corporate documentation
- Consistent "look and feel" corporate documentation
- Efficient documentation review and approval lead times
- Enables users to find documentation easily
- Future regulatory submissions by EDMS

With the growing tendency for distributed work groups (on-site, intersite, or even intercontinental), the benefits of implementing an EDMS are potentially great for small as well as large international organisations. A major factor, however, even sometimes viewed as a constraint, in planning the implementation of such systems is GMP compliance. The validation approach for an EDMS is not different from other Information Technology (IT) systems; setting the context for validation, emphasis should be placed on authorisation, document release, document status, and access rights. Standard packages would appear to be the way forward to minimise the validation effort. Bespoke programming and customisation should be minimised if not avoided.

REFERENCES

1. European Union Guide to Directive 91/356/EEC (1991), *European Commission Directive Laying Down the Principles of Good Manufacturing Practice for Medicinal Products for Human Use.*

2. U.S. Code of Federal Regulations Title 21, Parts 210 (last amended 1994), *Current Good Manufacturing Practice in Manufacturing, Processing, Packaging, and Holding of Drugs;* Part 211 (last amended 1995), *Current Good Manufacturing Practice for Finished Pharmaceuticals.*

3. GAMP Forum/ISPE (1996), *Supplier Guide for Validation of Automation Systems in Pharmaceutical Manufacturing,* Second edition, UK GAMP Forum and International Society of Pharmaceutical Engineering.

4. FDA (1997), *Electronic Records; Electronic Signatures,* U.S. Code of Federal Regulations Title 21, Part 11, Rockville, MD: Food and Drug Administration.

Case Study I

The Vendor's Role in the Validation of Electronic Document Management Systems

Sion Wyn
Activa Systems
Wales

Document management systems cover a wide range of applications, and the term *document* now covers more than the traditional paperwork to include electronic information. The information may be in various forms, including text, images, numerical information, or even audio and video clips. These may be combined in many ways into a single unit that can be viewed, edited, stored, and retrieved on demand. Indeed, they need not necessarily have traditional paper equivalents [1].

As an indication of the types of documents dealt with in pharmaceutical manufacturing, the EU Good Manufacturing Practice (GMP) guidelines [2], which covers documentation in chapter 4, make specific reference to the following critical types:

- Specifications
- Formulae
- Process and packaging instructions
- Procedures
- Records

The U.S. equivalent—21 CFR part 211 Subpart J—deals with a broadly similar class of documents [3]. The control of these key GMP and business critical documents is dependent on correct and consistent operation of any Electronic Document Management System (EDMS) used. Their validation is, therefore, of crucial importance.

The critical, strategic requirements for EDMS are threefold:

1. The systems must comply with regulatory requirements for the use of computer systems within pharmaceutical manufacturing—in effect, they must be validated [4].
2. The processes and operations performed by the systems must enforce, or enable, compliance with general regulatory requirements, such as document control and change control.
3. The systems must support and reflect effective and efficient business processes.

The first two requirements are closely linked, and will be dealt with in the following sections. The third requirement is beyond the scope of this book.

GENERAL REGULATORY REQUIREMENTS

The EU and U.S. regulations regarding document management are broadly in accord, and can be summarized as follows:

- There should be careful control of documentation preparation and design, review, and distribution.
- Documents should not be ambiguous—the title, nature, and purpose of the documents should be clear.
- Documents should be approved, signed, and dated by appropriate and authorised persons.
- Documents should be kept up to date, and there should be systems in place to prevent inadvertent use of superseded documents.
- Alterations to documents should be authorised and reasons for change kept. The amended information should not be lost. In summary, there should be a full audit trail.

Electronic Systems

As EDMSs are used to control compliance critical information, further specific requirements apply. The system's use must be fully documented; examples of SOPs that may be needed for an EDMS include Creation of New Documents, Review and Approval, Document Distribution, Document Change, Withdrawal, and Archiving. Procedures will also be required for system management functions, such as controlling user accounts, system maintenance, and backup and recovery.

The records stored must be accurate. For example, the user must be given access to the correct version of a document. In practice, this means the system must have been fully qualified and validated, with emphasis being given during validation planning to those areas that are of particular importance, such as the integrity of documents and access control.

Modifications to records should be controlled. As well as the electronic system providing change facilities, the documents must also be secure from unauthorised change (whether accidental or intentional). To this end, physical and logical security controls are required, and the use of passwords should be enforced. The system should maintain an audit trail of changes, deletions, and any other significant events.

Electronic Signatures

Because issues of document approval and authorisation are central in an EDMS, this topic will be briefly covered. A full discussion of the implications of FDA rules [5] and *Validation of Automated Systems* [6] is beyond the scope of this case study, therefore, the following discussion is based on generally accepted industry understanding.

Most EDMS implementations will be closed systems, that is, access is restricted to people who are part of the organisation using the system. Closed systems require *dual contemporaneous entry*. This is akin to using a bank card to obtain money—the card and a pass code are required. Two component passwords or a barcode plus a password are examples of dual contemporaneous entry.

The proposed rule requires certain procedural controls, for example, a registered list of systems incorporating electronic signatures, security controls, and training. Controls should also be built into the system, to verify data entry, for example, or location checks to verify that data has come from the expected source.

SYSTEM ARCHITECTURE

The distributed nature of the systems means that the network infrastructure on which the application is based must be fully qualified. The latest edition of the *GAMP Guide for Validation of Automated Systems* [6] includes information on the validation of network-based applications. Figure 1 shows the logical architecture of a typical EDMS.

A typical enterprise-wide, fully functional EDMS will have features to support the following general requirements [1]:

- Input (creation or capture)
- Indexing and profiling
- Retrieval and display
- Review and approval
- Storage and administration

In the context of pharmaceutical manufacturing, the following key features are typically required, and their correct operation must be assured as part of supplier product testing or user acceptance testing:

- Definable, and validatable, workflows for document processes, such as creation, change, review, withdrawal, and archival of documents
- Electronic, on-line reviews, with annotations
- Approval of documents on-line by binding electronic signatures

Figure 1. Example EDMS Architecture

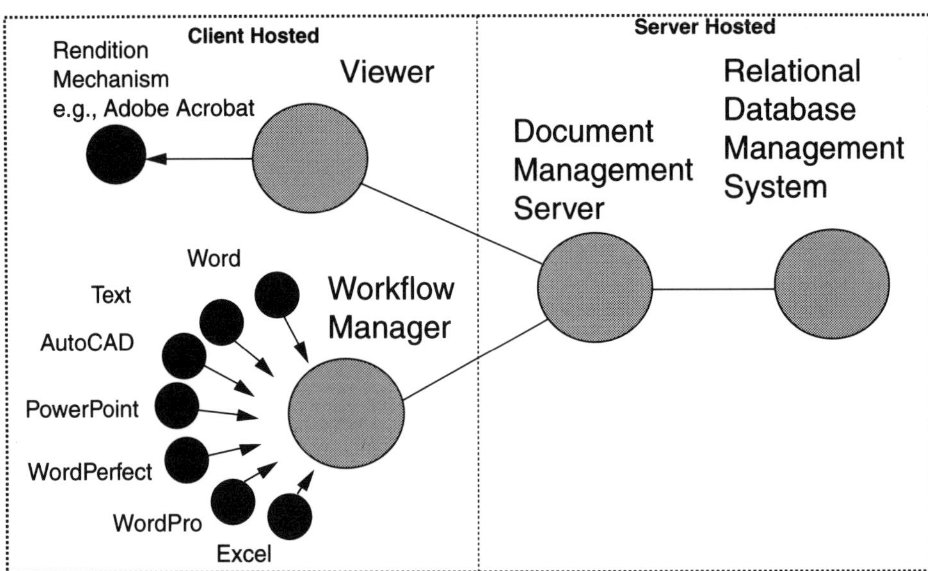

- Secure document change control with audit trail
- Secure read-only viewing, allowing access only to predefined versions of documents
- Controlled printing to mitigate the effects of uncontrolled paper copies

PROJECT AND VALIDATION LIFE CYCLE

Most major EDMS applications, especially those controlling GMP or business critical information will be based on the integration of preexisting products rather than bespoke development. For instance, referring to Figure 1, a solution could consist of an Oracle™ RDBMS, a Documentum™ Server, and Active Compliance™ Document Manager and Viewer.

In such a case, it would be expected that these core products would be fully tested and documented before release by the supplier, and that the validation activities required by the customer or user be limited to

- Requirement definition
- Supplier assessment
- Supplier monitoring and control
- System acceptance testing
- Performance Qualification (PQ)

In such cases, PQ would typically include checking the implemented workflows against business and process requirements, and the use of the system in the context of the controlling Standard Operating Procedures (SOPs). Disaster and recovery testing should also be addressed.

It is useful for a major EDMS application to distinguish between *customisation* and *configuration*, and to refer to the GAMP Guide [6] for guidance on different categories of software.

In the case of a GAMP category product—a standard software package, often called a canned or COTS (commercial off-the-shelf) configurable package in the United States—the core functionality will have been tested extensively by the supplier. Any *configuration* of the system should be addressed by the user PQ of the system, but the standard core package functionality does not need retesting.

In the case of *customisation*, usually the production of custom modules, each should be treated as GAMP category 5—custom-built or bespoke software. In such cases, a complete validation life cycle is necessary, as described elsewhere in this book, albeit on a smaller scale because the scope may be limited.

SUPPLIER LIFE CYCLE

As mentioned above, suppliers of EDMS components typically have a comprehensive product life cycle, aimed at producing a fully tested and documented product. The major part of the validation effort on EDMS will have typically taken place before delivery. Various suppliers may have different terminology, but the life cycle will generally be similar.

A typical supplier life cycle, such as that used by Activa Systems, and based on GAMP principles is shown in Figure 2.

Requirements and Specification

The requirements definition should encompass both functional requirements and the nonfunctional requirements enforced by both regulations and commercial considerations.

The functionality and features provided by the product are typically defined in a Functional Specification (FS) or its equivalent. This document is maintained up to date for each version of the product, and is the controlling

Figure 2. Typical Supplier Life Cycle

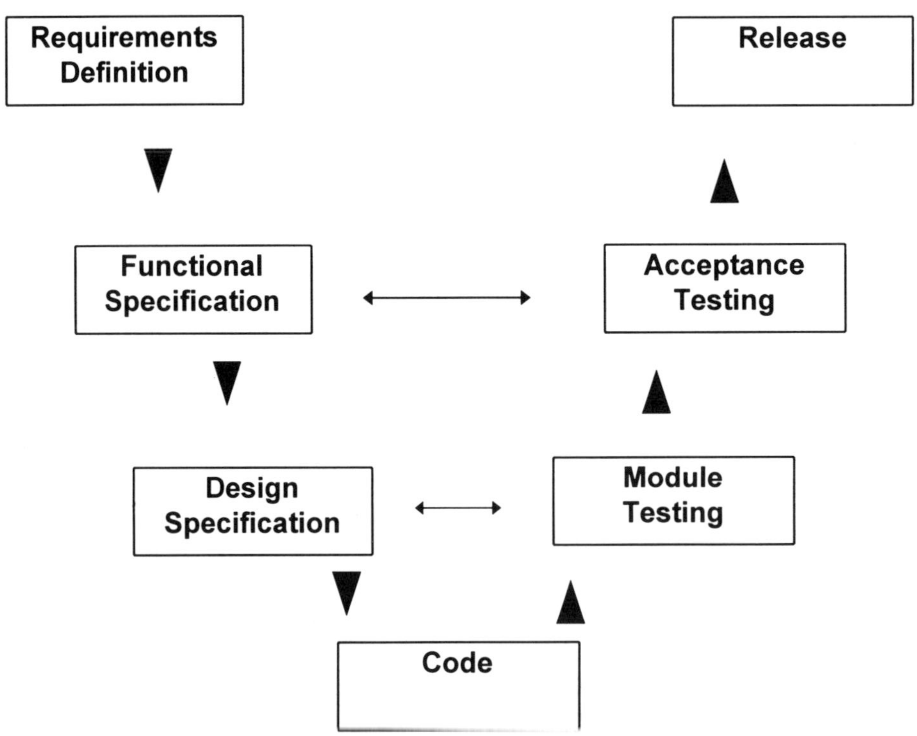

specification against which acceptance testing is performed. The Acceptance Test Specification is produced from the FS.

The FS will typically contain the following sections:

- *Introduction*
- *Overview,* covering key objectives and benefits, a high level description, and the main interfaces at the highest level
- *Product assumptions,* covering any design or implementation assumption, such as the use of standard packages, operating systems, or hardware
- *Functions and features,* describing the functions and facilities to be provided by the product, and defining configuration options and limits
- *Safety and security,* covering action in case of selected software or hardware failures, self-checking, input validation, redundancy, time-outs, and data recovery
- *Data definition* (sometimes a separate data definition document, such as a data dictionary, is produced)
- *Interfaces* to users and other systems
- *Nonfunctional attributes,* covering aspects such as reliability, redundancy, error checking, and expansion and enhancement possibilities
- *Glossary*

The supplier may choose numerous levels of design specifications, with the system typically separated into functional units, sharing common libraries wherever possible. This design breakdown would then be summarised in the highest level design specification. These functional units, or modules, are fully documented in individual design specifications, which become the controlling documents against which internal low level testing takes place, as test specifications are produced against them.

Implementation and Testing

All product software should be developed in accordance with formal coding standards, and independently reviewed, preferably as a team effort, to confirm its structural integrity. Inspection is often a very important part of product testing, and should be performed against checklists as well as against coding standards documents.

> *The earlier that errors are found, the lower are the costs of correcting the errors and the higher the probability of correcting the errors correctly* [7].

The purpose of testing is to find and resolve problems, not merely to confirm compliance of the product with specifications, a point that is particularly relevant to the regulated pharmaceutical environment. Challenging the software and formally testing expected error conditions, unexpected situations, combinations, calculations, input and outputs, and normal expected routes is, therefore, essential. Testing of the software is typically executed in two stages, although as explained above, a supplier may choose more levels of design and testing. The following, however, is a common model:

1. Module or unit testing
2. Acceptance testing, which includes integration testing, internal acceptance testing, and beta acceptance testing of each product version

Beta testing involves testing each version of the product on selected customer sites for an agreed-on period in order to build confidence in the software in end user environments. The product should not be released to customers for beta testing before the satisfactory completion of internal acceptance testing; all incidents and queries raised during this phase should be formally recorded, progressed, and closed. While beta testing can be a valuable source of information for both supplier and customer, it is not recommended practice for beta test software to be used in the live manufacturing environment, unless there are sufficient safeguards to ensure the integrity of GMP critical data.

For unit or module testing, white box testing concentrating on boundary values [7] is often performed, while for acceptance, the following should be covered:

- Volume testing (e.g, determining the level of continuous heavy load at which system performance degrades significantly, or fails)
- Stress testing (e.g., multiple simultaneous connections to document databases, multiple simultaneous workflows)
- Usability testing (e.g., GUI consistency, error message text, "help" messages)
- Security testing (e.g., attempt to subvert product or system software security features)
- Performance testing (e.g., response times under workload)
- Configuration testing including installation procedures
- Reliability testing
- Recovery testing, including introduction of corrupt data, and forcing invalid actions
- Documentation and procedure testing (e.g., testing accuracy of user, maintenance, and installation documentation)

When new product versions are created, a comprehensive test strategy is required, covering tests of new features and functions, complete product suite tests, and regression tests.

Regression Testing

Regression testsing is aimed at discovering the effect of newly introduced changes on previously tested and accepted software. The incorporation of new features, facilities, or new software components can often affect seemingly unrelated functionality.

A common approach is to define a set of regression test cases, and perform these periodically, to detect any regression problems. The vendor must decide what level of regression testing is required, and how often to perform it. Rerunning a full acceptance suite each time is not always a realistic option.

The trade-off is often between performing a large set of tests infrequently, or a smaller set more frequently. The former approach can lead to a significant delay before regression problems come to light, while the latter runs the risk of not covering all critical functions.

One approach is to define different sets of regression test cases to apply depending on the level of change applied. It has been suggested [8] that certain test cases are more effective at finding regression problems than others, and that, therefore, the success history of the individual test cases should be monitored and analyzed. For systems such as EDMSs where certain functions have very direct GMP significance, regression testing should concentrate on those areas.

Product Version Control and Release

A product version is a complete and controlled set of product items intended to provide specific, defined functionality. A product version could be for release to the customer, or for internal use only. A product release is a controlled set of product items distributed to customers, and identified by a unique reference or release number.

Typically for a major IT system, such as an EDMS, several categories of releases are defined, depending on the nature of the changes involved. Often major and minor releases are regarded as separate product versions, while maintenance and patch releases are not.

A typical scheme for generating a new and unique number for each product release would produce a release number with the following format:

Major.Minor[.Maintenance][.Patch] [Beta]

The first two digits indicate the product version and are mandatory. The other fields cover maintenance, patch and beta releases and are optional. In this example the types of release are defined as follows:

- *Major Release:* Major functional changes to the product.
- *Minor Release:* Functional change to some parts of the product.
- *Maintenance Release:* A number of bug fixes incorporated in the product.
- *Patch Release:* A small number of bugs (usually one) has been fixed and those fixes have been issued to a specific customer or customers. The patch number increases incrementally as further patch releases are issued. Each patch release includes patches made in prior releases.

REFERENCES

1. *Requirements for an Enterprise Document Management System* (1995), Black Forest Group, Association for Information and Image Management International.
2. *Guide to Good Manufacturing Practice for Medicinal Products* (1992), The Rules Governing Medicinal Products in the European Community, Vol. IV.
3. U.S. Code of Federal Regulations, Title 21, Parts 210 (last amended 1994), *Current Good Manufacturing Practice in Manufacturing, Processing, Packaging, or Holding of Drugs;* Part 211 (last amended 1995), *Current Good Manufacturing Practice for Finished Pharmaceuticals.*
4. Wyn, S. (1996), The Regulatory Requirements for Computerised Systems in Pharmaceutical Manufacture, *BCS/IEE Software Engineering Journal* (March).
5. FDA (1997), *Electronic Records; Electronic Signatures,* U.S. Code of Federal Regulations Title 21, Part 11. Rockville, MD: Food and Drug Administration.
6. GAMP Forum (1996), *Supplier Guide for Validation of Automation Systems in Pharmaceutical Manufacture,* 2nd Edition, available from the International Society of Pharmaceutical Engineering.
7. Myers, G.J. (1979), *The Art of Software Testing.* New York: John Wiley & Sons.
8. Humphrey, W.S. (1989), *Managing the Software Process,* Addison-Wesley.

Case Study J

Validating Engineering Management Systems

Peter Owen and Peter Gough
Eli Lilly and Company
Basingstoke, UK

An Engineering Management System (EMS) is a computer software package that is designed to address the day-to-day needs of the maintenance management of plant items in a manufacturing environment. These packages are designed for use in many industries and organisations; therefore, EMS packages generally are modular in design. Modular design allows for different options to be added and configured as required by different users. It should be noted that most EMS packages are proprietary and available for use under a licencing agreement; as such, the functions described herein are taken from a combination of documents that were produced during the validation of a number of EMS packages. The requirement for the computer validation of EMS packages is covered in the EC Guide to Good Manufacturing Practice for Medicinal Products, Annex 11, and U.S. 21 CFR Part 211, subpart D. Equipment used in the manufacture and processing of pharmaceuticals is required to be maintained at appropriate intervals to prevent malfunctions; it is also a requirement to keep records of the maintenance that is performed on specific plant items. This is referred to in the EC GMP in chapter 4, clause 4.26, and in 21 CFR Part 211, subpart D 211.67 and 211.68.

VALIDATION APPROACH

Eli Lilly and Company has developed a computer validation policy that covers the process of computer validation during development, implementation, and use of computer systems. The policy identifies the following 16 validation products that are a minimum requirement for a computer system. The policy has been developed to be in line with the life-cycle approach as required by the EC GMP Guide, Annex 11, clause 2 and 21 CFR 211.68(a).

1. Validation Plan
2. Current situation
3. Requirements definition
4. Preimplementation change management
5. Vendor requirements
6. Design
7. Security
8. Application software
9. Testing
10. Operation
11. Business continuity plan
12. Training
13. System acceptance
14. Postimplementation change control
15. Record retention
16. Periodic reviews

Many of these "deliverables" are generated during the normal course of a computer system project. This case study will discuss each of these deliverables and detail how they should be applied to the validation of EMS packages. Where appropriate, the relevant section of the EC GMP Guide will be indicated.

VALIDATION PLAN

A Validation Plan is required by Annex 11, clause 2, and is normally started during the requirement definition phase of a project. It should be combined with a project development plan, as it defines the activities throughout the project life cycle that will ensure that a project conforms to validation requirements.

It is very important in this document to scope the validation, as it may be possible to place certain items beyond the scope of the validation. These may include the following:

- Operating system software
- Terminal emulators
- Application programs, such as word processors

The rationale for exclusion may be that such systems have a large user base and are subject to a supplier's Quality Assurance procedures. The reliability of such systems has been demonstrated through standard and widely based usage in the marketplace. However, it should be noted that this rationale should be supported by documented evidence.

CURRENT SITUATION

The current situation deliverable helps to define the existing processes in place prior to the start of the validation by capturing the justification for the system. It will also help to establish the potential number of records the system will be required to handle and future expansion facilities for the system. It is important to understand the current situation, since it is difficult to define adequately the requirements for a new EMS without understanding the existing system. Estimates indicate that 80 percent of the functionality of an existing system will transfer to a new system. The current situation deliverable usually precedes the Validation Plan, and is typically the first product generated, since the information is closely linked to the project justification.

REQUIREMENTS DEFINITION

The primary purpose of the Requirements Definition is to define the basic needs or functionality of the system from the end user's perspective and in the user's language. This document may form part of contract document between the vendor and the client. It may also be used when comparing products from different vendors for "best fit" to the user's requirements.

Basic System Functions of an EMS

The basic requirements for an EMS are to store details of all plant items that require periodic or emergency maintenance, together with details of the actual maintenance jobs required and facilities to produce automatically details of maintenance requirements on a planned basis. To assist in these functions, the system should also be able to hold details of maintenance staff and stocks of spares/service items.

The basic system functionality can be broken down into five distinct areas:

1. Information requirements
2. Maintenance of static data
3. Generation of work
4. Analysis of completed and outstanding work
5. Configuration

Critical System Functions

The critical features of an EMS system may include the following:

- Ability to create work orders on the due date
- Ability to vary the scheduled maintenance period of the plant item depending upon its criticality
- To suppress specific jobs when more than one job for a specific plant item falls on the same due date
- To reschedule jobs at the correct time interval and to correctly warn of low stock levels
- Correct information user input in order to be able to present accurate information

The above are driven by a combination of the system clock, static data, and, in some circumstances, the correct input of work order completion for previous jobs.

From the above, it should be noted that the most critical operation on the system is accurate data input when reporting stock usage, plant downtime, etc. on work order completion. Without accurate information, the system cannot function correctly.

Information Requirements

The system should be able to record details of each plant item that is within the scope of the Maintenance Department. It should be able to record the interrelationships of plants to one another. These relationships exist where plants are built from other plant items, each of which may be recorded separately and may require differing maintenance requirements from the whole.

- Details of the maintenance required for each plant item and the time interval for repeated maintenance should be recorded together with maintenance instruction lists.
- The system should record details of the maintenance staff—their departments, skills, and availability—and use this information to plan maintenance tasks.
- Details of what parts are stored for each plant item should be recorded, as should lists of what parts are required to carry out specific maintenance tasks.
- Where stored parts may be assembled from other more basic parts that are also stored, then parts assembly lists should be held.
- On the completion of maintenance tasks, work completion details, including time taken, downtime, waiting time, and parts used, should be recorded and archived for analysis and stock control purposes.
- The details of main suppliers and secondary suppliers should be held for stored parts. It should be possible to raise purchase orders from within the system and to record supplier pricing and performance.
- The system should be capable of projecting future stock usage for planned maintenance and warn of possible low stock situations before they arise.

The system should be capable of analysing data on plant downtime, waiting time, maintenance time, part usage, and supplier performance in order that maintenance management may view the effectiveness of planned maintenance procedures on plant items and highlight troublesome plant items that may then be used to justify replacement. The system should also be capable of catering for unplanned maintenance tasks (breakdowns) in order that complete records of plant maintenance are retained.

Overview of Static Data

The core of an EMS is the static data and such data may include the following fields

- Type of work undertaken
- Craft skills employed
  - Employee name
  - Craft code

- Starting date
- Finishing date
- Average hours available
- Known absence periods
- Charge rates

- The departments serviced
- The priorities to be implemented
- Identification of any faults to be tracked
- Analysis headings for job delays
- The employees involved in maintenance work
- The plant items involved
- Interplant relationships
- The master work plan per plant item
- Security (who is allowed to do what)
- Checklist word processing (what checklists are required)
- Inventory management

Plant Register

Each plant item should be allocated a unique number. The format of this number should follow some logical structure to allow a visible hierarchy. Where plant items are related to each other in a hierarchical manner, the plant item number should reflect the relationship.

Maintenance of Static Data

The static data stored on the EMS are data that are set up at the initial installation of the system and are only updated when, for instance, an employee leaves, a new employee arrives, a new item of plant is purchased, a new maintenance procedure is put in place, and so on. The static data can also be said to include the basic stock control data (e.g., supplier's, inventory items and initial stock levels).

Generation of Work

The system should detail individual plant jobs, which may include the following:

- Skills required to complete it
- Stock items required to complete it
- Date the job is due
- Repeating frequency of the job
- Instructions required to carry it out

When a job becomes due, the system should automatically generate a report advising staff on where, what, and how to carry out maintenance tasks. This is the core function of the system—the ability to schedule work based on the availability of staff, their skills, job requirements, time constraints, maintenance interval, and stock items required. It is desirable to be able to plan ahead; therefore, the system should be able to record stock usage and project future stock requirements against current stock levels. This means that accurate stock levels can be maintained, which gives savings both in plant downtime and on excessive stock levels.

Analysis of Completed and Outstanding Work

The details entered after tasks are completed should provide information on

- Time actually spent on individual jobs
- Machine downtime
- Actual stock usage
- Resources used

As the system is used, actual times for maintenance jobs can be more accurately gauged and adjustments fed back to static job data. These data can then be used to improve scheduling accuracy.

Planned Maintenance Procedures

Where Planned Maintenance (PM) procedures have a GMP impact it is important to be able to include comments relating to items such as GMP checklists, critical features, and so on. It is important that the EMS outputs should cross-reference to the relevant Standard Operating Procedures (SOPs), IQs, OQs, and PQs in the PM procedures.

PREIMPLEMENTATION CHANGE MANAGEMENT

During the phases before implementation, it is important to define a method for the control of documents and changes to the system during development. It ensures that the most recent documents can be identified, previous versions are archived, and changes have been approved.

VENDOR REQUIREMENTS

Annex 11, clause 5, requires users to take reasonable steps to ensure that software has been produced in accordance with a Quality Assurance system. The vendor requirements deliverable, therefore, applies to vendor-provided products and services that may include all of the following:

- Computer hardware and software
- Operating procedures
- Maintenance manuals
- Operating manuals
- Support activities

The objective is to confirm that the vendor can support the validation of the system and that there is evidence of vendor-provided product quality. Generally, this activity will include a vendor assessment process. This activity should be initiated as early in the validation process as possible to determine if the vendor and the product can meet all of the validation requirements.

It very important when assessing an EMS vendor-supplied product to establish that the product has been under the control of the vendor's Quality Assurance procedures for the entire product life cycle. It is important to evaluate the relative risks regarding the vendor's capability, working relationships, experience, and customer base before committing to a contract.

When assessing the vendor of EMS systems, the following Quality Assurance activities should be assessed:

- Is the company ISO 9000 registered?
- Application software development methodologies
- Programming standards
- Formalised test procedures
- Change control procedures
- Software release processes
- Configuration management
- Documentation management
- Testing and acceptance
- Software metrics
- Client records and configuration management
- Help desk support activities and procedures

The most effective method of establishing if the vendor has an effective Quality Assurance process is an audit. This, however, is an expensive process. Due to the critical nature of an EMS system to a business, this is probably justifiable.

DESIGN

Certain features of an EMS's design are not generally available to the customer due to the fact that the vendor will regard such information as confidential and is not willing to divulge it. It has been our experience that it is possible to obtain access to this type of information if it is discussed before the placement of orders. This will most likely involve entering into formal nondisclosure agreements.

If this information is not available, this will somewhat restrict the scope of the validation. Where information is lacking, it should be established that the "common" use nature of many EMS packages will suffice in supporting its use.

Design efforts should be concentrated on providing the design documentation necessary or should be useful for the support activities of the end user technical support group. It is a requirement of the Annex 11 clause 4 to have a "written, detailed description of the system".

Another consideration is the disaster recovery plan, which may require the use of external software engineers to help with recovery. The availability of design documentation would certainly assist them in any recovery work that they may be required to carry out.

Design documents should include the following:

- Descriptions and Operation sequences
- Subsystem boundary definitions (interfaces between subsystems)
- Data flow diagrams
- System architecture block diagrams
- Physical input/output (I/O) layouts and configurations
- Database description (tables/files, indexing, linking, and field/column formats)
- Bill of materials and inventories for both hardware and software components

During the assessment of the vendor, it should be established that appropriate design documentation exists to support the validation of the system. When the information is held by the vendor, a reference/location/owner of the document should be provided so that it may be located when required.

SECURITY

The requirements for system security are referred to in the Annex 11, clauses 8, 13, and 14. An assessment of the risk to security and the method of implementation of the security measure for the items addressed should be made as part of the validation. Tables 1, 2, and 3 are sample assessments made for a typical EMS system. The risks involved can be devided into

- Physical security
- Procedural security
- Logical security

The tables document the perceivable security risks to a typical EMS package and the method of implementation of security measures for physical, procedural, and logical security.

APPLICATION SOFTWARE

When validating a system, one must identify and locate the following:

- Software source code
- Comments and annotations, if held separately from the source code
- Programming guidelines/standards used in the production of the source code

Software Possession

Where application software is considered proprietary in nature, as in the case of vendor-provided EMS packages, it is important to obtain statements from the vendor that their code would be made available to government regulatory agencies if requested during an inspection or investigations. The issue of source code availability may face legal obstacles if the software is considered proprietary or copyrighted. Escrow agreements for application software are designed to allow the client access to the source code under certain conditions. These may include

- Bankruptcy
- The vendor no longer supporting the product

TESTING

The requirements for testing are given in Annex 11, clause 7. During the assessment of the vendor, it should be established if software testing has taken

Table 1. Physical Security Assessment for a Typical EMS System

Aspects of Security	Perceivable Risk to Security	Implementation Method
I/O cabinets and panels	Access to the central processing unit (CPU) cabinet.	The CPU is located in a computer room that is controlled via card/ access codes.
Control rooms	Access to EMS terminals in the engineering workshop.	Workshop access is controlled via card/access codes.
Spare parts inventories	Spare parts are not kept for the EMS system.	Spares would be purchased when required as the system hardware is off-the-shelf (OTS) in nature. Software spares are available as part of the annual maintenance contract with Matrix.
Documentation libraries	Loss of documentation would cause inconvenience but would not stop the use of the system.	Use fireproof safes and dual storage of important documents. Covered by the EMS Operation Procedure.
Software media storage facilities, both off-site and local	If lost, backup tapes would incur a large amount of preparatory data entry on recovery from a system fault. This would entail an enormous amount of effort, but the system could be recovered.	Use fireproof safes and multi-location backup storage as described in the EMS Operation Procedure.
Programming or configuration terminals and keyboards	Programming/configuration is possible through all user terminals.	Physical access is possible, but password security would prevent logical access.
Development systems, process simulators, and system development tools	N/A, EMS is a proprietary product. The development facilities are not available are not available to Eli Lilly.	N/A
Other aspects of physical security not covered in the above points	Network security.	Covered separately.

place during the development of the package. A review should be made of the test specifications and test plans for the software ensuring they have been reviewed, documented, and approved for use.

When the EMS has been configured to meet the client's requirements, it is important to test the completed system. This will require that data are held on the completed system. It should be agreed if all data must be checked or if random sampling may be used in order to ascertain data integrity.

The following should be considered:

- How many of the records must be checked?
- Can automated testing be used?

Table 2. Procedural Security Assessment for a Typical EMS System

Aspects of Security	Perceivable Risk to Security	Implementation Method
Password modification, user account additions, modifications, and deletions	Access to the system by unauthorised or untrained personnel	The system administrator is the only person having access to password/ account modification/addition as per the EMS Operation Procedure.
Card/key control and distribution	Physical access to equipment	The EMS may be located in offices that have controlled access, such as the engineering or production offices. Access to these areas is generally controlled by site security procedures.
Cipher lock combination changes	Physical access to equipment by personnel no longer authorised to enter a controlled area	The EMS may be located in offices that have controlled access, such as the engineering or production offices. Access to these areas is generally controlled by site security procedures.
Removal of authority when personnel cease to work in an area	Physical access to equipment by personnel no longer authorised to enter a controlled area	The EMS may be located in offices that have controlled access, such as the engineering or production offices. Access to these areas is generally controlled by site security procedures.

Table 3. Logical Security Assessment for a Typical EMS System

Aspects of Security	Perceivable Risk to Security	Implementation Method
Access rights	Access to the system by unauthorised or untrained personnel	Personnel are given access passwords only to those parts of the system they are authorised and trained to use.
Verification of identity	Access to the system by unauthorised or untrained personnel	Each trained, authorised individual has his/her own, unique password.
Provision of authorisation	Provision of access rights to unauthorised individuals	Each individual must be both trained and authorised by his/her manager in order to apply for access rights. This is by means of a security form provided in the EMS Operation Procedure.

Automated testing will involve software that has been written to read data and check the data's integrity against predefined parameters. The whole subject of automated testing is a very complex area and requires thorough investigation before being initiated. Software-based automated test tools will require validation. Potentially, this could be as extensive as the validation itself and will raise its own issues and problems.

Once the test method is agreed on, then the following tests should be considered:

- Record completeness (all required fields as per procedures are filled in)
- References to other files/records are correct (referenced record exists)
- Internal structure links (record to record) are complete
- Data duplication (Does more than one copy of the same record exist?)
- Data conformity (In free format fields where procedures exist for company specific formatting, are data being entered in the correct format?)
- External references correct (When locations, serial numbers, part numbers, and so on reference objects external to the system, check that referred to objects exist.)

Event-driven functions must be tested by providing the correct external stimulus to initiate them. This may include clock-related report generation. Event-driven functions can be driven by simulating the events or by testing in operation under test conditions. Sequences of data, conditions, and events must be specified for each function test, together with the expected effects/results. For all of the above, pass/fail criteria should be specified.

Once the tests are agreed on, a test protocol for applying the tests should be produced. This protocol is not just for use once. It may be used on a periodic basis to ensure that the system is still performing as designed or when modifications and updates have been implemented. It should provide all the instructions for carrying out tests including the following:

- A list of tests
- Test procedures, including how failures are handled
- Acceptance criteria
- Documentation requirements before, during, and after each test
- Sequence of tests

Functional testing of the completed system may typically include the following:

- System security and access testing
- Work order scheduling

- Automatic reordering of spare parts
- Work order completion testing
- Work order reprint

OPERATIONS

All manuals and documents required for the operation of a system must be provided. Any logs recording system faults, maintenance, and so on must be maintained. This means locating and reviewing the following documents on a regular basis:

- System support procedures
    1. Start-up and shutdown of system
    2. Initialising programs
    3. Mounting tapes/disks
    4. Logbook usage for system start-up, backup, downtime, and archiving
    5. Backup of data and software
    6. Data archiving
    7. Adding and removing accounts and changing access privileges as described in the security procedures
    8. Making changes as per the postimplementation change control product.
    9. Conducting periodic reviews as per the postimplementation periodic review product
- Maintenance procedures
    1. Cleaning tape/disk drives
    2. Replacing any filter elements
    3. Cleaning printer carriages
    4. Replacing printer ribbons
    5. Running system diagnostics
    6. Checking voltages
    7. Calibration checks
    8. Electrical safety checks

- Service contract details
    1. What component serviced
    2. Date and time of service
    3. Reason
    4. Who requested?
    5. Who performed?
    6. Nature of service
    7. Who performed hardware test?
    8. How was hardware test performed?
- User manuals
    1. Proprietary
    2. Internal procedures for use of system
    3. Action required on alarms
- Vendor documentation (software and hardware)

BUSINESS CONTINUITY PLAN

The requirements for alternative arrangements in the event of a system failure are referred to in the Annex 11, clauses 15 and 16. The continuity plan is more commonly known as a disaster recovery plan or contingency plan. The impact of the system becoming unavailable in unforeseen circumstances on the customer's business must be evaluated. The impact of unavailability is for the customer's management to quantify. The plan to provide continuity in such an event is as minimal or as detailed as the customer dictates. It is important to consider the impact of data loss in this scenario.

Based on the customer's needs assessment, the business continuity plan should cover all critical systems, including identification of

- Installed hardware inventory that including all of the information required for the purchase of replacement equipment.
- Software inventory, including the version and revision numbers of all proprietary and application dependent software.
- Spare parts requirements and the location of those held as spares. Written assurances of supply and lead times on components not held locally.

- System recovery personnel. Those who are called in an emergency. List contact numbers, addresses, and specific responsibilities.
- Off-site location of archived software, should it be required
- Procedures for rebuilding the system software from archived material.
- Emergency operation procedures to continue operation during downtime and subsequent recovery periods.

Procedures for updating the system after a period of downtime from data produced by the previously mentioned emergency operation procedures.

TRAINING

List all documents and courses covering:

- How to operate computer equipment described in the user manuals and execute system support functions.
- How to perform actions that satisfy the procedures described in the operations product
- Programming standards (on in-house software)

Training material should be reviewed, where missing or falling short of requirements new training material should be produced. Make sure that all procedures referenced in the validation package are addressed in the training material so that all personnel having responsibilities placed them are aware and capable of carrying them out.

SYSTEM ACCEPTANCE

The system acceptance validation product will provide evidence that the validation described in the Validation Plan has been satisfactorily carried out. This should involve a summary report of the validation work performed and the results obtained. The use of a checklist to ensure that all validation deliverables have been completed is recommended. The report should conclude with the justification for acceptance of the system being "validated". The report should be formally signed off by management and the Quality Control unit; the system may only be implemented after this formal sign-off.

POSTIMPLEMENTATION CHANGE CONTROL

The importance of change control is indicated in Annex 11, clause 11. Thus, it must be possible to audit all postimplementation changes to the system. A change control procedure should include the following:

- Nature and type of changes permitted or prohibited
- Prechange request notification
- Criteria and requirements for testing and evaluations necessary to demonstrate that changes do not adversely affect system performance
- Responsibilities and procedures for formal authorisation to implement changes
- Documentation of system performance
- Postchange review and approval authorisation
- Postchange notification of implementation completion (i.e., acceptance of change in operation)
- Postchange documentation retention

Change control records should include the following:

- Unique change identifier
- Origination date
- Requester name
- Identification of component or software module to be changed
- Description of change
- Reason for change
- Change implementor
- Identification of systems and documentation affected
- Test plan
- Test results
- Formal review and approval documentation

Proprietary software product updates must be checked at two levels. The first is to make sure that installation is as per the supplier's instructions (i.e., checking dipswitch settings, option settings, etc.). The second check is to make sure that the changed software operates as expected according to the testing product for retrospective verification. This should include the reexecution of all or part of the original test protocol.

RECORD RETENTION

It is a requirement that all of the records (documents, files, software, etc.) referenced in this file should be available for inspection just as any other company asset is. Procedures should be in place or created so that the following may be achieved:

- Protection of information regardless of media (include storage of copies in an off-site building to protect against fire, etc.).
- Definition of retention period.
- Classify documents according to company requirements.
- Specify who is responsible for the maintenance of each record.
- Location of all media (files, disks, etc.)
- Provision for record security.
- Provision for updating record media, should existing media become obsolete or should media reach end of life (a point safely prior to the manufacturer's specified degradation period). Obsolescence could also be considered.
- Provision for disposal of records after the designated retention period has expired.

PERIODIC REVIEWS

Annex 11, clause 17, requires the recording and analysis of errors to enable corrective action to be taken, hence, a system of postimplementation periodic reviews should be in place. This should include the following:

- Schedule to determine the frequency of periodic reviews.
- Schedule for items to be reviewed at review time.
- Responsibilities by group and job function for initiating the periodic reviews.
- Report of the review process, including the following:
    1. System identification
    2. Reviewer name(s)
    3. Date of review
    4. Date of previous review
    5. Summary of review findings
    6. Action plans to address outstanding or open issues
    7. File report in validation package

- A formal review of the report should occur and the signature(s) of the reviewing personnel should be filed with the report on a separate form.

The review should include the following:

- Self-audit of the system (check it is all there)
- Examine maintenance logs, system logs, and so on.
- Changes since last review (software updates, documentation updates, etc.—audit)
- Security measures
- Verify correct software loaded
- Check spares and procedures comply with continuity plan
- Check training plans (are they up to date with system changes?)
- Preventative and corrective maintenance check
- New software adheres to standards
- Interview end users for comments

CONCLUSION

The validation of an EMS should follow the life-cycle model in the same way as all computer system validations. The "Static Data" are critical to the use of an EMS package, and particular emphasis should be placed on the input of data and checking of this data to satisfy the requirements of the Annex 11, clause 10.

The ability of proprietary configurable software to meet the required validation standards varies considerably. A key element of validation effort will involve the vendor and the vendor assessment process. The software and the vendor should be investigated thoroughly prior to implementing or purchasing the software. Too often, the validation is only considered once the system has been delivered and installed.

ACKNOWLEDGMENTS

We would like to acknowledge the work done and the assistance provided by Mr. William Spragg of Eli Lilly, Mr. Chris Ruffell of Eli Lilly, Mr. Martin Gatsby of Optimal Ltd, and Mr. Tim Cronin of Tritec Ltd who assisted in the validation of our EMS packages.

REFERENCES

1. *Guide to Good Manufacturing Practice for Medicinal Products* (Rules and Guidance for Pharmaceutical Manufacturers, Part Four).

2. U.S. Code of Federal Regulation Title 21, Part 211 (last amended 1995), *Current Good Manufacturing Practice for Finished Pharmaceuticals.*

3. GAMP Forum (1996), *Supplier Guide for Validation of Automated Systems in Pharmaceutical Manufacture,* 2nd ed. UK GAMP Forum and the International Society of Pharmaceutical Engineering.

Case Study K

Validating Building Management Systems

Terry R. Lucy
Glaxo Wellcome Operations
Dartford, England

The objective of a Building Management System (BMS) is to centralise the monitoring, operation, and management of a processing building or unit. The rationale for installing such a system is that critical process and building environmental parameters, such as room pressures and temperatures, can be maintained and recorded. Another benefit of installing a BMS is that energy is used in a more efficient manner and costs are, thereby, reduced. In the process of meeting these objectives, the BMS has evolved from a simple relay and timer-based system to a totally integrated system using modern microelectronics technology. However, software must be written by the BMS vendor to drive the controllers. If failure of the BMS could, on review, effect patient safety, then regulations [2,3] dictate that this software must be validated.

The BMS market has typically been at the lower specification end of the control system spectrum, because user requirements from such a system are typically

- Low cost
- Reliability
- Background running

This leads to a more tried and tested system being used, as computing speed is not of great importance. Typical control within the building takes place over minutes rather than the milliseconds required by some processes.

An Environmental Management System is a system that optimises the operation, temperature, and processes of an HVAC (Heating, Ventilation, and Air-Conditioning) system within a process building or unit. An Environmental Monitoring System for a new building is essentially a subset of the BMS, the only difference being that the Environmental Monitoring System is configured only to monitor data points and not to control. Indeed, it would be possible that the BMS and Environmental Monitoring System could be on identical control hardware platforms. The aim of the monitoring system is to provide a feedback of plant conditions that is independent of the BMS.

PLANNING

The first task is to decide if computer system validation is required. The purchasing company should have a procedure in place to cover this activity. The elements of this procedure should include the following:

- Identify system
- Define system extents
- Set up a review team
- Undertake a review
- Document decision
- Sign off by Quality Assurance

The review team would normally consist of a

- User
- System expert
- Quality Assurance representative

The following seven points should be considered by the team:

1. The user company policy.
2. The main function(s) performed by the BMS.
3. Where relevant or known, the main hardware and software components.

4. The impact of an unnoticed computer system failure on patient safety, product quality, and business interruption.
5. Any control measures, both existing and proposed, that would reduce the impact of an unnoticed system failure.
6. Computer systems that are not controlling critical processes related to sterile parenteral products and whose critical functions are regularly and independently verified will not require validation.
7. Some parts of computer systems, or software components of systems, may be regarded as "industry standard".

A justification for not validating must be approved by Quality Assurance. For a flowchart of the process, see Figure 1.

During this activity, it should be remembered that computer system validation (CSV) is not the only solution. Points for the team to consider are as follows:

- Identify critical functions.
- Only validate these functions if possible.
- If not feasible, consider the economics of installing independent monitoring on these critical elements.
- Document this decision.
- Have Quality Assurance approve the decision.
- Have a calibration system in place for any critical instrumentation.
- If all of these alternative strategies fail, consider replacing the system.

It is important to remember that the installation of independent monitors should only be undertaken when CSV is demonstrably not practicable. Where the system is critical, such as on an autoclave, it may be more economical to replace the control system, rather than try to validate it.

Now, let us assume that from this procedure CSV is required. The next task is to plan how the CSV is to be undertaken. This plan is a crucial document. From experience, the best method to create the plan is to set up a small team, consisting of the user, system expert, and Quality Assurance representative.

This team has the same composition as the review team mentioned previously. The team should determine what the crucial functions are. This is especially important for a BMS, as it is likely that only a part, often a small part, contain critical functions that impact on Good Manufacturing Practice (GMP). Also, the plan must include what documents are required, when they will be produced, and by whom.

Figure 1. Decision Tree

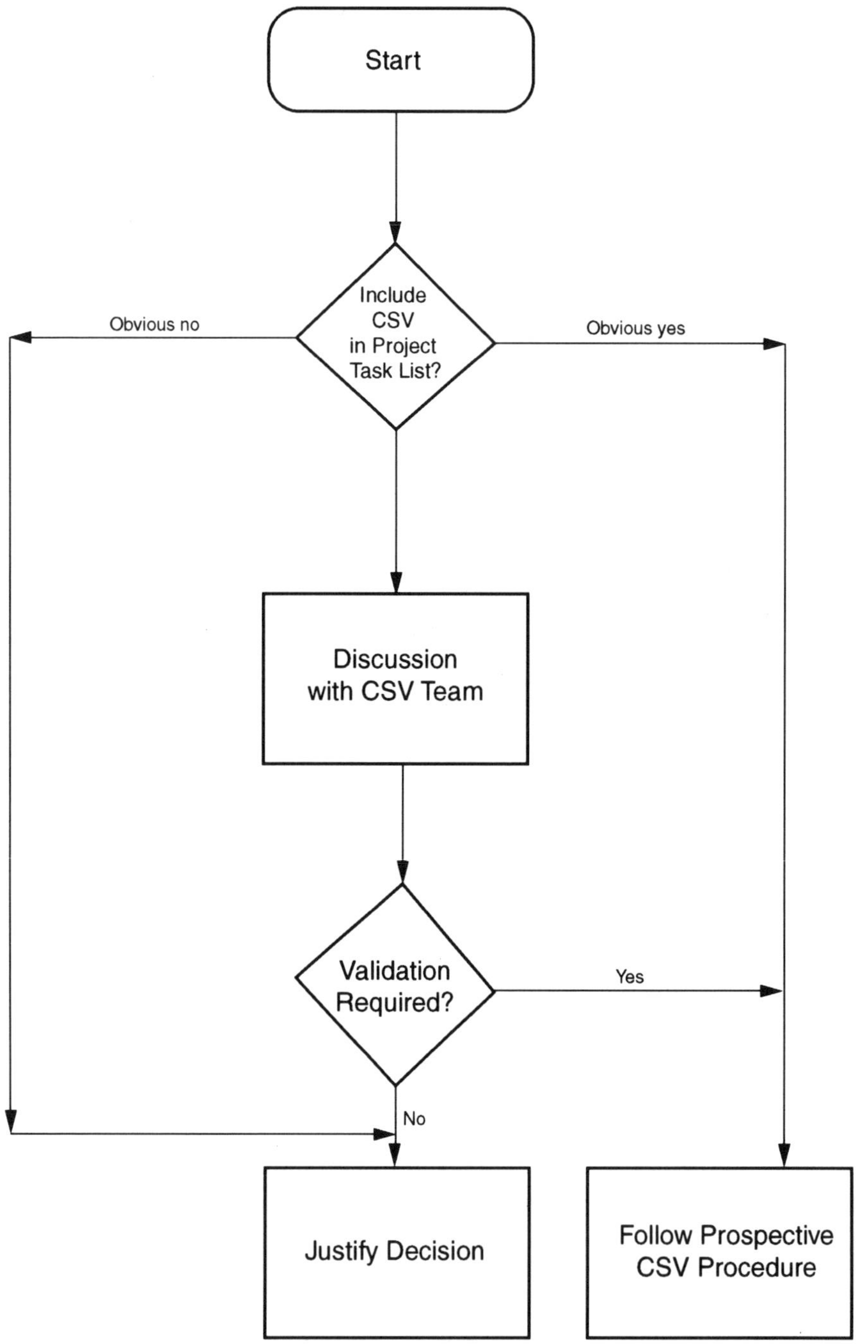

Because the BMS tends to be a hybrid system, the team should consider carefully any "industrial standard" software used within the system. The consideration of "industrial standard" software by the team can, in the author's experience, considerably reduce the amount of CSV effort involved, although it must be justified in the plan.

"Industrial Standard" software has been divided into five categories by the Good Automated Manufacturing Practice (GAMP) [1]:

1. *Operating Systems:* Established, commercially available, operating systems that are used in the pharmaceutical industry and can be considered validated as part of a project (e.g., DOS, Windows, etc.).
2. *Standard Instruments, Controllers, and Smart Instrumentation:* These are driven by nonuser programmable firmware (e.g., microcontrollers, bar code readers, and weigh scales).
3. *Standard Software Packages:* These are canned or COTS (commercial off-the-shelf) configurable packages in the United States (e.g., Lotus 1-2-3, Microsoft Excel, and other spreadsheet packages).
4. *Configurable Software Packages:* These are custom configurable packages in the United States (e.g., Distributed Control Systems [DCS], Supervisory Control and Data Acquisition [SCADA] packages, Manufacturing Execution Systems [MES], some Laboratory Information Management Systems [LIMS], and Manufacturing Resource Planning [MRP II] packages). Some BMSs fall into this category. The system and its hardware platform should be well known and mature before being considered in this category, otherwise category 5 should apply.
5. *Custom-Built or Bespoke System:* The full life-cycle model approach must be followed for all parts of the system.

Typically, a BMS is a mixture of categories 1, 2, and 4. It is important that the Validation Plan for the whole system identifies the validation extents.

SUPPLIER AUDIT

The BMS tends to be at the lower end of the control spectrum; the next activity, therefore (i.e., that of Supplier Audit), is also an important task. As BMS vendors generally supply to the construction industry, they have little experience in GMP and the resulting requirements for CSV. GAMP [1] gives the following guidance:

Summary of an Accreditation Procedure

Software supplier accreditation is the prospective examination of the methods and working practices of a supplier to establish its capability to produce software of a quality acceptable to the customer.

Organisation

The accreditation team consists of two or more people covering the roles of

- User representative (expert in process/business): This person must be briefed on the auditing technique prior to the audit, and will assist in the audit by having a detailed knowledge of the type of system to be installed.
- An expert in the type of software system for which the supplier is being considered: This person's role will be to have enough knowledge to judge the quality of the system. To assist in the audit, this person will be briefed on the auditing technique prior to the audit.
- Software audit coordinator (who must not be a member of the supplier's organisation): This person acts as the lead auditor.

Scope

The procedure should only consider aspects of the software supplier that impact on software quality. Other aspects of supplier accreditation (e.g., commercial evaluation) are not included. Source Code Review of "standard software" should be undertaken on software were the quality system used to create it is not known or is found to be unacceptable.

Procedure Flowchart

A flowchart indicating the activities of the accreditation team is given in Figure 2. The following sample supplier's assessment questionnaire can also be used by the accreditation team.

Sample Supplier Assessment Questionnaire

1. Are you registered to BS 5750, ISO 9000, or TickIT? If so, which parts and when? By whom?
2. What project team structure do you use? Who is responsible for software Quality Assurance?
3. How do you establish user requirements?

Figure 2. Audit of Suppliers

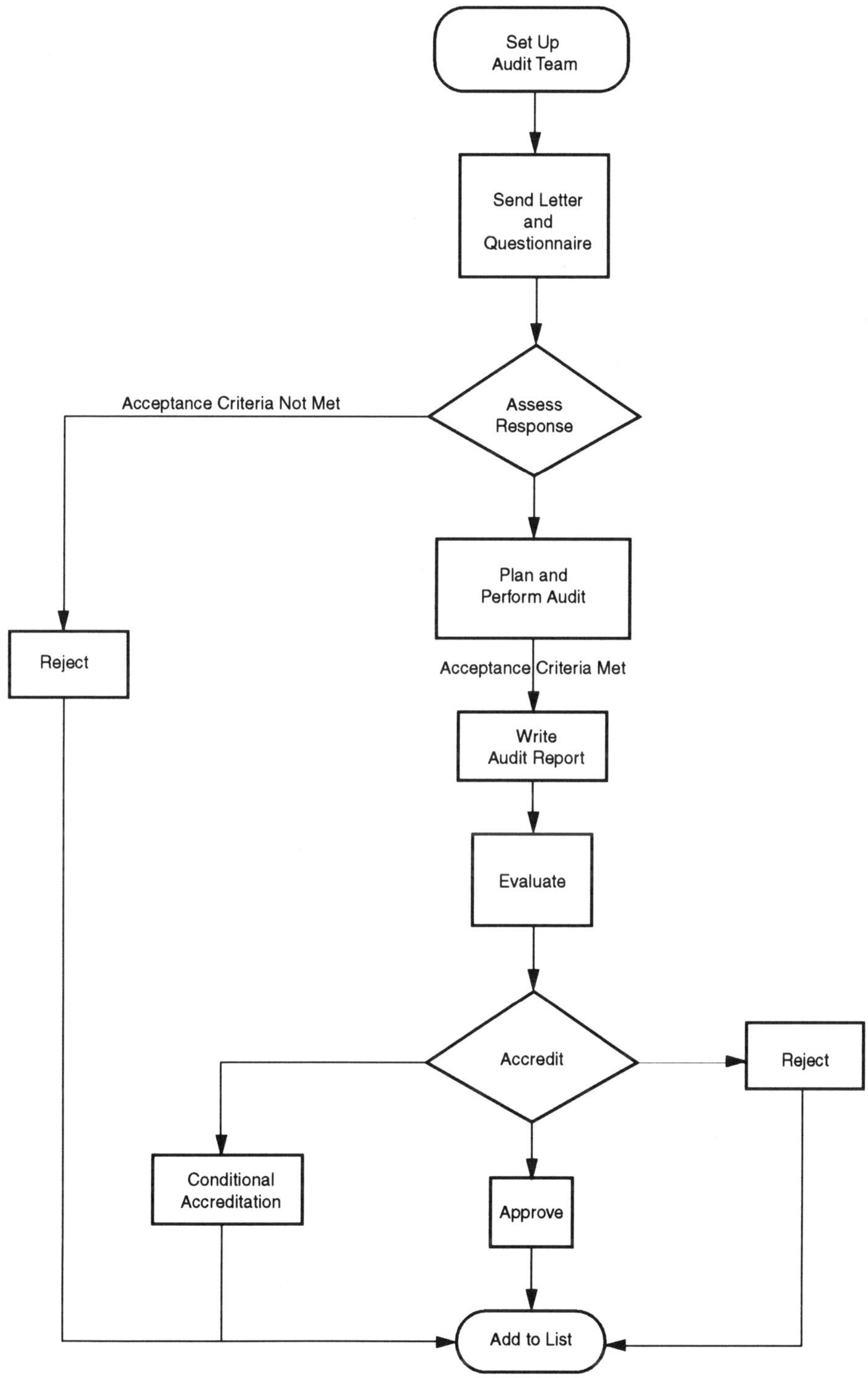

4. Is a quality plan in place for every project? Who compiled and approved it? How do you ensure compliance?
5. What development life cycle and methodologies are used for developing the system?
6. What are the products/deliverables for each phase of the life cycle?
7. How do you ensure that the user requirements are addressed?
8. Describe the document review techniques used, and how the reviewers are qualified for the task.
9. What test strategies and levels of testing are used for verifying that the computer software will meet its requirements?
10. What tests would you perform for each level of development?
11. How do the developers satisfy themselves that their testing is effective?
12. Who are the approval signatories for each document type produced on a project, and how are they qualified to approve the documents?
13. Please describe any change control procedures used during development and how proposed changes are approved and by whom.
14. Please describe any fault reporting procedures used on a project. (A fault is an error discovered in an approved product/deliverable.)
15. Do you use subcontractors for any part of software development?

SYSTEM SPECIFICATION

Normal documents (i.e., User Requirements Specification [URS] and Functional Design Specification [FDS]) are required. However, as the BMS is designed as part of the building design, it is not unusual for these specifications to be part of the building package. If this proves to be the case, then it is not necessary to rewrite these specifications. The recommended strategy is to create a map or index document that references those parts of the building package that are relevant to the CSV requirements for the identified critical functions. The Functional Specification is a crucial contractual document. Its contents typically contain the following information:

- *Control areas:* The areas of control and monitoring required for a specific building will vary depending on the type, the process involved, and other factors, such as humidity requirements.
- *Field instrumentation*

- Temperature range
- Exposure to corrosion
- Vibration
- Hazardous area requirements, if any
- Index of protection (IP rating) for hosing down
- Accessibility
- Calibration requirements
- Maintainability and spares

- *Outstations:* The location of outstations should take account of local instrumentation and area network requirements.
- *System controller and networking:* The controller should be capable of overseeing the networked system with response times suitable for the process controlled. The presentation of data that takes into account the variety of users on the system and the various levels of technical information required. Records and presentation handling will have to satisfy many statutory bodies, such as the UK Medicines Control Agency (MCA) [3] and the U.S. Food and Drug Administration (FDA) [2].

  The presentation of data may include the following:

  - Dynamic mimic displays
  - Graphical trend plots
  - Printed reports
  - Spreadsheets for processing data
  - Audible and visual alarms

DESIGN AND DEVELOPMENT

The BMS is generally a standard system configured to the user's requirements; therefore, little original design and development is required. However, as mentioned before, as the supplier has little knowledge of GMP, careful supervision is required to ensure that the configuration work and code testing are independently reviewed and documented. Another aspect to consider is how the "standard modules" are to be configured. A simple recompiling of source code elements may be required. If, however, special code needs to be written (e.g., to give a special function), then full validation of this element will be required.

SYSTEM BUILD

Build is normally part of the construction process. The supplier should install the system with supervision from the user. It should be remembered that, generally speaking, standard components from the vendor's range will be used so that no special build is required. However, sometimes marshalling and display cabinets will be required. Special care must be exercised with regard to the more modern components of a BMS that contain firmware. Design Qualification (DQ) on these components should be undertaken.

PREDELIVERY TESTING

It is recommended that as much factory testing should be carried out as soon as possible. This may be limited to a simulation of the controlling elements (i.e., the building is obviously not in place at this time). Full testing can occur only once installation in the process building is complete. The extent of Predelivery Testing should be specified in the Validation Plan. Often, the successful outcome of this testing is linked to stage payments and, therefore, should be carefully documented.

ON-SITE TESTING

Normal Installation Qualification (IQ) and Operational Qualification (OQ) procedures must be followed (e.g., the creation of test protocols and subsequent testing). It should be remembered that the GMP elements of this testing may be only a small part of the overall system. Therefore, these CSV elements should be combined with general testing. These tests should be uniquely identified and then a report created that summarizes these results with any conclusions as to whether the testing has been successful. Full account must be taken of the above Predelivery Testing. Again, the Validation Plan should define what retesting will be required. This can normally be limited to those critical functions that relate to GMP. It should not be underestimated how long this activity may take. Several (six) months is not uncommon. It should be noted that Performance Qualification (PQ) (i.e., testing the environment in all zones of the building) is normally carried out by operations. The overall Validation Plan for the project should give details of the requirements and the testing to be carried out.

Typically, the tests required would consist of the following:

- Check instrument calibration
- Wiring integrity tests
- Communication tests from outstations to main processor

- Loop function tests
- Mimic screen checks and moving from one screen to another using menus and function keys
- Running control algorithms
- Check functions with some degree of challenge testing for critical functions
- Alarm testing and subsequent control action

It is good practice for the BMS *not* to control the process (i.e., an alarm will not stop production). Relevant parameters identified at the process design stage should be printed out by the system for every batch. This report is attached, electronically for the most modern systems, to the batch report. It should highlight any deviations from the required parameters (e.g., high temperature or humidity). It is for the qualified person to decide on review of the batch documentation as to whether the batch is to be passed for sale or to be reworked.

REPORTING

The standard Validation Report is required. Due to the nature of the BMS, as mentioned above, it is likely that the majority of the report will only comment on and make reference to other documents. It is normally the case that these documents are too large to be conveniently attached to the report. It is important, therefore, that the location of these documents is referenced and is suitably accessible.

RETROSPECTIVE VALIDATION

It is the author's experience that retrospective validation of a BMS is virtually impossible, as the suppliers have little experience in the requirements of GMP. The only options that are sensibly available are as follows:

- Use alternative methods, such as independent monitoring.
- Scrap the system and replace with new.

CASE STUDY

A leading pharmaceutical manufacturer decided to upgrade its grinding and blending facilities for finished active drug substances by constructing a purpose-designed facility in a new building. The site was chosen as it was close to new, primary manufacturing facilities. The site is relatively new, with a site-wide BMS. The system consists of a central monitoring room, and a satellite station in each building. The new grinding and blending building could, therefore, be an extension to the existing site BMS. Because this was a primary facility, completed in 1987, no CSV on the BMS has been undertaken.

However, when an assessment was carried out as part of the overall validation exercise for the facility, it was found that a malfunction of the BMS could, under certain circumstances, lead to a loss of room pressure differential and, therefore, the possibility of cross-contamination. CSV of the BMS software was, therefore, required. As a first step, as required by procedures in place, an audit of the supplier was undertaken. The initial questionnaire was received. This indicated that there may be problems with the vendor's quality systems. However, due to the critical nature of this existing software to the project, it was decided that they would send in the audit team. This was undertaken some weeks later, and their concerns were confirmed. The supplier not only did not have a quality system in place, he did not know what one was! The audit report rating was "to impose a documented quality system on the supplier for any new contracts awarded." A subsequent review by the project team and their Quality Assurance section responsible for CSV compliance concluded that the existing software that was installed was unvalidatable, as it was uncertain as to the quality system that had been employed in its creation; in essence, to validate it would have meant the reverse engineering of the software and, from this activity, re-creating the required specification documentation from scratch. From this work, full IQ and OQ protocols would have needed to be created and carried out.

They were then faced with three choices:

1. Do not install the BMS system, but use manual control.
2. Rewrite the existing software so that it could be validated.
3. Install independent monitors on those critical control elements.

Item one was impractical, as the BMS was already installed by the contractor by this time, and item two would have been too expensive to justify, judged against item three. They then again reexamined the system to identify the critical elements. This turned out to be only the room differential pressures. It was decided that independent pressure indications and recorders would be installed. Retrospective validation of the existing software could then be eliminated. This decision, with all of the above reasoning, was documented and "signed off" by their Quality Assurance compliance department. It should be noted that to ensure compliance with the regulations, it is important that if you use this approach, a metrology system is in place that regularly checks the calibration of these independent devices. This calibration must be traceable back to national standards.

So what was the outcome of this exercise? Well, the above vendor was appalled at his accreditation rating. This was especially true when it was pointed out to him that if he continued in this manner, he would sell no more systems to the pharmaceutical industry. They, and other pharmaceutical companies, worked with the supplier to help him develop a quality system that meets other requirements. About 18 months after the first audit, he was reaudited and gained the accreditation "use but minor corrective action required." The supplier subsequently made the requested changes and was moved to "use for the production of BMS software."

The pharmaceutical company now plans to use this vendor to supply a BMS system for a new secondary manufacturing building to be used to make a variety of tablets. This system will be validated and, as such, no independent monitoring system is planned. The supplier is contracted to supply a large part of the validation documentation package and carry out the required testing.

REFERENCES

1. GAMP Forum (1996), *Good Automation Manufacturing Practice (GAMP),* Version 2. The Hague, Netherlands: International Society of Pharmaceutical Engineering.
2. U.S. Code of Federal Regulations Title 21, Part 210 (last amended 1994), *Current Good Manufacturing in Manufacturing, Processing, Packaging, or Holding of Drugs;* Part 211 (last amended 1995), *Current Good Manufacturing Practice for Finished Pharmaceuticals.*
3. European Union Guide to Directive 91/356/EEC (1993), Computerised Systems, Annex 11 of *Guide to Good Manufacturing Practice for Medicinal Products.*

Case Study L

Validating a Manufacturing Resource Planning (MRP II) System

Kate Samways
Rhône-Poulenc Rorer
Dagenham, UK

Manufacturing Resource Planning (MRP II) systems are many and varied—from discrete to process manufacturing—running on anything from a Personal Computer (PC) to a mainframe. To be able to claim that an MRP II system is validated, the environment in which it functions must also be validated and maintained in a state of control. In many instances, the realisation that the application software needs validating leads to the realisation that so does the hardware and operating system on which it runs and the network over which it is distributed. Often, this is the first system (business) to be validated, necessitating the implementation of a controlled infrastructure. Other case studies address the validation of that infrastructure—the hardware (AS/400, PC, peripheral devices, etc.), operating systems, and networks. This case study addresses the application software—the MRP II software itself. The validation of MRP II systems is relatively new (1990s) and is now receiving regulatory scrutiny. (There have been several 483s that specifically mention aspects of MRP II, e.g., stock control.) It may be expected that there will be an increased focus of attention on these systems in the coming few years to bring them more in line with the existing focus on systems associated with automated equipment and Distributed Control Systems (DCSs).

Validation should not be thought of as a task separate from other tasks in a project to implement something new. It is an integral part of the process. With this in mind, it is not surprising that any description of the process of validating an MRP II system resembles an MRP II implementation plan.

OVERVIEW OF THE MRP II PROCESS

MRP II systems assist a business in calculating demand for product (forecast plus customer orders), plan the manufacture according to the available capacity (manufacturing rooms, equipment), acquire materials in line with that manufacturing plan, and ship product to customers by the due date. The system must take into account all lead times—purchase, Quality Control testing (both raw material and product), and manufacturing. It will use lead time data and capacity data (facility availability, e.g., 8 hr/day; machine operating speed, e.g., 5000/hr; labour) to calculate a schedule to which product should be manufactured. An MRP II system is usually interfaced to both an Accounts Payable and an Accounts Receivable module of financial application software. MRP II systems may also be interfaced to other operational systems, such as a LIMS (Laboratory Information Management System) and an MES (Manufacturing Execution System). A schematic of an MRP II system is presenetd in Figure 1.

ELEMENTS TO BE CONSIDERED

There are many elements to be considered; the major ones are listed here [2]. Each is dealt with in turn in the remainder of this case study.

- Project Team
- Education
- User Requirements Specification
- Validation Plan and Validation Report
- System selection and Supplier Audit
- Design
- Testing, qualification, and reporting
- Procedures

Figure 1. Overview of the MRP II Process

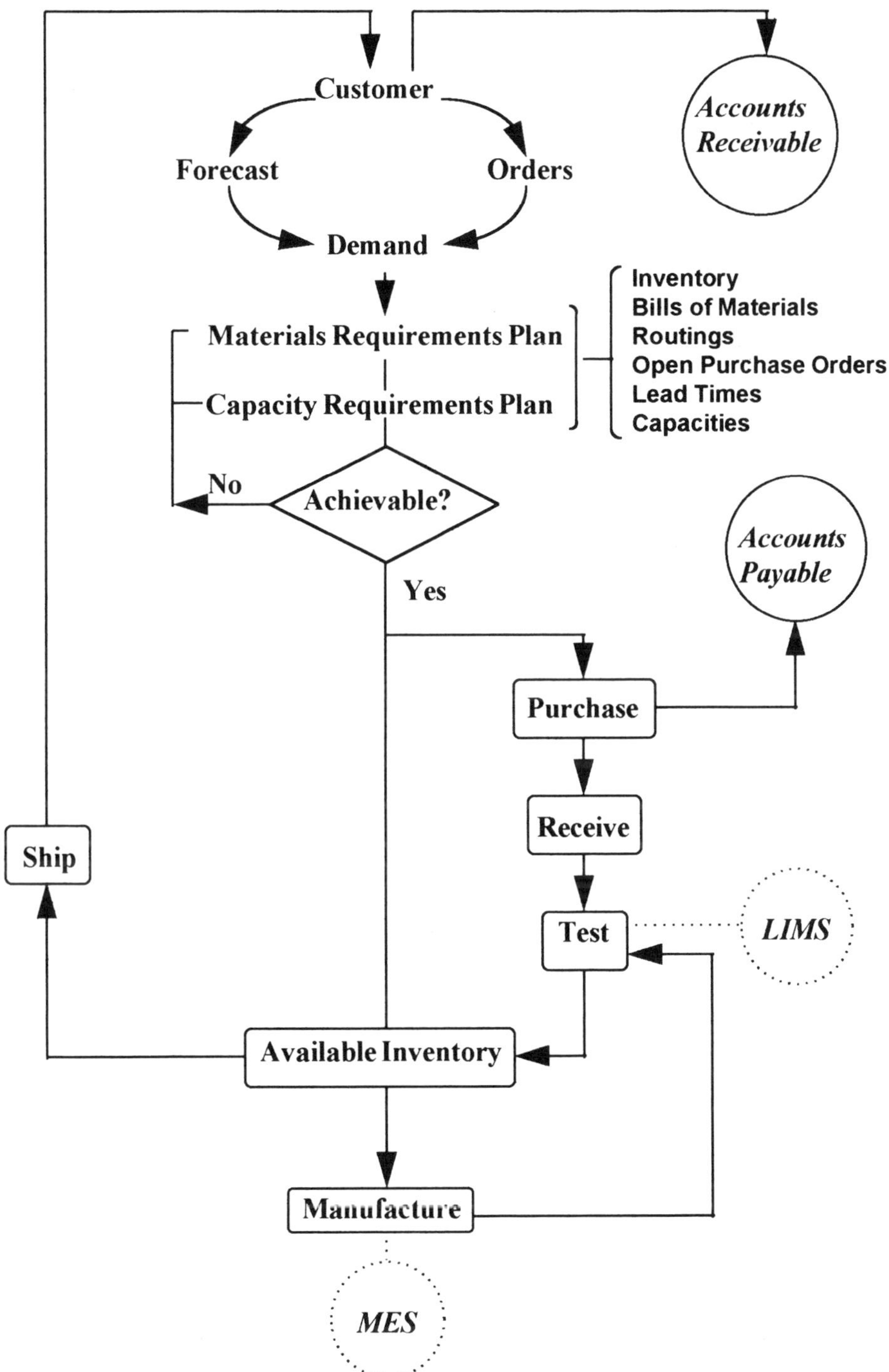

- Training
- Cutover
- Maintenance of the validated state

PROJECT TEAM

The MRP II implementation team will be multidisciplinary. One of the team members must be assigned to ensure that the "validation tasks" are completed appropriately (i.e., to the nominated standard, on time, in the correct sequence, and with correct approvals where appropriate). Depending on the size of the organisation and the complexity of the implementation, it may be necessary to appoint a validation team led by the assigned member of the MRP II implementation project team or it may be sufficient for the implementation project team to assume the workload. Whichever structure is most appropriate, those assigned to ensure the validation is completed must be trained to a level of competency [4].

The project team will need a project plan! The project plan will certainly detail all of the implementation tasks. It is the project team's choice whether the project plan also includes the details of the validation tasks/milestones. If the project plan contains only the high level "validation tasks", there must also be a detailed Validation Plan timetable. This plan must be overlaid on the implementation project plan timetable to ensure that all of the tasks are completed in the appropriate sequence and to ensure that the validation effort does not extend the implementation period. Implementation and validation are integral parts of the same process and, therefore, run concurrently. If we accept that project management costs are approximately 15 percent of the project cost, then validation, typically, adds a further 4–8 percent to the project cost. (It may be higher if this is the first business system to be validated and the infrastructural procedures are not in existence (see "Education" and "Procedures").

EDUCATION

The implementation team, even if most of them are not directly assigned to validation, must understand the requirements for validation and how the validated state will be achieved and maintained. Education, therefore, may well be necessary at several levels:

- An overview of validation for the implementation team
- The scope of the validation in relation to the functionality of the MRP II application software

- In-depth education for the validation team, if this is the first major system to be validated

During this phase, it will become clear that a number of "how to" guides will be necessary (e.g., how to write a User Requirements Specification [URS], a Design Specification, a Validation Plan, a test protocol, a Qualification Report, etc.). It is often possible to use already published guidelines such as Good Automated Manufacturing Practice (GAMP) [1] to assist, but it may also be necessary to adjust these generic guidelines to suit your business culture (corporate, global, multinational) and publish them in-house as Standard Operating Procedures (SOPs). These procedures are part of the infrastructure of systems management.

Without these standards with which to work, the validation effort will fail. With them, consistency in approach and content will be achieved and all the required elements will be covered.

USER REQUIREMENTS SPECIFICATION

The URS will be an approved document and must include *all* the functional and nonfunctional requirements. It should include all the *musts* and the *wants* (i.e., all the functions regarded as mandatory and all the functions regarded as "nice to have"). Each requirement should be uniquely numbered and identify whether this requirement has Good Manufacturing Practice (GMP) impact [3]. While care should be taken to avoid including a suggested design in the URS, it may be necessary to include some constraints (e.g., must be IBM compatible, must be able to be used in a cleanroom environment), which then limits the design choices. The numbering of the requirements allows cross-referencing to the Design Specification and, subsequently, to the test protocols and test scripts.

It has been assumed for this case study that the limit of the scope of the qualification testing is those features that impact GMP. However, an organisation may determine that the testing includes financial features of the system, in which case these should also be identified within the URS. It is best done at this point, as the Performance Qualification (PQ) will be based on the URS.

VALIDATION PLAN AND THE VALIDATION REPORT

Validation Plan

Following in-house approval of the URS, a first, high level Validation Plan can be written and approved. It is usually not possible at this stage to identify the detail of the qualification protocols; that will come when the Conference Room Pilots are completed and the design has been finalised.

The first version of the Validation Plan should identify, at least in principle, what tasks will be undertaken (e.g., a Supplier Audit); the deliverable documents and to what standard they will be produced; the personnel involved in completion of the "validation tasks"; a broad outline of the expected qualification protocols and the standard to which they will be executed; and the general acceptance criteria including those for qualification testing, training, and procedures.

When the Conference Room Pilots are completed, how the system will be used will be known. At this stage, it will be possible to update the Validation Plan to version 2, with the qualification protocols itemised and assigned to specific individuals for preparation, approval, and execution and full knowledge of the required procedures and training.

Validation Report

When each of the qualification protocols has been executed and reported on, the Validation Report can be prepared. The Validation Report will summarise the overall results of the qualification testing, identify the resolution for any discrepancies and draw a conclusion as to the suitability of the system for use. There are several possible conclusions:

- Pass (i.e., everything is satisfactory)
- Conditional Pass (i.e., the system may be used under certain conditions or with the introduction of some additional procedures or controls)
- Fail (i.e., there were sufficient adverse results to make use of the system unsafe from a GMP, or business, point of view)

SYSTEM SELECTION AND SUPPLIER AUDIT

With the URS approved, the MRP II system must be selected. The Request for Proposal (RFP) needs to contain not only the URS but also the

- Contact person
- Confidentiality requirements
- Timing
- Quality system requirements
- Cost constraints
- Purchasing terms and conditions

The RFP should request the following from a prospective supplier:

- A function by function response to the URS
- Cost (with breakdown)
- Training and support recommendations
- Timing
- Description of the quality management system
- Recommended customisation if the standard software does not meet the URS

Responses to the RFP must be evaluated: (1) for the product, to determine how closely it is matched to the URS, and (2) for the prospective supplier, to determine whether he produces a quality product and how well he will be able to support the implementation and maintenance of the product throughout its life.

The evaluation of the supplier as part of the response to the RFP will help to determine which supplier to target for a full audit. The response to the RFP alone will not suffice. A full Supplier Audit will confirm the responses contained in the RFP and serve to give assurances that the quality of the work done is adequate and that a written and approved Quality Management System is used.

It should be recognised that the audit will be the first one in a programme of audits of this supplier during the life of the software that is purchased from the supplier. The frequency of follow-up audits will depend on a number of factors:

- How well the supplier performed at the initial audit
- How frequently software is updated
- Whether the supplier will change technologies and, therefore, need to change the Quality Management System.

Certification to a recognised quality standard (e.g., ISO 9001/ISO 9000-3) does not necessarily assure that the supplier will meet your requirements. It does give some measure of assurance that the supplier has a Quality Management System in place that should assist the conduct of the audit.

With the advent of schemes to certify products, to adopt codes of practice for the development of software, and to conduct joint audits, it may become easier to make choices of product and supplier and minimise the need for each company to audit multiple suppliers and to audit at least one company on multiple occasions.

DESIGN

The design documentation has a number of elements:

- Hardware
- Operating platform
- Network over which the system is distributed
- Application software (MRP II)

Other case studies address the first three items; this case study addresses the application software.

MRP II systems have an enormous amount of functionality; some with GMP impact, some not; some you will need to use, other parts you will ignore as not useful to your business. To discover this in sufficient detail to achieve a successful implementation, it will be necessary to conduct a number of Conference Room Pilots (i.e., experiments that allow you to model the business process). Until it can be established how best to use the software in support of the business process, it is not possible to finalise the design. This series of Conference Room Pilots could also be considered to be a form of prototyping or configuration.

It will be helpful in the long term, if decisions made during the Conference Room Pilots are documented with the reasons for those decisions. Many MRP II packages allow choices in their setup that fundamentally affect the functional responses of the system and, without documented reasons, justification for the choices can be lost. This will help future change control. The design documents themselves require only how the system meets the requirements and need not include why.

For purchased packaged software, provided the supplier supplies both User Reference Manuals and Logic Manuals and the standard functionality meets the business requirements, a simple approach can be taken to the design documentation. In these conditions, it would be sufficient to identify the menu and option and/or programme that performs the function required, together with a brief description and a reference to the relevant parts of the User Reference and Logic Manuals.

Where it is necessary to make in-house modifications, these would have to follow a standard development life cycle and include a detailed design specification. It must be possible to code the change from the detailed design. Unit and Integration Testing must be conducted and documented.

At completion of the Conference Room Pilots and, thus, the design documentation, it is possible to identify the business and application procedures that must be produced to ensure that the system is used correctly. This will be a large task, not only in writing them but also in getting them approved and used in the training process.

TESTING, QUALIFICATION, AND REPORTING

Testing may be considered in two parts:

1. Unit and Integration Testing
2. Qualification

Qualification may itself be considered to be in three phases, each of which requires reporting on:

1. Installation
2. Operational
3. Performance

Unit and Integration Testing

Unit and Integration Testing is the responsibility of the supplier—whether that supplier is internal to your business or a third party. It is the documented testing that shows that each discrete piece of code functions as intended and, when programs are integrated, that the functionality is as expected (specified).

That the supplier carries out unit and Integration Testing must be one of the points addressed in the Supplier Audit. This must include establishing exactly what the supplier does, how, to what standard, and how it is documented. Other case studies in this book address the detail of unit and Integration Testing.

If the supplier does not do or does not document the unit and Integration Testing, the wisdom of doing business with him or of acquiring this software must be seriously considered. Alternatively, a detailed plan to test the structural quality of the software would have to be put in place by the customer.

Qualification

In considering what qualification to do, take into account all of the hardware, the operating systems, the network over which the system runs and all of the peripheral devices. Other case studies deal with these in more detail but, from the software point of view, it may include category 1 (operating systems), category 2 (smart instruments, e.g., bar code readers), category 3 (database management software), category 4 (the MRP II application software) and category 5 (custom-built) software. More details on how to deal with these categories are given in the GAMP Guide [1].

Focussing now on the MRP II application software, it is clear that there will be several qualification protocols. The scope for each one must be carefully considered and may approximate to the functional modules of the software (e.g., purchasing, inventory management, customer order management, shop floor control) or to business processes (see Table 1).

When developing protocols and test scripts, consider the origin of the data. For example, a business typically has a Financials package in place with supplier master records (for Accounts Payable) interfaced to a purchasing module (probably within the MRP II package) and customer master records (for Accounts Receivable) interfaced to a customer order management module (also probably within the MRP II package). To ensure the traceability of purchases and sales, it is necessary to test the interfaces to ensure the data are not corrupted.

Table 1. Data Elements That Should Be Considered in Validating an MRP II System

Lot Information	**User**
Lot Number	Name (and Password)
Lot Status	Security Access
Dates (e.g., expiry, receipt, issues)	**Item**
Quantity/Potency	Item Number
Conversion Factors	Item Notes
Lot Notes	Location (including storage conditions and cycle counting
Quality	Type
Purchase Order	Quality
Purchase Order Number	Shelf Life and Retest Days
Supplier Lot Number	**Shop Order**
Dates	Shop Order Number
Transactions	Quantities
Bill of Materials	Receipt Date
Items	Transactions (e.g., issues, receipts)
Quantity Per	**Customer Orders**
Units of Measure	Customer Order Number
Conversion Factors	**Supplier**
Work Centres	Quality Approval
Yield Factors	
Approval	

Installation Qualification (IQ)

The first phase of qualification—installation—may be jointly shared between the customer and the supplier. In any event, it must include not only installing the software to the supplier's instructions but also reviewing the availability and completeness of installation procedures—including those for change control and maintenance.

Operational Qualification (OQ)

OQ is that phase of the testing which shows that each piece of functionality works independently. It will include challenge testing (i.e., testing for data input at and outside the allowable boundaries), for example, ensuring that inventory transactions cannot result in an inappropriate quality status being applied to a resource/lot/location. It will not include testing for, say, alpha characters in a numeric field; this will have been done by the supplier (internal for a modification or the third-party supplier) as part of unit testing. OQ may be conducted on test hardware of an exactly similar nature to that which will be used in the "live" mode, loaded with an exactly similar operating system.

Performance Qualification (PQ)

PQ is the testing that shows that when the system is used with the mix of activities in the sequence that best supports your business, it consistently functions as expected. To be able to do this, all of the business processes must have been considered and all of the procedures defined.

In practice, it may be that the tests you define as necessary for PQ have actually been conducted at OQ in the sequence that best supports your business process. In this circumstance, there is no need to repeat the test.

PQ must be conducted on the "live" hardware and all software (irrespective of application type) that is intended to run on this machine/network must be loaded. It is usual to include in the scope of the PQ other activities, such as training and where a parallel run is required, this can also be included. Both of these points will be considered later in this case study.

Qualification Reporting

Each qualification protocol will have a corresponding report. Each report will summarise the results of the execution of the tests conducted as part of that protocol, identify the resolution for any discrepancies found and draw a conclusion. Hopefully, each passes unconditionally but there may be a range of results leading to an overall conclusion, when the Validation Report is written, of a conditional pass for the whole application.

PROCEDURES

As for any system, it is tempting to underestimate the time required to develop, write and approve the standard operating procedures (SOPs) required to support the use of an MRP II system. Some of these procedures will be general in nature and relate to the Information Systems infrastructure; others will relate to the business processes and to the use of the MRP II application itself.

"How to" Procedures

There must be a set of "how to" procedures to act as the reference standards for a number of the activities associated with software implementations and validation. It may be possible to use published guidelines for some of these or it may be necessary to customise them for your particular business. Examples of "how to" procedures necessary are as follows:

- Write a URS
- Write a Validation Plan
- Write a Design Specification
- Write a Qualification Protocol and Test Script
- Plan and conduct User Training
- Audit a supplier
- Manage documentation
- Develop applications

The "Standard" List

Additionally, there is the "standard" list:

- System access and security
- Backup/recovery/archive/retrieval
- Incident reporting
- Change control
- Maintenance
- Periodic review
- Contingency Plan

It is worth considering some of these in more detail here; others are addressed elsewhere.

System Access/Security

Apart from any site policy for systems access and security, it is necessary to address who may grant authority for access to each function within the MRP II system. One approach is to assign each menu (option or suboption) to the manager who "owns" that functional department (e.g., create purchase orders belongs to purchasing, receiving goods against a purchase order belongs to warehousing, creating bills of materials belongs to manufacturing, etc.). Then for each job type, create a profile of the options required to perform that job. For each menu/option/suboption in the profile, have the "owner" approve its inclusion in this access profile for this particular job type. Once this is in place, a new user with a particular job type can be granted access to the system (after suitable training!) with the already approved profile on the written authority of his departmental manager. As MRP II systems are functionally rich, there are multiple job types who use the system and many individual users. Therefore, this task should not be underestimated. As each user should have a unique USERID, each user access profile must be maintained. Often, this is delegated to the Information Systems department who must be in receipt of the written, approved authorisation request before updating any user profile.

Change Control

Change control needs to consider changes to

- Hardware
- Software
- Processes, and any interrelationship between them
- Planned and unplanned (emergency) changes
- The magnitude of the change

This latter item refers mainly to software. It may be feasible when implementing the fix for a single "bug" to conduct an impact analysis and limited testing; for a new release of the MRP II software, it will probably be more cost-effective to update test scripts as necessary (and perhaps, write a few new ones) and reexecute the OQ and PQ.

Periodic Review (Audit)

There may be a site policy on when and how to conduct periodic reviews (audits) of systems. However, each application subject to the policy will need its own specific checklist of things to be considered. For an MRP II system, the periodic review checklist should include the following:

- Review of business and application procedures for continued relevancy, accuracy, and expiry

- Review of training records to ensure that all of the user access profiles have a corresponding training record
- Review of access authorisations to ensure user access profiles have the corresponding written authorisation
- Review of audit trails for changes to key data, such as bills of material and resource master records
- Review of key audit reports, such as lot traceability and recall reports
- Review of the incident log to ensure that all "bugs" have been resolved satisfactorily (or are in process) according to the change control procedure.

Contingency Plan

The Contingency Plan identifies the actions to be taken in the event that the main system fails to function for a period of time and how the business will be managed during this emergency. While the system is nonfunctional, can the business continue to function using manual records? The Contingency Plan should detail how to manage this situation and how to record any actions taken (e.g., increments and decrements to inventory, placing purchase orders, filling customer orders).

The actions taken to bring the system back into use may involve a "temporary" solution (e.g., bringing an alternative computer on-site, loading the software and running, whilst the original computer is repaired or replaced). In this circumstance, consider what testing is needed to give assurance that the "temporary" solution is functioning in a controlled manner (i.e., is it validated?). Also consider the change control procedure to be followed to bring the repaired or new hardware into the system, how data will be recovered, and the system "cutover" from the temporary solution to the permanent one.

Business and Application Procedures

Finally, there are the business and application procedures. These relate quite specifically to

- The business processes to be used (e.g., how to route a manufacturing order through the plant)
- How to use the application to record something in the system (e.g., how to use the option to decrement inventory)

There are, of course, many business and application procedures that will be identified during the course of the Conference Room Pilot and that must be written and approved prior to user training. The writing of these procedures is best delegated to those who have the appropriate functional experience. They may be members of the project team or the task can be delegated to some of those who participated in the Conference Room Pilots.

USER TRAINING

There are four elements to be considered here:

1. Training plan
2. Training materials
3. Functional training
4. Training records

Training is usually considered to be part of the PQ.

Training Plan

The training plan details who will be trained to do what and demonstrates the timetable for that training. As MRP II systems are functionally rich and there are many job profiles and many users to be trained, the training plan is a critical feature of the implementation plan. Without it, not only the implementation will fail but also the overall validation, because a requirement of PQ is that all of the users be adequately trained *prior* to using the system "live".

Training Materials

Training sessions cannot be conducted without adequate preparation, and consideration must be given to the

- Objectives of this training session
- Structure of the session (the lesson plan)
- Data to be used
- Preparation of the database
- Training manual
- Training facilities

Functional Training

It is best to train users in small groups (no more than 10 people) and for each to have his own terminal for the hands-on sessions. After initial training in the basic functionality of the system, training sessions should be structured around the business processes. This allows cross-functional groups to interact in a "test" environment and helps to confirm that procedures (both business and application) are correct and appropriate.

Training Records

Training records are inspectable records. They must demonstrate who the trainer was, who were the trainees, and in what functions/processes/procedures they were trained. It will be necessary to keep these records up-to-date to account for any new users being granted access to the system at any time after the initial implementation and to account for any change to the functionality permitted for any user profile.

CUTOVER

In "cutting over" from the test system to the live system, it is necessary to show that the two are exactly similar. If this cannot be demonstrated, then none of the OQ and PQ is valid. It is also necessary to put in place a procedure to ensure that the data loaded to the new, live system have integrity. Whether the data have been keyed in afresh or converted from a previous system, it will be necessary to ensure that they are accurate. If they have been converted, then the conversion process/program itself must be validated.

In some circumstances, it may be decided to run a new system in parallel with the old system for a period of time. For MRP II systems, this is an enormous burden and should be considered carefully before being undertaken. It may be better to decide to monitor particular business processes for a defined number of iterations instead. In any event, if a parallel (or limited parallel) run is included in the project, make it part of the PQ. To achieve this it will be necessary to show that

- The OQ has been completed satisfactorily
- Procedures are approved and user training is completed. Then cutover can occur, the parallel run conducted and the PQ report written up. In this case, the PQ report includes the equivalent of the "cutover report".

If there is no parallel run, the PQ should be completed and reported on, the Validation Report should be approved and then cutover can occur. In this circumstance, there is NO alternative system to use. Therefore, it is essential that OQ and PQ have been appropriately completed successfully, the data load procedures have been followed and the data integrity has been reviewed. In the absence of a parallel run, *cutover is the "point of no return"*!

After a defined period, a cutover report should be produced to confirm the following:

- That the system is working as planned and expected
- The continued integrity of the data
- The set-up of the libraries, the job schedules, and so on

MAINTENANCE OF THE VALIDATED STATE

Once validated and implemented, the MRP II system must be maintained in a state of validation. There must be in place a policy and procedure for the periodic review (audit) of the system, change control, and incident reporting. It must be demonstrated that all relevant procedures are followed and in date, that change histories are available, that incidents are resolved and that training is up-to-date. The change control procedures will be critical for this aspect of maintaining an MRP II system.

REFERENCES

1. GAMP Forum/ISPE (1996), *Supplier Guide for Validation of Automated Systems in Pharmaceutical Manufacture,* version 2.0. UK GAMP Forum and the International Society of Pharmaceutical Engineering.
2. Samways, K.A. (1995), *The Validation of an MRP II System,* ISPE European Computer Systems Validation Seminar, 20–21 September, Zurich.
3. *Rules and Guidance for Pharmaceutical Manufacturers* (1993), The Orange Guide. HMSO. Crown Copyright 1993.
4. Samways, K.A., Sattler, L.M., Wherry, R.J. (1996), Computerised System Validation: One Company's Approach to Assigning Tasks and Responsibilities. *Pharmaceutical Technology* (August): 45–49.

Case Study M

Validation of Computer Systems in Analytical Laboratories

Ludwig Huber
Hewlett-Packard GmbH
Waldbronn, Germany

Computers are widely used in analytical laboratories for instrument control, data evaluation, and data management, and are subject to all validation and verification activities. Verification and validation activities to assess computer systems used in analytical laboratories cover all life-cycle phases, from Requirements Specifications, design, development, and manufacturing to installation and operation. In this case study, users of computer systems will find guidelines on

- How to define user requirements and Functional Specifications (FSs)
- Which type of documented evidence the vendor should provide to prove that the system was developed according to recognized standards

- How to validate and document software developed in the user's own laboratory
- How to proceed in cases where vendors do not give evidence of validation
- How to qualify a computer system at installation and for operation
- How to evaluate computer systems in analytical laboratories retrospectively
- How to ensure an ongoing performance control during routine analysis

This case study does not cover verification activities during development at the vendor's site. This is described elsewhere [1].

A computer system, as used in an analytical laboratory, consists of computer hardware, peripherals, and software to perform a task. It can perform different tasks:

- Instrument control, data acquisition, and data evaluation
- Laboratory information management

Figure 1 shows an example of a complex computer system that includes computerized analytical instruments for the collection and evaluation of

Figure 1. Computerized Laboratory

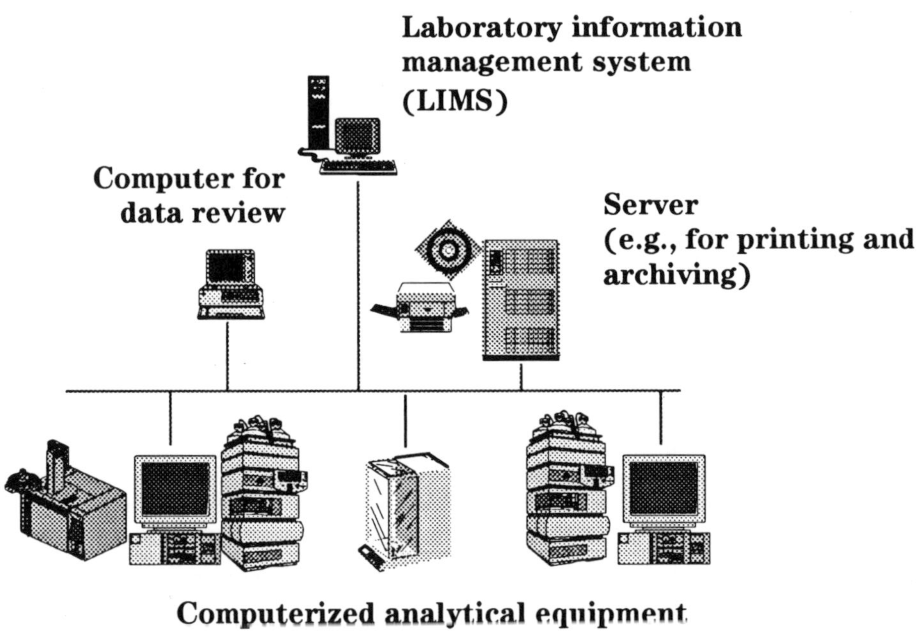

data, servers for data review and centralized archiving, and a laboratory management system.

On a computer used in analytical laboratories, we generally find three different software categories.

1. *System software,* such as operating software (DOS® or UNIX®), drivers, and file management, supplied by software vendors. These are supplied with the computer in a machine-executable format that cannot be modified by the user and is not unique to any one user's system. The correct function of this software is verified whenever an application runs under the system software.
2. *Standard application software,* for example, off-the-shelf chromatography software, generally supplied by an instrument vendor. The correct function should be verified during and at the end of development. The user must perform acceptance testing prior to use.
3. *User specific application software,* written by the user or by a third party for a specific user to meet the specific functional needs in the user's laboratory. Examples are macros to customize a system for specific user needs. This software must be validated prior to and during routine use.

OVERVIEW OF VALIDATION STEPS ASSOCIATED WITH COMPUTER SYSTEMS

Figure 2 illustrates the validation steps in an analytical laboratory from a user's point of view. For a specific project, validation activities should follow a 10-step validation plan.

1. The user requirements are set. These describe the analysis problem and include instrument performance requirements for a specific analysis task.
2. From the user requirements, the type of analytical equipment, and computer system, the functions and Functional Specifications are derived.
3. The user then selects a standard instrument and appropriate options.
4. A vendor should be selected who develops hardware and software equipment in accordance with a quality assurance system, for example ISO 9001.[1]

1. Steps 2 to 4 are sometimes called the Design Qualification. The user should verify that the design of the computer system meets the requirements and that the vendor meets the vendor qualification criteria.

Figure 2. Validation Life Cycle

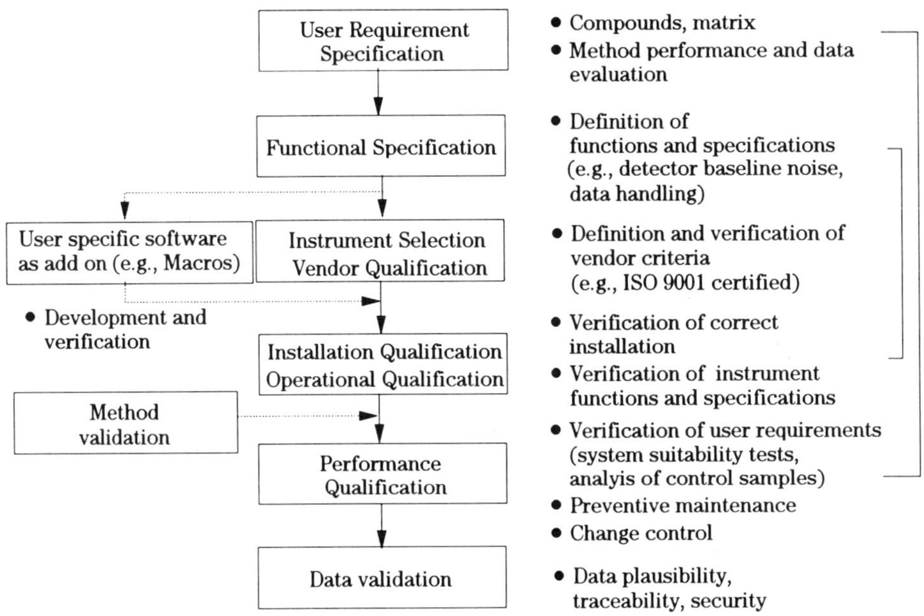

5. If the standard software supplied by the vendor does not cover all of the user's requirements, user specific software is developed as an add-on macro, either by the user, the vendor, or by a third party.

6. The modules are installed and put together as a system. Correct installation and operation should be verified against Functional Specifications as defined by the user, a process that is called Installation Qualification (IQ) and Operational Qualification (OQ).

7. The proper functioning of analytical methods should be verified on the new system. This covers testing of significant method characteristics, for example, limit of detection, limit of quantification, selectivity, and linearity. If the method has not been validated or if its scope did not cover the new instrument, the method should be either newly validated or revalidated.

8. The performance of the complete system should be validated against the User Requirements Specifications. The system combines the instrument hardware, computer hardware and software, and the analytical method. In chromatography, it also includes a column and reference standards for calibration. This validation, usually referred to as system suitability testing, tests a system

against documented performance specifications for the specific analytical method. Analytical systems should be tested for suitability prior to and during routine use, practically on a day-to-day basis.

9. When analyzing samples, the data should be validated. The validation process includes documentation and checks for data plausibility, data integrity, traceability, and security.
10. A complete audit trail that allows the final result to be traced back to the raw data should be in place.

Table 1 lists in chronological order the steps that a user of computerized analytical equipment can follow for the entire validation process.

The type and degree of validation of a computerized analytical system depends on its complexity. For example, the functions of a simple, computer-controlled system, with little or no flexibility regarding data input or

Table 1. Recommended Validation Steps with Examples

Step	Explanation	Examples
Define user requirements	Criteria: compounds, matrix, detection limit, precision, selectivity, accuracy, concentration range, qualitative or quantitative, throughput, regulatory requirements	Analysis of phenoxy acid herbicides in drinking water, detection limit: 0.01 μg/L, qualitative and quantitative information, electronic archiving of data, 30 samples/day Method and equipment: solid phase extraction and high performance liquid chromatography (HPLC)/diode array detection Computer for data evaluation
Define Functional Specifications	Define intended equipment hardware, software, and system functions and operational limits	HPLC: binary gradient, flow rate range 0.2 to 2 mL/min, diode-array detector with 10-mm path length, baseline noise less than or equal to $\leq 4 \times 10^{-5}$ AU, computer for integration, quantification, peak purity check, interactive and automated spectral library search, qualitative and quantitative report, system suitability testing and archiving of method parameters with raw data file
Select and qualify vendor-purchased equipment	Develop criteria for vendor selection and check if criteria are met	Quality system, availability of validation documentation, local support and response time, reputation and experience; information through documentation available from the vendor

Continued on next page.

Continued from previous page.

Step	Explanation	Examples
Develop user specific software	Macro, spreadsheet	Customized reporting; statistical evaluation
Qualify modules and systems prior to routine use	Installation Qualification, Operational Qualification	Check if shipment complies with purchase order. Test equipment (e.g., test the precision of amounts and retention times)
Validate methods (optional, if the methods are not already validated)	Specify validation parameters and acceptance limits Define and execute validation experiments	Limit of detection, limit of quantification, selectivity, linearity, precision, accuracy, ruggedness
Assure ongoing performance	Develop and implement schedules and procedures for periodic preventive maintenance, for calibration, and for initial and ongoing Performance Qualification	Calibration of balances; calibration of ultraviolet grating for wavelength accuracy; exchange of lamps; system suitability testing; analysis of quality control samples and evaluation of results using control charts
	Develop and implement procedures for error detection, recording, and handling	ROM check at system boot up; automated shutdown of pump if leak is detected in an autosampler or detector
	Develop procedures for change control	Authorize changes to user-written software
Assure validity, security, integrity, and traceability of data	Develop and implement security relevant procedures	Limited system access through user-specific passwords; data file integrity through checksum or other routines

evaluation, can be verified by executing holistic tests [2] and by comparing the test results with anticipated results. On the other hand, a more complicated computerized system with on-line databases and extensive flexible data evaluation requires complex validation.

ASSESSMENT OF THE NEED FOR VALIDATION AND THE VALIDATION PLAN

Before validation can begin, management should assess whether the system requires formal validation. Criteria to be considered are whether the system will be used in a regulated or quality standard environment and how critical the data generated by the system are. Examples of such environments are as follows:

- Good Laboratory Practice (GLP)
- Good Manufacturing Practice (GMP)
- ISO Guide 25
- European Norm EN 45001

When the decision has been made about the need for a system validation, sufficient resources should be allocated. For larger projects, the recommendation is to form a validation team consisting of Quality Assurance personnel and technical experts. All validation activities at the user's site should follow a Validation Plan.

USER REQUIREMENTS AND FUNCTIONAL SPECIFICATIONS

Requirements Specifications define how the system will be used. For an analytical system, these can include the following:

- The type of compounds and matrix
- The expected limits for detection and quantitation
- The expected precision and accuracy
- The number of samples in a given time frame and mode of operation: manual or automated
- The type of information: qualitative and/or quantitative
- The type of information calculated from original data, printed in the report and stored on electronic media
- Archiving of data

From the Requirements Specifications, the user can derive the instrument type and its minimal Functional Specifications. For example, if an instrument is scheduled to run overnight, the number of samples should be specified so that the system can inject automatically. The UV/visible detector's baseline noise specification can be determined from the specified detection and quantitation limit of an HPLC analysis. The required data evaluation will determine the demands on the evaluation software.

The next step is either to select an existing system for the analysis task or to purchase a new system. When a new system is purchased, it is often purchased not just for a specific analysis but also for use in general applications in the laboratory. In this case, the Requirements Specifications should include a representative mix of the anticipated applications, and the FSs should be set such that the instrument can handle all of the requirements. Next the user should look for an instrument on the market that best meets these requirements. If the selected system does not provide all of the functions, for example regarding software, the user can decide whether to develop these himself.

RESPONSIBILITIES OF VENDORS AND USERS

New software and computerized systems in analytical laboratories are usually purchased from a vendor. A frequently asked question is who is responsible for the validation of such a system: the vendor or the user? The Organisation for Economic Co-operation and Development (OECD) states clearly in consensus paper number 5: "It is the responsibility of the user to ensure that the software program has been validated" [3]. This is also the practice of the U.S. Food and Drug Administration (FDA) as specified by Ron Tetzlaff, a former FDA investigator: "The responsibility for demonstrating that systems have been validated lies with the user" [4]. However, it is obvious that product quality cannot be achieved by testing in a user's laboratory. This must be incorporated during design and development. Therefore, the OECD makes a further statement in a new consensus paper [5]: "There should be adequate documentation that each system was developed in a controlled manner and preferably to recognized quality and technical standards (e.g., ISO 9001)". Furman et al. [2] from the U.S. FDA also make it clear: "All equipment manufacturers should have validated their software before releasing it."

- The vendor is responsible for assuring that the system is developed, tested, and supported according to proper development and change control procedures.
- The user is responsible for the entire validation. One part of this overall validation process is to obtain documented evidence about the proper development according to documented standards. To have this assurance, a vendor assessment program should be developed that may include formal written procedures for the selection, evaluation, and qualification of vendors.

One criteria for vendor qualification should be whether the vendor has a documented Quality Assurance program that follows recognized quality standards, for example, ISO 9001. This registration is usually sufficient for those laboratories that must comply with ISO 9001 or with a laboratory accreditation standard, such as ISO Guide 25 or EN 45001. However, it is the author's experience that regulatory agencies do not always accept such third-party evaluation or successful registration according to ISO 9001, or the equivalent, as proof of a vendor's qualification. They expect vendors to have other proof of qualifications, such as documented familiarization of their staff with software development practices, GLPs and cGMPs, procedures for software backup, archiving and periodic integrity checks, a software tracking and response system, or references from internal or external users of the system. Frequently, additional documents are requested, such as development validation certificates and an assurance by the vendor of accessibility to the source code by regulatory agencies.

VALIDATION OF NEWLY PURCHASED SYSTEMS WITHOUT EVIDENCE OF VALIDATION FROM THE VENDOR

If a vendor is not able or willing to provide documented evidence of validation, the user should consider selecting another vendor: This recommendation is easy to follow if there are a number of competitors for the same or similar products. If this is not the case, for example, when special software for an emerging technique is required, a user may purchase the software anyway, but should evaluate the vendor and perform more thorough testing and keep more detailed documentation. For example, for an evaluation of the vendor, checklists can be sent to the vendor with questions on the following topics:

- The company (history, size, financial status, number of employees)
- The organization (Quality Assurance department)
- Certifications (ISO 9001)
- Hardware and software development (quality and technical standards)
- Testing and verification of life-cycle phases (reviews of Requirements Specifications, design, code inspections, are there release criteria for the phases?)
- Source code (guaranteed accessibility to regulatory agencies, where stored, escrow account)
- The product (how many sold to the target industry?)
- Security (how are unauthorized changes prevented? do disaster plans exist?)
- Support (response, language, phone, on-site, modem, support plan existing)
- Handling of failures and enhancement requests (formal procedures)
- Change control (who initiates and authorizes changes, version identification, and revision history?)
- People qualification (training programs)
- User documentation (what is archived for how long?)

- Customer training (topics, frequency, next location)
- Equipment hardware (how are specifications verified?)

A detailed checklist for vendor qualification has been developed by the author [1]. If the answers to the checklist are not satisfactory, a direct audit should be considered.

If no documentation of performance testing can be obtained from the vendor, the user should evaluate the system retrospectively. Detailed test cases with well-characterized test data sets and known results should be developed to evaluate the correct functioning of all software programs. In the case of completely computerized analytical systems, the analysis results with reference standards or quality control samples should be compared with known results from the standard or sample. Besides this holistic test, it is recommended to verify the performance of each individual subsystem. Such checks should include the proper response of the equipment to inputs from the computer. The tests should also check the system's error-handling capabilities. The system should recognize and display any wrong entries, for example, entries that are out of the system's operating range. Another simple test would be to check how the program responds when alphanumeric data are entered into fields that are designed to accept numerical values. In addition, the mathematical formulas should be verified with alternative methods of calculation.

VALIDATION OF USER–CONTRIBUTED SOFTWARE (e.g., MACROS)

Application software developed by the user should be fully validated and documented by the user. Such software may be a stand-alone software package (e.g., for statistical data evaluation), or it may be an extension to purchased standard software (e.g., a macro to enhance functionality). The development and validation of such software should follow a documented procedure, and the source code should be available. The effort involved in validation depends very much on the size and complexity of the program. The development of large programs should follow the software development life cycle and can take several months or years. Validation can take several weeks and the documentation will be extensive. On the other hand, the validation of small programs can be done in a few hours and the documentation may be only a few pages. The development, validation, and documentation of such small programs requires the following steps at minimum:

1. Describe the problem, how the problem is solved currently, and how the newly developed program will solve it.
2. Identify responsibilities for development, test, and approvals.

3. Describe the task and the system requirements (hardware, system software, standard software).
4. Describe the program in terms of the functions it will perform.
5. Document formulas and algorithms used within the code.
6. Write and document the code in such a way that it can be understood by other people whose knowledge and experience are similar to the programmer's. Print the code.
7. Develop test cases and data sets with known inputs and outputs. Include test cases with normal data across the operating range and at the boundary, and some unusual cases with incorrect inputs. The results should be calculated by the new program and also by using alternative methods. The development of an automated test procedure that can be executed as often as possible is recommended. Test procedures and results should be documented, reviewed, and signed off.
8. Develop user documentation with information on how to install, test, and operate the program.
9. Describe and implement procedures for data backup and security routines for limited access to authorized people.
10. Develop a procedure to authorize, test, document, and approve any changes to the software and documentation.

For combined systems, vendor-updated software revisions may be critical, especially if the updated version supplied by the vendor will have an effect on the interface between the vendor's and the user's software (e.g., if the meaning of a macro command has been changed). The user should obtain information from the vendor on how the updated version may affect the interface. The user should also test his or her software after it has been integrated into the vendor's updated standard software. More details about Standard Operating Procedures (SOPs) for developing and validating simple, as well as complex, applications software developed in the user's laboratory are found elsewhere [1].

PREINSTALLATION

Before the instrument arrives at the user's laboratory, serious thought must be given to its location and space requirements.

- A full understanding of the new equipment must be obtained from the vendor well in advance: required bench or floor space and environmental conditions, such as humidity and temperature, and, in some cases, utility needs, such as electricity and compressed gases for gas chromatographs.

- Care should be taken that all of the environmental conditions and electrical grounding are within the limits as specified by the vendor and that correct cables are used.
- If environmental conditions may have an influence on the validity of test results, the laboratory should have facilities to monitor and record these conditions, either continuously or at regular intervals.
- Any special safety precautions should be considered (e.g., for radioactivity measurement devices), and the location should also be checked for any devices generating electromagnetic fields nearby.

INSTALLATION

Once the instrument arrives:

- The shipment should be checked by the user for completeness.
- It should be confirmed that the equipment ordered is what was in fact received. Besides the equipment hardware, other items should be checked (e.g., correct cables, other accessories and documentation).
- The documentation should be checked for completeness (operating manuals, maintenance instructions, SOPs for testing, safety, and validation certificates).
- For more complex instrumentation, wiring diagrams should be generated, if not obtained from the vendor.
- An electrical test of all modules and systems should follow.
- The impact of electrical devices close to the computer system should be considered and evaluated if a need arises. For example, when small voltages are sent between sensors and integrators or computers, electro-magnetic energy emitted by poorly shielded nearby fluorescent lamps or by motors can interfere with the transmitted data.
- When complex software is installed on a computer, the correctness and completeness of the installed program and data files should be verified. Vendors can assist this process by supplying installation reference files and automated validated verification procedures. In this case, the integrity of each file is verified by comparing the cross-redundancy check (CRC) of the installed file with the

checksum of the original file recorded on the installation master. Modified or corrupt files have different checksums and are, thus, detected by the verification program. Verification reports include a list of missing, changed, and identical files.

The installation should end with the generation and sign-off of the installation report, in pharmaceutical manufacturing referred to as the IQ document. The hardware and software should be well documented with model, serial, and revision numbers. For larger laboratories with lots of equipment, this should be preferably a computer database. Entries for each instrument should include the following:

- In-house identification number
- Name of the item of equipment
- The manufacturer's name, address, and phone number for service call; service contract number, if available
- Serial number and firmware revision number of equipment
- Software with product and revision number
- Date received
- Date placed in service
- Current location
- Size, weight
- Condition, when received (e.g., new, used, reconditioned)
- List of authorized users and responsible person

It is recommended to make copies of all important documentation: one copy should be placed close to the instrument; the other should be kept in a safe place. An identification sticker should be put on the instrument with information on the instrument's serial number and the company's asset number.

LOGBOOK

An electronic or bound paper logbook should be prepared for each instrument in which operators and service technicians record all equipment-related activities in chronological order. Information in the logbook can include the following:

- Logbook identification (number, valid time range)
- Instrument identification (manufacturer, model name/number, serial number, firmware revision, date received, service contact)

- Column entry fields for dates, times, and events (e.g., initial installation and calibration, updates, column changes, errors, repairs, performance tests, quality control checks, cleaning, and maintenance plus fields for the name and signature of the technician making the entry).

OPERATIONAL QUALIFICATION AND ACCEPTANCE TESTING

After the installation of hardware and software, the hardware should be calibrated, where required. An operational test should follow, a process that is referred to in pharmaceutical manufacturing as OQ. The goal is to demonstrate that the equipment's hardware and software operate "as intended" in the user's environment.

For a computer system in an analytical laboratory, OQ can mean, for example, verifying correct communication between the computer and other hardware. As part of the product documentation, vendors should provide operating procedures for the tests, limits for acceptance criteria, and recommendations in case these criteria cannot be met. The documentation should also include algorithms for critical calculations and procedures on how to verify the algorithms in a user's environment. If the user finds the tests recommended by the vendor inappropriate or insufficient, the user can design and perform other or additional tests.

Chemical standards used for instrument calibration or qualification tests should be traceable to national standards.

The documentation of testing should include the following:

- The description and unique identification of equipment
- Test items
- Acceptance criteria
- Summary of results
- The date
- Names and signatures of persons who performed the tests

The instrument should be labeled with the calibration and qualification status, indicating the dates of the last and next calibration and OQ.

QUALIFICATION OF SOFTWARE

The correct functioning of software loaded on a computer system should be checked in the user's laboratory under typical operating conditions. During the equipment hardware test, as described in the previous section, many software functions are also executed, such as instrument control, data acquisition, peak integration, quantitation, file storage and retrieval, and printing. Therefore, after successful completion of hardware tests, it can also be assumed that the software operates as intended. There are two situations where software verification independent of the equipment hardware may be necessary:

1. If not all critical software functions are executed during the hardware verification
2. If a verification of the software functions should be done without a need for equipment testing

This is the case after a change on the computer system, for example, if a new operating system has been installed or if new hardware, such as CD ROMs or a hard disk, has been installed on the computer system.

The following paragraphs describe a procedure for the verification of important chromatography software functions without injecting a sample (Figure 3). The concept has been described in detail elsewhere [1]. It is very generic and can also be used to test and verify the correct functions of other software packages.

Well-characterized test chromatograms derived from standards or real samples are stored on disk as a master file. Chromatograms may be supplied by the vendor as part of the software package or can be recorded by the user. This master data file goes through normal data evaluation from integration to report generation. Results are stored on the hard disk. The same results should always be obtained when using the same data file and the same method for testing purposes.

Preferably, tests and the documentation of results should be done automatically, always using the same set of test files. In this way, users are encouraged to perform the tests more frequently, and user specific errors are eliminated. In some cases, vendors provide test files and automated test routines for verification of a computer system's performance in the user's laboratory. Needless to say, the correct functioning of this software should also be verified. If such software is not available, the execution of the tests and the verification of actual results with prerecorded results can be done manually.

Successful execution of such a procedure ensures that

- Executed program and data files are loaded correctly on the hard disk.
- The current computer hardware is compatible with the software.
- The current versions of the operating system and user interface software are compatible with the ChemStation software.

Figure 3. Verification Process of Chromatographic Software

Generate Master Data

1. Generate master chromatogram.
2. Develop method for evaluation.
3. Generate master result.
4. Save results electronically and on paper.

Verification

1. Select master chromatogram and method.
2. Run test (manually or automatically).
3. Compare new results with master data.
4. Report verification results.

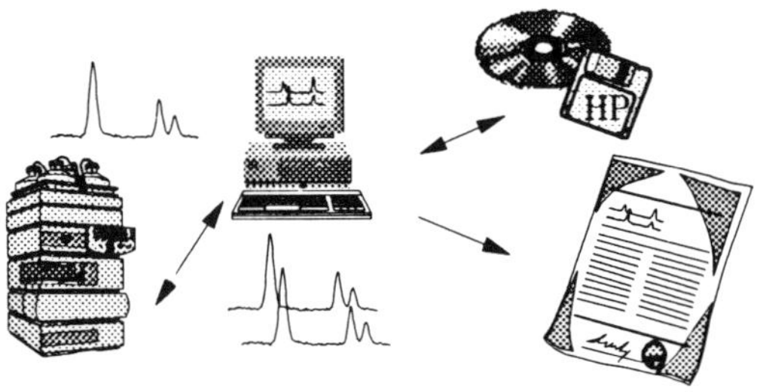

Test items

- Data transfer
- Data acquisition
- Integration
- Quantification
- Storage
- Retrieval

- Data are correctly transferred between the equipment and the computer (if this feature is supported by the system).

ROUTINE MAINTENANCE AND ONGOING PERFORMANCE QUALIFICATION

When the installation is complete and the equipment and the computer system are proven to operate well, the computerized system is put on routine analysis. Procedures should exist that show that *"it will continue to do what it purports to do."*

Each laboratory should have a quality assurance program that is well understood and used by individuals, as well as by laboratory organizations, to prevent, detect, and correct problems. The purpose is to ensure that the results have a high probability of being of acceptable quality. Ongoing activities may include the following:

- Preventive instrument maintenance
- Performance verification and calibration
- System suitability testing
- Analysis of blanks and quality control samples
- Ensuring system security

Preventive Maintenance

Operating procedures for maintenance should be in place for every system component that requires periodic calibration and/or preventive maintenance. The idea is to replace critical maintenance parts before they have a negative effect on the quality of analytical data.

- Critical parts should be listed and should be available at the user's site.
- The procedure should describe what should be done, when it should be done, and what the qualification of the engineer performing the tasks should be.
- System components should be labeled with the date of the last and next maintenance.
- All maintenance activities should be documented in the instrument's logbook.
- Suppliers of equipment should provide a list of recommended maintenance activities and procedures (SOPs) on how to perform the maintenance.

All maintenance activities should be recorded in a maintenance logbook. To make this more convenient, modern equipment includes electronic maintenance logbooks, where the user enters the type of maintenance and the equipment records this activity together with the date and time.

Calibration

Operating devices may become miscalibrated after a while (e.g., the temperature accuracy of a gas chromatography [GC] column oven or the wavelength accuracy of a UV/visible detector's optical unit). This can have an impact on the performance of an instrument. Therefore, a calibration program should be in place to recalibrate critical items of an instrument.

- All calibrations should follow documented procedures and the results should be recorded in the instrument's logbook.
- The system components should be labeled with the date of the last and next calibration.
- The label on the instrument should include the initials of the test engineer, the form should include his/her printed name and full signature.

System Suitability Tests and Quality Control Sample Analysis for Ongoing Performance Qualification

The analysis of standards or Quality Control samples with the construction of Quality Control charts (Figure 4) has been suggested as a way to incorporate quality checks on results, as they are being generated. Such tests can then flag those values that may be erroneous for any of the following reasons:

- Reagents are contaminated.
- GC carrier gas is impure.
- HPLC mobile phase is contaminated.
- Instrument characteristics have changed over time.

For an accurate quality check, Quality Control samples are interspersed among actual samples at intervals determined by the total number of samples and the precision and reproducibility of the method. The control sample frequency will depend mainly on the known stability of the measurement process—a stable process requiring only occasional monitoring.

Control samples should have a high degree of similarity to the actual samples analyzed; otherwise, one cannot draw reliable conclusions on the measurement system's performance. Control samples must be so homogeneous and stable that individual increments measured at various times will have less variability than the measurement process itself. Quality Control

Figure 4. Quality Control Chart with Warning Lines and Control Lines

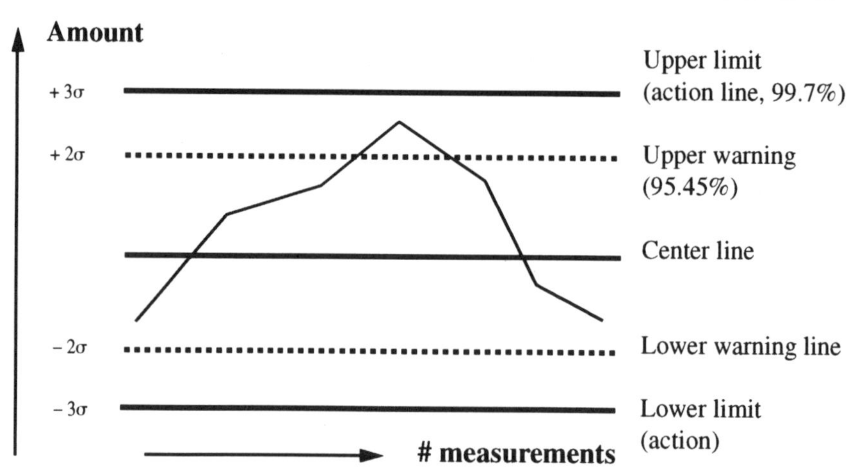

samples are prepared by adding known amounts of analytes to blank specimens. They can be purchased as certified reference material (CRM) or may be prepared in-house. In the latter case, sufficient quantities should be prepared to allow the same samples to be used over a longer period of time. Their stability over time should be proven and their accuracy verified, preferably through interlaboratory tests or by other analysis methods.

The most widely used procedure for the ongoing peformance control of equipment through Quality Control samples involves the construction of control charts for these samples. These are plots of multiple data points versus the number of measurements from the same samples using the same processes. Measured concentrations of a single measurement or the average of multiple measurements are plotted on the vertical axis, and the sequence number of the measurement is plotted on the horizontal axis. Control charts provide a graphical tool to demonstrate statistical control, monitor a measurement process, diagnose measurement problems, and document measurement uncertainty. The most commonly used control charts are X-charts and R-charts as developed by Shewart. X-charts consist of a central line representing either the known concentration or the mean of 10–20 earlier determinations of the analyte in control material. The standard deviation has been determined during method validation and is used to calculate the control lines in the control chart. Control limits define the bounds of virtually all values produced by a system in statistical control.

Control charts often have a center line and two control lines with two pairs of limits: a warning line at $\mu \pm 2\sigma$ and an action line at $\mu \pm 3\sigma$. Statistics predict that 95.45 percent and 99.7 percent of the data will fall within the areas enclosed by the $\pm 2\sigma$ and $\pm 3\sigma$ limits. The center line is either the mean or the true value. In the ideal case, where unbiased methods are being used, the center line would be the true value. This would apply, for example, to precision control charts for standard solutions.

When the process is under statistical control, the day-to-day results are normally distributed about the center line. A result outside the warning line indicates that something is wrong. Such a result need not be rejected, but documented procedures should be in place for suitable action. Instruments and sampling procedures should be checked for errors. Two successive values of the Quality Control sample falling outside the action line indicate that the process is no longer under statistical control. In this case, the results should be rejected and the process investigated for its unusual behavior. Further analyses should be suspended until the problem is resolved.

Change Control

Software has one distinct advantage over hardware: it does not change its performance characteristics over time. Theoretically, there should be no need to revalidate software as long as the hardware and environmental conditions do not change. However, almost 100 percent of all software written will be changed following its release for use. There are three reasons for a software change:

1. To correct errors
2. To adapt software to changes in its operating environment
3. To enhance the software (e.g., to add functionality)

In addition to software changes, there may be hardware changes to a computer system. The processor may be upgraded, the system may get additional disk space, or new memory chips may be installed. All software and hardware changes to a computer system may influence the performance and correct functioning of the system and may need a reverification or revalidation. A control system should exist that describes what should be revalidated after a change to the system. Procedures should be available for changes to a system purchased from a vendor as well as for software developed in-house.

Software developed and validated by the user should also be revalidated by the user. Principally, software redevelopment and testing should follow the same procedure as for newly developed software. Procedures should include information on who authorizes changes, who executes the changes, and who can finally release the changed version. Compared to new software, the amount of testing can be reduced through intensive reuse of previously developed test files and test procedures.

If computer systems are upgraded with new operating systems or when new hardware is added, the user should thoroughly document the upgrade and perform acceptance testing as for a new system. The use of existing test files and automated procedures can make this process very efficient.

If the user purchases a software upgrade, the supplier should prove that the upgraded version has been validated. A declaration of validation or an equivalent document shipped with the upgrade is adequate as proof. The vendor should also provide information on

- System requirements for the upgraded version
- How to install the upgrade
- What the changes are
- If the new software may have on impact on any macro program written by the user

The installation should be documented and the user should perform an acceptance test.

REFERENCES

1. Huber, L. (1995), *Validation of Computerized Analytical Systems*. Buffalo Grove, IL. Interpharm. Hewlett-Packard part number 5959–3879.

2. Furman, W.B., Layloff, T.P., and Tetzlaff, R.F. (1994), Validation of Computerized Liquid Chromatographic Systems. *J. AOAC Intern* 77 (5): 1314–1318.

3. OECD (1992), *Compliance of Laboratory Suppliers with GLP Principles*. Series on Principles of Good Laboratory Practice and Compliance Monitoring, Number 5, GLP consensus document, environment monograph No. 49. Paris: Organisation for Economic Co-operation and Development.

4. Tetzlaff, R.F. (1992), GMP Documentation Requirements for Automated Systems: Part III, FDA Inspections of Computerized Laboratory Systems. *Pharm. Tech.* (May): 71–82.

5. OECD (1995), *The Application of the Principles of GLP to Computerized Systems*. Series on Principles of Good Laboratory Practice and Compliance Monitoring, Number 10, GLP consensus document, environment monograph No. 116, Paris: Organisation for Economic Co-operation and Development.

Case Study N

Validating Laboratory Information Management Systems

Nick Townsend
Beckman Instruments (UK) Ltd.
High Wycombe, UK

John Bianculli
Beckman Instruments Inc.
Fullerton, CA, USA

Laboratory Information Management Systems (LIMSs) are specialized database applications intended to meet wide-ranging laboratory information management requirements, including laboratory sample and test tracking, manual and automated result capture, result verification, review, and reporting (Figure 1). Most systems provide an audit trail and numerous other features to ensure data integrity and aid compliance with laboratory quality assurance guidelines such as those specified by Good Manufacturing Practice

Figure 1. Typical LIMS Data Flow

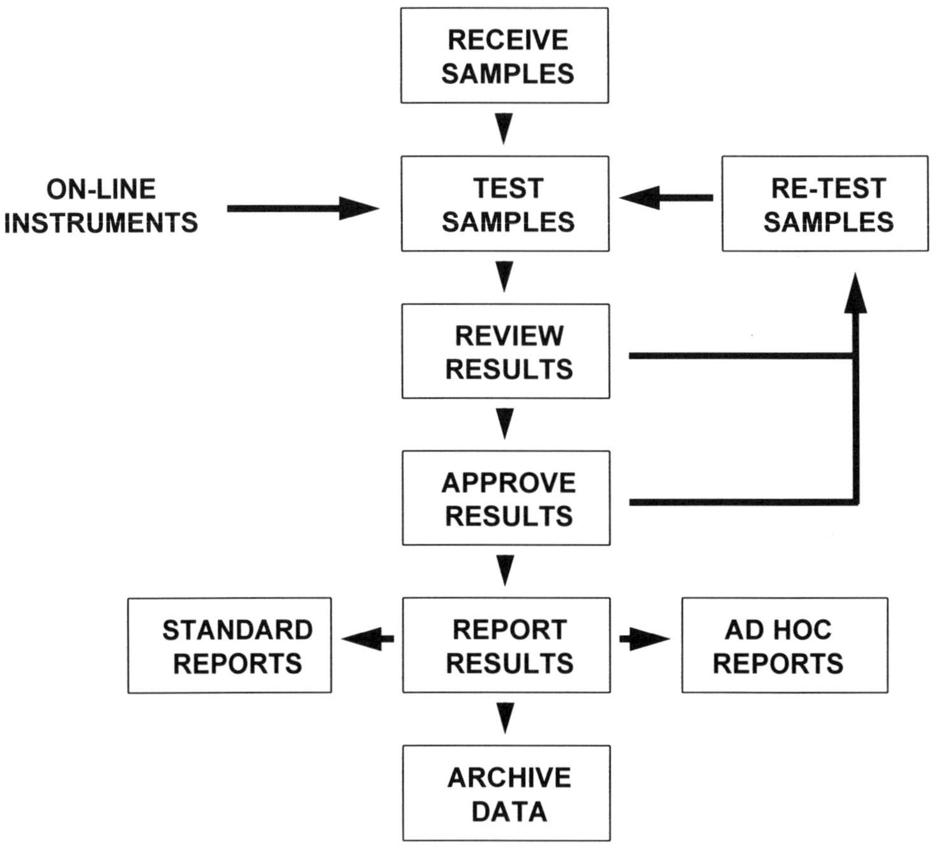

(GMP). LIMSs are increasingly found at the heart of company R&D and manufacturing processes. The key drivers being increased productivity, automation, and regulatory compliance.

Some LIMSs are highly *configurable* software systems, consisting of a standard application program core and a standard commercial database (e.g., Oracle™), to which can be added a customer specific "layer." The configurable layer allows the system to be adapted to meet customer requirements (Figure 2). Database tables, fields, the relations between the tables and fields, screen layouts, menus and reports, and so on can all be configured without compromising the obvious advantages of a standard application program and database core that is regularly updated by the supplier.

The application program core is normally manufactured in the supplier's development center. Following an order, the configured portion is usually designed and implemented close to the customer in the supplier's local office, or even in situ on a customer site (Figure 3).

Figure 2. Components of a Configurable LIMS

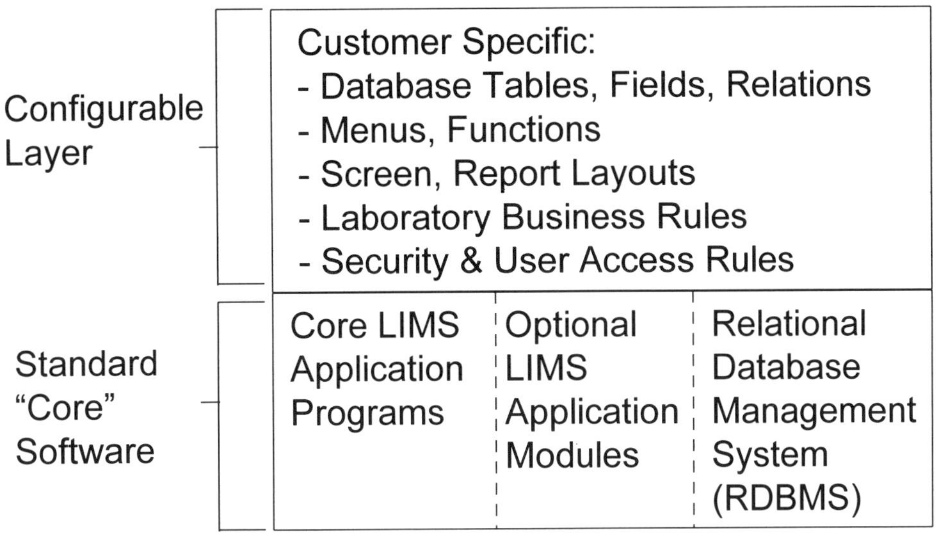

HISTORICAL PERSPECTIVE

From the perspective of a LIMS, there has been a gradual shift in focus of customer requirements over the past 12–15 years. In the early 1980s, when LIMS technology was in its infancy, customer requirements were focused on improving system functionality in areas to aid compliance with emerging laboratory "best practice" quality guidelines. As a result, LIMS manufacturers responded by providing more secure systems in terms of user access controls, improved database security, and comprehensive audit trail features to monitor system use and "document" changes to important data. Additionally, new product features were required to automate some of the wider demands of regulatory compliance, such as

- Routine scheduling of instrument calibration and maintenance
- Automated chromatography instrument analogue/digital interface validation
- Method revision control
- Chromatography system suitability
- Analyst training records

In the late 1980s/early 1990s, LIMS customers became aware that regulatory pressure was shifting focus toward ensuring supplier software quality and the techniques used to validate computer systems.

Figure 3. Delivering a Configurable LIMS

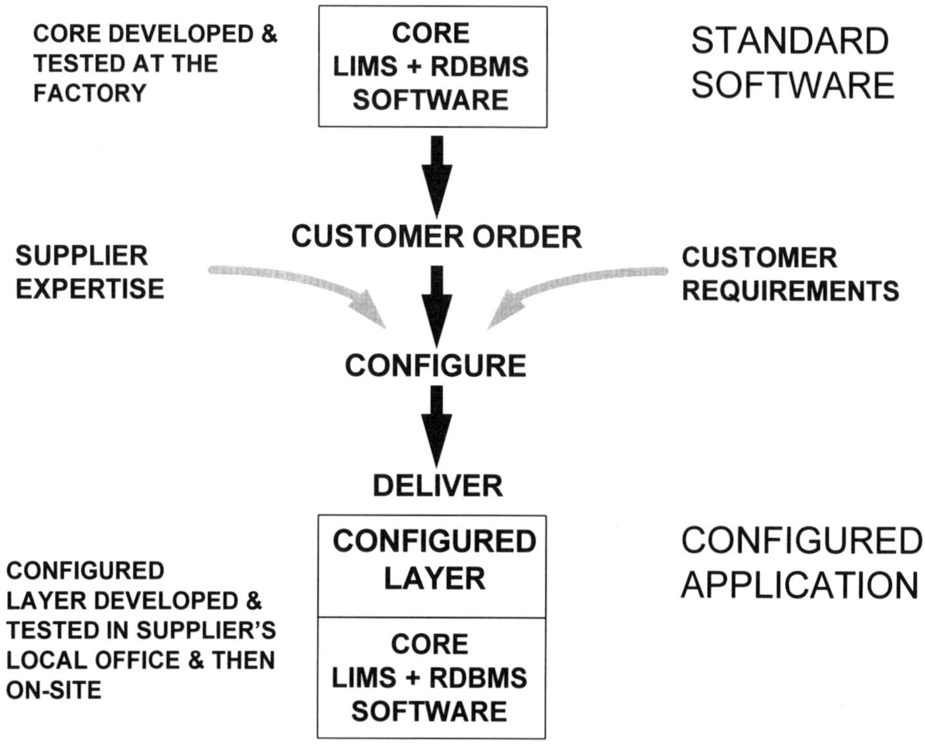

DEVELOPING A QUALITY CAPABILITY

When the first commercial LIMSs emerged, most suppliers, like many established software developers with their roots in the late 1970s, had no formalized quality system in place for software design, development, testing, distribution, and ongoing support. Design documentation was not comprehensive and often completed retrospectively. Testing was done on a largely unstructured, best effort basis. The importance of program revision control was understood, but poorly enforced. Bug fixes were patched into the software as discovered; new features were added almost at the whim of a particular programmer or to suit the needs of sales and marketing hungry to outflank a competitor to win an order!

By the mid 1980s, some suppliers recognized the need for some form of Quality Management System. Products were becoming more and more complex, the installed system base was growing and there were the first indications from LIMS customers that software quality would be scrutinized more closely in the years to come. Quite simply, adopting a quality system appeared to make good business sense and some suppliers worked to adopt the ISO 9001 standard.

The move toward a formalized quality system provides interesting and unique *challenges:*

- *The importance of the Vendor/Supplier Audit:* The organization must be educated about the reasons for, and the importance of, Vendor Audits. The quality system must be made clear and simple to follow in order to improve the efficiency of Vendor Audits and minimize the risk of misunderstandings.
- *How to use "today's" technology with "yesterday's" standards:* Computer software engineering is fast moving and the evolution of quality standards does not keep pace. The implications of using the latest fourth generation language tools, client/server technology, and Graphical User Interfaces (GUIs) must be carefully thought through.
- *Configuration management:* As software applications become more complex, careful control of source code, modification process, program libraries, and so on requires strict discipline and control.
- *Quality certification is not the final goal!* A significant challenge for any organization is to ensure that adherence to the quality system continues beyond the point of certification! Too much self-congratulation can lead to "collective relaxation", allowing the opportunity to be caught off-guard.
- *Learn to work with your customers:* Suppliers must learn to be open with their customers. Experience shows that the most valuable insights into quality system deficiencies come from the supplier's customers.
- *Testing is important!* The organization must learn to view early and comprehensive testing as a benefit and not a unpleasant chore.
- *Change the way you do business:* In many instances, suppliers must be prepared to change the way they do business. Often, this means better planning, "documenting before doing," and revising traditional estimates for typical project completion times to take into account new testing protocols.
- *Find tools to assist validation:* While implementing a quality system, suppliers realized the importance of developing protocols and tools to assist their customers with on-site validation. Significant effort must be focused on finding appropriate solutions and new validation tools.

- *Find one standard!* Multinational suppliers are faced with the (ongoing) challenge to find and work to one internationally recognized standard appropriate to the nature of their business.

THE VENDOR/SUPPLIER AUDIT

Regulatory guidance and common sense now make it common practice for the LIMS customer to audit the supplier. Often, audits are performed by prospective customers before system purchase. If not, many regulated customers audit the supplier after system purchase. An increasing number will reaudit supplier facilities on an ongoing basis to verify continued ability to meet their validation requirements.

Each LIMS customer has a number of validation-related objectives that can be met by auditing their LIMS supplier. Obviously, the customer must determine whether the audited organization has appropriate policies and procedures able to support minimum quality and documentation requirements. If these are in place, meaning the system can be validated, the next issues are commonly related to how much effort will be required to perform the validation. If the supplier has excellent procedural and control mechanisms in place, the effort required by the LIMS customer to validate the system can be minimized.

Two fundamental business drivers are as follows:

1. The high level of "design" in daily business activities
2. The longevity of LIMSs in customer laboratories

Often, the approach to managing these well is the implementation of an ISO 9001 quality system, with appropriate inclusion of ISO 9000-3, which provides quality guidelines specific to software. The ISO quality system requires that the supplier undergo regular external audits from a certified body. It is also necessary to perform frequent internal audits (e.g., monthly), so that on an annual basis all areas of the quality system are audited. Support for customer audits performed at a supplier's facility is simply another level of scrutiny, and the ISO quality system and its implementation throughout the business is the primary focus of the audits.

A typical audit may have the following structure:

- *Supplier's organizational structure:* Defines roles and responsibilities. This is always relevant, and introducing the organization at the beginning helps clarify further discussion.
- *ISO 9001 quality system:* Scope and details of supplier's quality system. This is fundamental to the audit process and provides a basic understanding of the approach to quality throughout the organization.

- *Software development life cycle:* Highlights the processes the supplier uses to define, develop, and test software products. Closely tied to the quality system.
- *Tour of the supplier's facility:* Provides an opportunity to relate what has been discussed so far with the actual personnel and equipment employed to realize software products and services.
- *Response to auditor questions:* Auditor(s) generally prepare a script of questions to cover during the audit. An opportunity is provided to respond to questions not yet answered by preceding audit discussion topics.
- *Surveillance of quality records:* The "core" of the audit activity—auditor(s) focus on quality records. The objective is to verify that topics discussed above are actually being performed as discussed and documented.

The makeup of the audit will probably vary from customer to customer. Prospective customers will often focus most carefully on "product" features and related processes. Since a configured LIMS relies on a functional core, it is reasonable that a careful examination of the procedures and processes used to develop the core should be conducted. Existing customers will tend to focus more on issues pertinent to their particular situation. This may be documentation regarding their system implementation, software revision's updates, or perhaps a review of technical support records related to requests for assistance they have made. Certainly, more mature customers who reaudit a supplier will tend to focus more on these types of issues rather than the general assurance that the supplier's organization will meet overall validation-related requirements.

Of course, different customers will have different motives and capabilities for performing audits. Highly experienced auditors will tend to be more "nuts and bolts" oriented, and often use their experience to zero in on potential areas of concern. Less experienced auditors may approach an audit as a necessary evil. In this situation, the audit itself is the milestone on which to focus, rather than the audit results.

While suppliers may appreciate "getting off lightly" with less demanding audits, those that are more detailed and focused can provide the supplier with several benefits. First, audit observations tend to help focus on actual or perceived inadequacies in the quality system and its implementation. Since the audit is being conducted to help support the customer's LIMS validation, observations generally tend to point out potential improvements the supplier can make that support the customer's validation objectives. Second, audit observations can often help us to "predict the future." With many emerging validation requirements, suppliers have the opportunity to discuss with auditing customers the potential to do certain things, well before they become requirements. The issues covered by the Good Automated Manufacturing Practice (GAMP) framework is an example of one source of information suppliers could have been aware of well before they are defined as required by their customers.

Although suppliers must make a significant resource commitment to support customer audits, in the big picture the overall effect is a "win-win" situation. Suppliers are able to demonstrate a good understanding of software validation, especially in highly regulated environments, that supports their customers' needs. In turn, feedback is given, typically in a constructive manner, which allows suppliers to improve business practices, making them stronger and more responsive for their overall market.

DESIGN AND DEVELOPMENT CONSIDERATIONS

Any validation activity has at its core a determination that the system being validated is meeting its intended purpose accurately and reliably. With a LIMS, the intended purpose is broadly stated as "laboratory data management", but specific requirements are often difficult to define. When preparing to develop a new LIMS functionality, a supplier must often derive specific functionality requirements from a variety of sources as summarized below:

- *Existing customer wishes:* Specific enhancements to existing product features improve functionality in the laboratory.
- *Prospective customer functional requirements:* Overall product features, often including "non-LIMS" functionality. LIMS knowledge is sometimes limited, resulting in overly general requirements specification.
- *Popular computer technologies:* Emerging computer trends and technologies will likely replace existing functionality or allow significant new features.
- *Internal LIMS implementation personnel:* Product features provide greater LIMS functionality.
- *Internal technical support personnel:* Software simplicity reduces support required and provides rapid corrections to product problems.

These different sources frequently have opposing views of what is "most important." New customers want to take advantage of the latest technology as soon as possible. Existing customers, with their LIMS operating in validated production, are often more cautious and need to assure lack of system downtime. LIMS implementation staff will generally want greater capabilities and flexibility and are often willing to forego simplicity to obtain new features faster.

During the requirements gathering and evaluation process, a supplier should always consider new functionality in perspective with the existing installed base.[1] Typical customers have their LIMS installed for seven years or more, and the supplier will usually provide major and minor software revisions during this period. Therefore, downward compatibility is a major driving force in shaping what new features are implemented and how. Effective delivery of compatible software revisions allows the customer to implement and revalidate new software revisions with the minimum effort possible.

Ultimately, the result of the requirements gathering phase should be a formal Requirements Specification. From a marketing perspective, this document typically addresses the business need for a proposed new functionality. It should then go into detail about what functionality is required and what specific features and benefits are expected. In addition to the staff members who prepare the document, the supplier's management should also formally approve the Requirements Specification. This provides an opportunity for the entire organisation to review the proposed requirements and address any concerns there might be at the beginning of the process.

BUILDING THE CORE SYSTEM

Unlike most "physical" products that have a large manufacturing, storage, and delivery component, software products are almost all a result of "design" activities. In fact, LIMS "designers" include both product development staff who develop the core product software and the LIMS implementation consultants who realize complete systems by configuring the core product to meet individual laboratory requirements. These activities are, by far, the largest cost and quality drivers in a LIMS implementation. Core product software development is discussed in this section; LIMS implementation is discussed in the next section.

Product design starts with the formal Requirements Specification discussed earlier. It is the role of Product Development staff to realize a formal product design from the defined requirements. The formal product design considers each requirement and defines technical details and corroborating information to describe how each requirement may be realized. An important factor is often the need to support multiple software platforms and

1. One useful vehicle Beckman Instruments has successfully employed is a "flash fax" feedback system. During requirements analysis, or even early in the design process, it is not uncommon to have questions about exactly how a feature should work, or how its implementation might affect existing customers. In these cases, Beckman Instruments sends faxes to potentially affected customers (for example, those who have an option they are planning to update), giving them background on the issues and requesting their feedback. Beckman Instruments has found this system particularly time effective for receiving feedback on specific details of customers' requirements.

technologies. To meet the requirements of different target markets, LIMS products may be required to execute on more than one server operating system, support multiple core relational database management systems, and have a client/server option required to support multiple versions of Microsoft Windows™ and a variety of network protocols. This is a significant challenge, and product design must address this situation as efficiently as possible.

Development staff usually meets the challenge by effectively segregating platform-specific items from the overall body of software product, maximizing the proportion of platform-independent programming. The remaining programs should be well segregated and deal with platform-specific issues, such as disk input/output (I/O), network interfacing, database access, on-screen display, and so on. When the specific areas are well understood, development and subsequent testing activities need thoroughly consider the vast majority of programs only once. Remaining platform-specific items must then be accounted for on a platform-by-platform basis. This approach provides for thorough verification and validation testing throughout the development life cycle, without a need to exhaustively retest common code sections. A retrospective review of reported software problems strongly supports this approach.

Some suppliers have traditionally relied on the "waterfall" method of software development, which embodies a series of sequential steps from requirements, to design, development, testing, and release. More recently, they may have had to make methodology adjustments to support a more responsive, quality-oriented software development methodology. Software projects usually now employ more cross-functional team members and rely on overlapped work activities to speed the overall progress without adversely affecting quality results.

The ISO quality system defines a number of procedural mechanisms to manage the software design and development process. These are essential if adequate control of the software development and testing process is to be accomplished. The major control mechanisms include the following:

- *Programming standards:* With a number of programmers, thousands of interrelated source programs, and multiple platform considerations, having adequate programming standards is essential. These include standards for code design, adequate commenting, and modification logging to ease long-term capability to support and enhance programs. Supplier programming standards provide a basis for ongoing software program interoperability and consistency from programmer to programmer and revision to revision.
- *Source code control:* A variety of programmers are usually involved in the efforts of any software release. They often reuse existing programming to provide enhancements or build new programming that will interoperate with existing programming. With backward compatibility in mind, it is essential that there be tight control of

what versions of source code are used and ultimately end up in the product. Programmers should follow a rigorous method of source code control to meet these objectives.

- *Unit testing:* Often termed "white box testing," development staff should employ programmatic unit testing techniques on a number of core routines. These are generally low level routines that are widely used throughout the supplier's system. Routine testing of these routines from release to release should improve the confidence that fundamental operations of the system are maintained from revision to revision.
- *System testing:* A supplier that has been established for many years will have probably amassed a collection of thousands of automated test cases that contain tens of thousands of checkpoints. These test cases individually provide testing on various components of the system, often termed "black box testing". In total, the thousands of test cases should provide rigorous testing of virtually all LIMS functionalities. These test collections are a fundamental test of a supplier's requirements for downward compatibility. As new software features are developed, new test cases should be created and verified, ultimately supporting ongoing testing for subsequent software revisions.

During the core product design and development process, it is not uncommon that a supplier will need to better understand particular product requirement details. Rather than relying solely on in-house experience, a supplier will often effectively use external sources to gather "real-life" information. These sources include the following:

- Prototyping/focus group input
- User group meeting presentations and feedback
- Flash faxes to existing customers requesting specific details and examples
- Customized development with eventual inclusion in standard product

Based on experience, established suppliers will have found it much more desirable to understand and implement features properly the first time, rather than having to modify them after initial implementation. The former approach is more work for the supplier but has obvious advantages.

Though programming standards and practices include a high degree of testing, a LIMS supplier should also rely on formal alpha and beta testing phases in their product development life cycle that should be coordinated by their Quality department. Alpha testing is testing of a completed product, prior to general release, by the supplier's own personnel. Beta testing is testing of a completed product, prior to general release, on actual customer systems.

Alpha testing is generally the first in-house opportunity to operate new software revisions in a nondevelopment environment. The focus of alpha testing is twofold. From a more structured viewpoint, a supplier will attempt to exercise new or corrected features to verify their capabilities and also to determine any "rough edges" in the implementation that might not work well in production. In a less structured sense, a supplier will also test that the entire system, new features and old, continues to operate consistently and predictably.

Beta testing is a continuation of these activities but is installed at customer sites. This provides a much greater opportunity to perform "variety" testing in different environments and configurations than in the supplier's own facility. Again, when a variety of platforms and technologies are supported suppliers will find that beta test customers provide a useful and efficient way to expand testing.

During alpha and beta testing, problems should be reported using a formalized system involving Test Incident Reports (TIRs). Each TIR will be recorded and tracked by the Quality department and responded to by Product Development. Internal procedures monitor changes to programs to correct TIRs, so that during the testing process changes can be implemented and verified while still maintaining strict source code control.

The duration of alpha and beta testing will primarily depend on

- Discovery rate and severity of TIRs
- Adequate coverage of all modules to be tested

As with any complex software system, a LIMS supplier will not expect to detect and discover every software problem during testing. The rate at which TIRs are reported will generally decrease substantially throughout testing. Near the end of testing, it may often take days of effort to discover software problems. Typically, at this stage, quality and development staff will review the status of a product and recommend whether to continue testing or end testing and freeze product in preparation for shipment. The supplier's management will properly act on the recommendation based on the data presented.

When a decision is taken to release the LIMS product, the supplier's Product Development department will generally have the responsibility for packaging the software into standard distribution software sets relevant to the various platforms released. Once prepared, each of these should undergo one more complete verification runs of the supplier's test cases, as before the start of alpha testing. This final verification testing should be performed to assure that the software changes made as a result of TIRs from alpha or beta testing have not caused a software change or failure throughout the system.

Once test case verification is complete, the product distribution software sets will be frozen and moved to distribution systems, where further changes are not possible. "Manufacturing" of the software (i.e., copying to distribution media) is normally performed using an automated procedure that essentially copies and verifies the frozen distribution software set(s) without the ability to modify them during the process.

SYSTEM IMPLEMENTATION

When a LIMS supplier's sales department receives an order, there then follows a sequence of events that depends on the degree of configurability of the LIMS and the preferred implementation approach of the supplier. Some LIMS are "fixed format," providing little or no configurability, requiring minimal implementation effort from the supplier, provided that the customer is prepared to modify laboratory practices and business rules to "fit the LIMS." Other LIMS products provide a significant degree of configurability using fourth generation language (4GL) tools. Some suppliers of configurable systems may intend these tools for customer use only. Other suppliers may prefer to "own" the implementation, configure the LIMS for the customer, and hand over a fully configured system. In the latter case, the LIMS configuration tools can then be used to extend the system as and when customer needs dictate.

In the case of a configured system, the typical activities and procedures that follow the receipt of an order are summarized below:

- Order review and acknowledgment
- Assignment of a supplier and customer project team
- Preparation of a project plan and agree dates for meetings and key milestones with the customer
- Agreement of software license and support contract documentation
- Site inspection
- Review of customer requirements and supporting documentation
- Preparation of Functional Specification documentation and test protocols
- System configuration, perhaps using an iterative process with periodic review meetings with the customer
- Preparation of bespoken add-on software *(if any)*
- Configured system testing
- Preliminary acceptance of the configured system (supplier's office)

- Approval of system test results
- Review of proposed deliverables
- Review of remaining proposed project timetables

- On-site installation, testing, and familiarization training
- Data loading
- Formal training
- Final (contractual) acceptance testing
  - Final review of configured system and any bespoken add-on software testing
  - Receipt of all project deliverables
  - Acceptance of overall project against key milestones
- Formal project handover to technical support

In former years, the implementation process was usually conducted on a rather more informal basis than is expected by LIMS customers today. Configuration work was often carried out using a largely undocumented, prototypical approach in which customer laboratory representatives periodically met with suppliers to build the system on a "try it and see" basis. While this approach usually delivered a perfectly functional system, configuration specific testing and documentation was less than adequate for modern, regulated environments.

In the 1990s, the need for a more formalized, documented implementation approach emerged for the following reasons:

- There is ever-increasing attention paid to the delivery of projects on-time and on-budget.
- Purchasing and contracts departments have a clearer understanding of the nature of software projects. Project deliverables are carefully identified and milestones are set for their delivery.
- Regulatory pressure has increased the attention paid to detail and the scope of documentation supplied with the configured software system. There is increasing awareness of the need to scrutinize testing of the configured system and not just the core application.

In response to customer needs, some suppliers are now providing a more formal planning approach to project implementation and now expect to formalize the requirements in a formal Functional Specification (FS) that clearly defines the scope and capabilities of the system to be implemented. This approach does not hamper or remove the benefits of prototyping, rather it provides an opportunity for both the customer and the supplier to clarify project expectations. This preliminary specification effort is a significant effort with significant cost. It is common for prospective customers who have already made a significant investment in a formal requirements specification (typically a Request for Proposal [RFP]/Quotation) to ask why there is a need to develop a new specification. Because the system being implemented is based on a product with fixed capabilities, it is essential to recognize that a general Requirements Specification must be "translated" into an FS specific to the system being implemented. In any event, having a well-defined project scope helps the supplier and their customers to

- Improve their ability to schedule and meet project milestones
- Better schedule resources—of key importance for project success
- Reduce the overall time to implement a system by reducing or eliminating "creeping elegance" that often occurs when the project scope and objectives are not clearly documented

HANDOVER TO TECHNICAL SUPPORT

Upon project completion, which is normally considered to be the contractual acceptance of the LIMS installation, the supplier's implementation team will usually "hand the system over" to a technical support department. This department is usually required to

- Provide a telephone hot line for assistance
- Provide remote system maintenance, perhaps by modem
- Supervise software update distribution and installation
- Operate a formalized technical support call logging and problem escalation procedures

Additionally, the Technical Support department may provide the LIMS supplier's training services and assist with alpha and beta testing programs.

As might be expected, after completion of an installation, the incidence of questions and problems directed to the hot line generally reduces over time, with potential "hot spots" occurring when new software updates are distributed or a customer decides to expand the LIMS.

As is no doubt common to all suppliers of specialized software for regulated environments, there are many challenges faced by LIMS Technical Support departments. Some examples are as follows:

- The need to maintain personnel skills and equipment for a variety of hardware, operating system, and database platforms
- The need to encourage the user base to move to the latest versions of LIMS software in a timely fashion to minimize support

overhead, while being sensitive to the logistical difficulties this may cause the supplier's customers

- How to provide effective support of bespoken add-ons to the core software and interfaces to third-party systems
- Providing effective support while at the same time allowing customers to modify installed systems using powerful 4GL configuration tools

Good management of the technical support "system" and its key processes are fundamental to the ongoing success of the installed LIMS customer base and the supplier's reputation. In addition to providing effective technical support, the Technical Support department has an important role to play by

- Generating invaluable information for the Quality and Product Development departments of system problems through the problem tracking and escalation system
- Documenting and processing customer complaints and other feedback through the ISO 9001 quality system
- Carefully staging and monitoring software updates in the field, especially in the initial stages of release of a new revision of software
- Developing good customer relations and dialogue, thereby encouraging free flowing and constructive input into the ongoing product development process.

LIMSs typically serve customers for many years, and there is a unique opportunity to develop a strong customer/supplier relationship. Established suppliers know the importance of this relationship and understand how to overcome support challenges such as those given above. Most LIMS suppliers also understand that providing effective technical support services is a major driver to securing repeat business from a customer and additional business from new customers by being able to quote happy reference sites.

SUMMARY

In the last 15 years, commercial LIMSs have evolved from simple sample and test tracking systems to become complex applications capable of managing almost all aspects of laboratory work. Furthermore, a modern LIMS is expected to integrate with and play an ever-increasing role in enterprise automation. More than ever before, customers are selecting a LIMS based on their regulatory compliance features and the quality of the product development and implementation service.

Suppliers have had to change their thought processes and codes of practice to meet the business challenges imposed by the increasingly important role played by their systems. System validation, historically a "minor" objective, has emerged as a significant component of LIMS implementation. Fundamentally, this means a move away from the largely unstructured, undocumented practice of the early 1980s to embrace fully the principles of modern software engineering and quality management. Suppliers have recognized a need to change both their product development activities and system implementation services to meet the validation challenge. Overall, these changes have been and continue to be implemented under the umbrella of the ISO 9000 quality system. This provides a "win-win" situation for the supplier and its customers, by simultaneously supporting the LIMS customer's validation requirements as well as improving overall how suppliers conduct their business.

AUTHORS' APPROACH

This case study described the validation issues relating to a LIMS vendor based on the experiences of the Laboratory Automation Operations division of Beckman Instruments Inc. (Fullerton, CA), a supplier of laboratory automation products, including Chromatography Data Systems (CDSs) and LIMSs. In particular, it described, from a historical perspective, how companies develop and implement laboratory automation systems, the reasons why they should choose to implement a quality system, and the challenges they may face.

Beckman Instruments has a long history of involvement with regulated industries and specializes in supplying laboratory instruments, software, services, and supplies for the life sciences, including the pharmaceutical, biotechnology, and clinical markets. Beckman Instruments' business necessitates that it carefully monitor and respond to regulatory trends and the evolving requirements of its customers. The input received during biannual LIMS user meetings over 12 years has provided invaluable information and has been a sensitive indicator of customer needs.

Beckman's Laboratory Automation Operations division produced its first quality manual in 1988 and began to control software manufacturing processes by documented procedures. The structure of the quality system was largely "home grown" but based on sound software life-cycle development principles taken from Good Manufacturing Practices (GMPs) and Pharmaceutical Manufacturers Association's (PMA) interpretations of regulatory requirements with respect to computer systems [1]. In addition, Beckman Instruments has been offering a customer audit service for several years and developed protocols required to provide Installation Qualification (IQ) and Operational Qualification (OQ) services for its clients.

In 1991, a Beckman Instruments corporate directive required all business units to work toward achieving ISO 9001 certification. The quality system their software group already had in place provided an excellent platform for ISO 9001, and by 1992, ISO 9001 certification had been achieved.

When first implemented, the ISO 9001 quality system was adequate to document current practices. However, the system has since undergone significant revision, reflecting changes and improvements in Beckman Instruments' business processes. More recently, the company has focused on ISO 9000-3, which provides a series of guidelines specific to software product development.

ACKNOWLEDGMENT

The authors should like to thank Peter Berthrong, Beckman Laboratory Automation Operations QA Manager (retired), for his contribution of information concerning the historical Quality Assurance perspective, and increasing our overall understanding of LIMS Quality Assurance processes.

REFERENCE

1. PMA's Computer System Validation Committee (1986), Validation Concepts for Computer Systems Used in the Manufacture of Drug Products. *Pharmaceutical Technology* (May): 24–34.

Case Study O

Validating Medical Devices and Their Automated Manufacture

Bob Paige and Guy Wingate
Eutech Engineering Solutions Ltd.
Billingham, UK

A medical device is an instrument, apparatus, appliance, material or other article, whether used alone or in combination, together with any software necessary for its proper application, which

a) *is intended by the manufacturer to be used for human beings for the purpose of:*

i. *diagnosis, monitoring, treatment, alleviation of disease,*

ii. *diagnosis, monitoring, treatment, alleviation of or compensation for an injury or handicap,*

iii. *investigation, replacement, or modification of the anatomy or of a physiological process, or*

iv. *control of conception; and*

> *b)* *does not achieve its principal intended action in or on the human body by pharmacological, immunological, or metabolic means, even if it is assisted in its function by such means* [1].

The definition's reference to software extends the scope of medical devices to include those based on programmable technology. Such devices can be extremely complex and consist of a large number of programmable elements. Figure 1 provides a schematic overview of a medical device's healthcare service: the delivery, control, and/or monitoring of medical treatment.

Medical devices require both product and process validation. Product validation is necessary to assure that they are designed and assembled consistently to assure a high quality of service. Process validation is necessary to assure that they are produced under a compliant regime of Good Manufacturing Practice (GMP). Particular validation requirements are laid down by European Directive 93/42/EEC [2] and the U.S. Code of Federal Regulations Title 21, Part 820 [3]. Some medical device manufacturers in Europe additionally seek CE marking, which is a quality standard given to organisations who successfully pass a quality inspection by a regulatory agency.

This case study discusses the particular issues affecting the automated manufacture and validation of a medical device involving the management and coordination of a number of suppliers:

Figure 1. Automated Medical Device Delivery

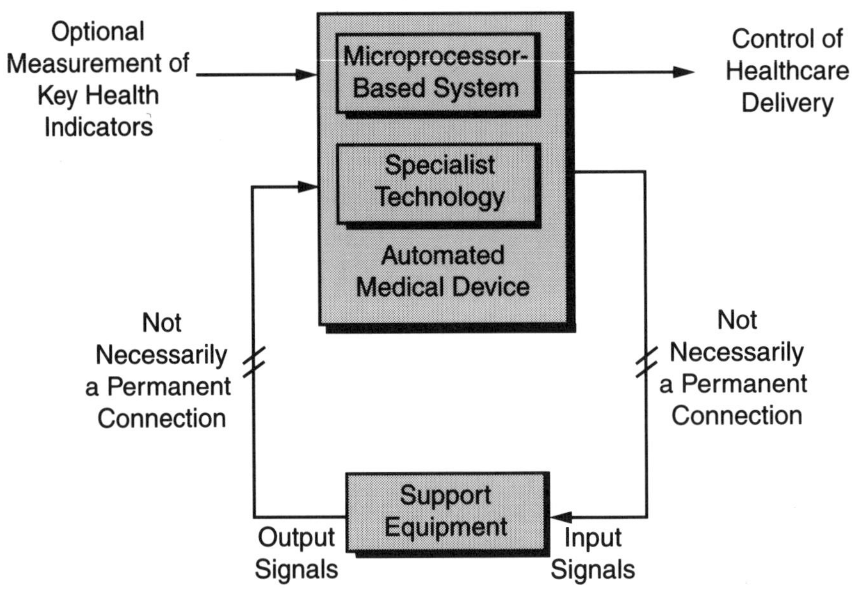

- One medical device designer
- One technology development designer
- Two supporting equipment designers
- One medical device manufacturer
- Four manufacturing process lines

VALIDATION PLANNING

The coordination of suppliers is vital, and, to this end, a Validation Master Plan is often produced, referencing a number of Validation Plans for each element of the automated medical device. Suppliers should be encouraged to produce their own Quality Plans in response to the Validation Plan for their portion of the system, so that any inconsistencies and ambiguities can be identified and corrective actions instituted before change becomes too inconvenient and expensive.

The selection of suppliers is often limited because only one or two suppliers will generally have the capability to provide a particular item of technology used in the medical device or in its manufacture. It may not be the case, therefore, that the supplier to be used has any experience in validation. Indeed, many suppliers supporting medical devices are small organisations and have a limited opportunity to develop an in-house validation capability. If this is the case, then training should be given to ensure that the supplier has no misunderstandings about the expectations made by GMP regulators. Care must be taken not to always take capability "sales-speak" at face value. The use of external validation consultants and/or the UK GAMP Guide for supplier validation can prove useful in training mechanisms [4]. Most suppliers are keen to pick up new skills and will welcome the chance to enhance the competency of their staff.

Because of such uncertainties, each supplier should be audited at the start of the project to establish whether a Quality Management System (QMS) exists that will support the validation of the equipment or process. Where none exists, an agreement must be reached with each supplier as to what quality measures will be used. This should be outlined by each company in their Quality Plan. In our case, we decided that all companies concerned should comply with the UK GAMP Guide, as this outlines validation documentation that is suitable for the U.S. Food & Drug Administration's (FDA's) requirements and may also be used to support the European Union's CE mark accreditation (see Table 1). The device was to be released in both the American and European markets.

A particularly important area to be addressed during planning is the consistent use of terminology. The GAMP Guide [4] includes a lexicon of

Table 1. CE Marking and Validation Documentation Relationships

Annex III, Section 3 of the European Union's Medical Device Directive [2] holds the key area that maps CE onto computer validation requirements.

EU Directive 93/42/EEC, Annex III, Section 3	Validation Documentation
The documentation must allow an understanding of the design, manufacture, and performance of the product and must contain the following items in particular:	
A general description of the type, including any variants planned	User Requirements Specification
Design drawings; methods of manufacture envisaged; in particular sterilisation; and diagrams of components, subassemblies, circuits, etc.	Drawings, Hardware Design and Software Design Specifications
The description and explanation necessary to understand the above mentioned drawings and diagrams and the operation of the product	Functional Specifications, Operator's Manual
A list of the standards referred to in Article 5, applied in full or part, and descriptions of the solutions adopted to meet the essential requirements if the standards referred to in Article 5 have not been applied in full	Validation Plan, Supplier Quality Plans
The results of the design calculations, risk analysis, investigations, technical tests, etc., carried out	Results of clinical trials; Threats & Controls; FMEA, Software Structural Analysis; IQ, OQ, and PQ tests; and Fundamental Science Document
A statement indicating whether or not the device incorporates, as an integral part, a substance as referred to in Section 7.4 of Annex I and data on the tests conducted in this connection	Relevant to medical device as a whole; not directly applicable to its automation
The clinical data referred to in Annex X	Clinical trial report
The draft label and, where appropriate, instructions for use	Relevant to medical device as a whole; not directly applicable to its automation

validation terminology that can prove to be a useful reference in this respect. Some practitioners prefer to include specific terms associated with a validation project and their definitions in the Validation Plans.

Intellectual property rights (IPR) should also be agreed to as part of the validation planning exercise. Particular elements of the automated medical device or its manufacture may be confidential to individual suppliers. Contracts must clearly define the terms and conditions affecting the supplier's rights.

DESIGN

Design documentation will consist of Hardware and Software Design Specifications for equipment and process definitions for process lines. Where a feasibility study has been carried out on a certain technology, a fundamental science document will be generated to summarise the technology on which the medical device is to be based. Fundamental science reports will examine the use of specialist hardware and programming and the ability of these technologies to provide the necessary functionality. The use of particular technologies may be inhibited because they are deemed as unvalidateable or because the validation is too expensive. A justification of the validation approach to be used for different technologies must be documented and made available for inspection by GMP regulatory authorities. It is highly unlikely that GMP inspectors will be experts in the technologies being used; therefore, a step-by-step argument supported by validation evidence should be developed so that the inspectors can walk through the validation exercise to check its integrity.

Early on in the design phase, a Threats and Control Analysis (also known as a Hazard Study) should be carried out, embracing the complete system to be built. This should ensure that all threats are covered by the existing designs or procedures to be written. The report will be part of the validation documentation and will make recommendations on what redesigns and what procedures are necessary.

Near the end of the design phase, a Failure Modes and Effect Analysis (FMEA) should be carried out to ensure that the hardware of the medical device and the supporting equipment cannot fail in an unsafe way. The report will be part of the validation, and any recommendations on redesign should be carried out before testing.

SOFTWARE PROGRAMMING

Software written for the medical device and any automated manufacturing equipment should be prepared in accordance with established industry Good Programming Practices. In particular, programs should be well structured and commented, and include headers giving details of version and change control. A Source Code Review (sometimes known as a Software Structural Assessment) should be conducted to verify the adoption of Good Programming Practices and verify any critical algorithms, such Fast Fourier Transforms (FFTs) on Digital Signal Processing (DSP) microchips, error handling by the software, and fail-safe or graceful degradation scenarios.

ASSEMBLY

It is not uncommon for a company to design a medical device prototype and then have it built by a company specialising in electronic manufacture. Where this happens, as in our case, a number of suitable companies should be considered for the project and those short listed, audited for capability. Selection would depend on the quality system in place, previous experience in medical device manufacture, control of subcontractors, level of testing supplied, and the amount of in-house technical support available. It is advisable to ensure that a legal agreement, Quality Plan and User Requirements Specification (URS) are employed to secure production standards for the device.

There might be a need with some prototype medical devices to reorganise the circuit board components in order to obtain a layout that will allow easy automatic assembly. Any changes must be noted in the Hardware Design Specification, and the new board must be checked against the prototype for functional equivalence. The FMEA report should be consulted to see if there are any critical components on the circuit board. If so, the manufacturer will have to make special arrangements to ensure that component traceability exists from supplier to circuit board to user.

A typical six-step manufacturing process for a medical device would be as follows:

1. Build circuit board. This will usually be done by automatic machines.
2. Check circuit board. The electronic manufacturer should have in-house expertise to program an automatic "in-circuit" tester for the board that ensures all components are in the correct place and that measures the correct value.
3. Load a test program into the device and place in a heat cycling oven. The heating profile and testing time should be agreed on between manufacturer and customer. It is important that the oven is temperature calibrated with a supporting certificate.
4. Load the current version of the validated software into the device.
5. Test the device on a suitable automatic test system.
6. Pack and ship to customers.

It is advisable to use a colour-coded labelling system to keep track of the test stages. In our case, a yellow spot was added after successful heat cycling with test software loaded, and a green spot half covering the yellow spot once the validated software had been loaded and the board tested successfully; no device can be shipped unless both spots are present. The manufacturer will be expected to supply a certificate of conformity for the devices produced, packed with each batch.

Assembly of the medical device may be partially completed by suppliers before final assembly by the device's registered manufacturer. In such situations, the registered manufacturer is entirely responsible for the work and is expected to assign their own Quality Assurance staff to monitor and perhaps witness supplier assembly.

QUALIFICATION

The medical device and all supporting equipment and processes covered by Validation Plans will each require a test specification. These will be generated by reading through the URS, Functional Specification, Threats and Control Analysis, and (where appropriate) the FMEA for each unit and determining which functions require testing. Critical areas should be examined very carefully, and a demanding set of tests drawn up to check each key area. If an automatic testing system is designed to test the medical device during manufacture, as in our case, the tests will need to check both the pass and fail routes of every test by using test medical devices with known hardware faults introduced.

The tests will be broken into Hardware Acceptance Tests (or Installation Qualification), System Acceptance Tests (or Operational Qualification), and Equipment Tests (or Performance Qualification). According to the size of the unit, all tests may be in one test document, or there may be three separate qualification documents. A test document will define the test philosophy and how the tests should be run. Each test will have a title, a reason for the test, an outline of any test equipment required, a description of the test, data to be recorded, and the test acceptance criteria. Calibrated test equipment must be supported with calibration certificates.

Each supplier will be responsible for generating its own test specifications, so it is important to ensure that all suppliers use the same standard for the test document. In our case, we insisted on GAMP for all nine test specifications.

Another point to remember is that where a software test harness is written to help test a medical device, this must be subject to validation (i.e., it must have functional, design, and test documentation to support it).

ENVIRONMENTAL TESTS

Apart from qualification testing, a medical device should undergo a number of environmental tests, as outlined in standards such as BS 2011 (British standard for environmental testing), CISPR 11 (limits and methods of measurement of electro-magnetic disturbance characteristics of industrial, scientific, and medical [ISM] radio frequency equipment), and BS 4826 (British standard for packaging electronic equipment for transport).

Typical tests that might be carried out on a medical device under environmental testing are as follows:

- Temperature operating range test
- Humidity operating range test
- Pressure operating range test
- Drop test
- Bump test
- Impact test
- Vibration test
- Damp heat test
- Transport packaging test
- Radio frequency radiation test
- Radio frequency immunity test
- Reliability test

These tests would be carried out on the final manufactured product by a company specialising in this field.

REPORTING

Potentially, the number of validation documents associated with a medical device can be great because each subsystem of the device is subject to its own validation life cycle (see Figure 2). It is very important to collate these documents. They must be managed, otherwise it is likely with the large number of participants that some will be lost, which will severely compromise the validation. In our case, an agreement was reached, at the beginning of the project, as to what validation documents would be generated by which supplier. This information was recorded in a live Document Tracking Report containing the title of document, reference, who was responsible, required date, current status, and issue date. It was issued every 4 weeks and proved invaluable with over 100 documents under control. The Document Tracking Report ended with a document library index.

Once the Document Tracking Report shows that all validation documents called for by a corresponding Validation Plan are present, all of the documents are reviewed and a Validation Report is generated, concluding on whether or not the automated medical device is suitable for its intended

Figure 2. Validation Documents

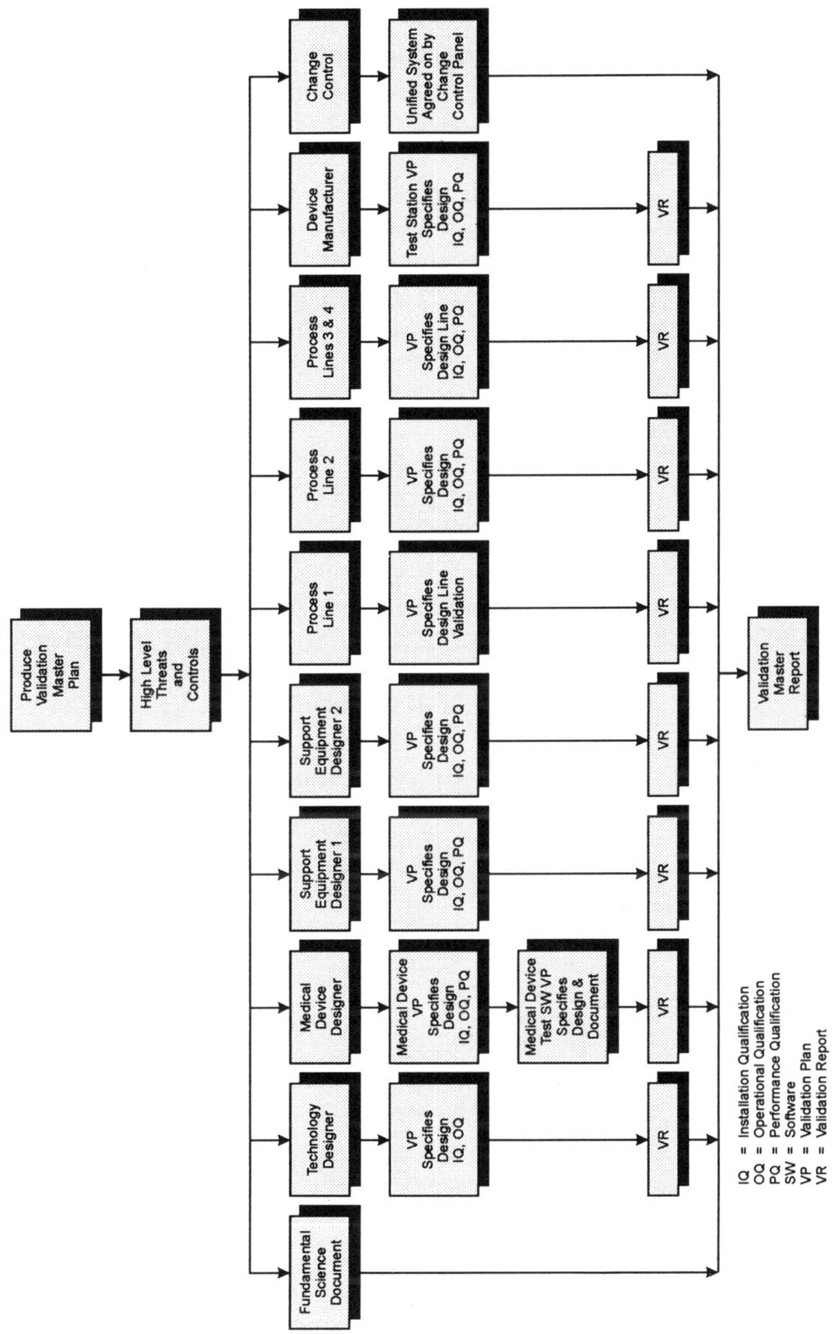

purpose. Any outstanding issues must be discussed, and either corrective actions raised or justification for taking no action must be made. The Validation Report should be periodically reviewed to check that the results of any changes, corrective actions, or regulatory requirements have not altered the validated status of the medical device. If additional validation is required, then this should be planned and completed as soon as reasonably practical. Any aspects of the additional validation that directly impact its safety should be addressed immediately.

When the project comes to the end, and all Validation Reports have been completed, each report must be reviewed to ensure nothing is outstanding and that all parts of the project are satisfactory for use. This information is covered by the Validation Master Report, which should be the last validation document to be written of the validation suite.

CHANGE CONTROL

Change control must be established for the validation project and ongoing support of the medical device. Each supplier associated with the project is likely to have its own particular change control practice. These must either be linked and coordinated, or a single change control procedure to be used by everybody must be enforced, to ensure effective logging and management of changes. In our case, a single coordinated change control procedure was established with all suppliers. Any supplier can make a change request, but it can only be authorised by all concerned parties. Once authorised, it may be carried out under the quality system of the supplier, with the test results being sent to all parties for approval.

The medical device itself must also be subject to change controls. It should be given a serial and version number. All embedded software must also be under version control.

CONCLUSION

Managing a large number of suppliers adds greatly to the administrative complexity of validation. This case study has identified some of the important issues. Other issues will arise on particular projects. The key to success is establishing a partnership between suppliers and the device's registered manufacturer. A team effort is required. Without it, validation is extremely difficult, if not impossible, to achieve.

REFERENCES

1. United Kingdom Medical Devices Regulations (1994), Regulation 2(1): SI 1994 No. 3017. This UK regulation implements EU Directive 93/42/EEC.
2. European Directive 93/42/EEC (1993) concerning medical devices—Class IIb, Parts III and V.
3. U.S. Code of Federal Regulations Title 21, Part 820, *Good Manufacturing Practice for Medical Devices*.
4. UK GAMP Forum (1996), *Supplier Guide for Validation of Automation Systems in Pharmaceutical Manufacture*, 2nd Edition, International Society of Pharmaceutical Engineering, The Hague, Netherlands.

Index